makeup makeovers in
5   10   15   20 minutes

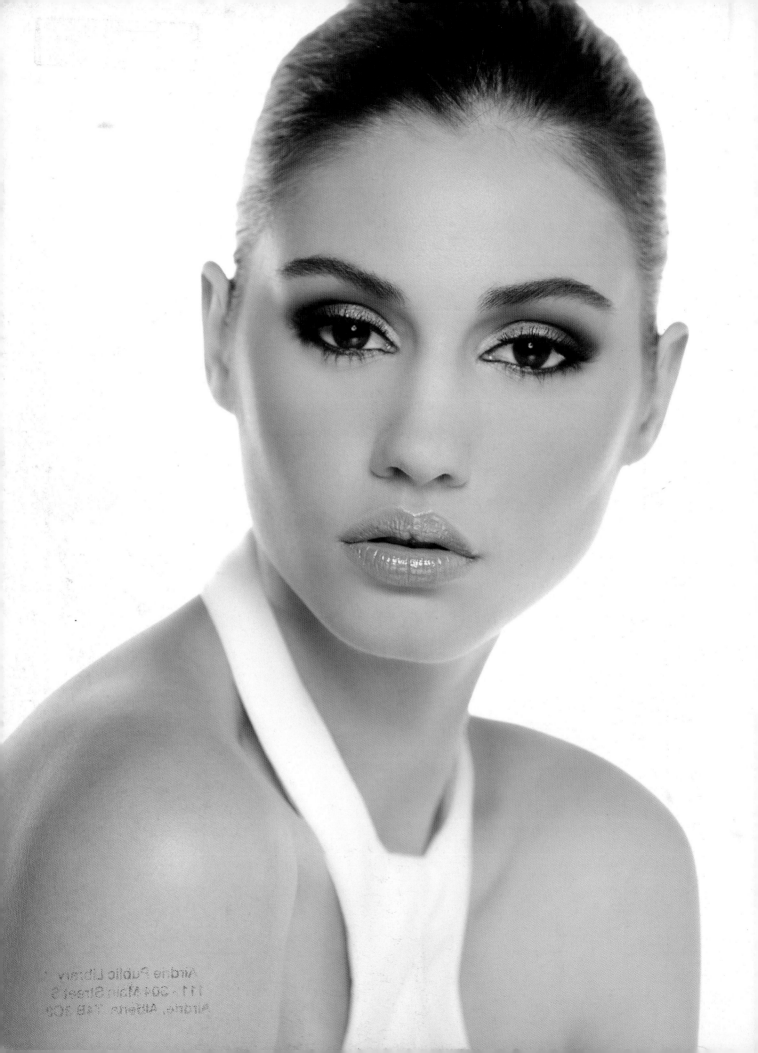

makeup makeovers in
5   10   15   20 minutes

expert secrets for stunning
transformations

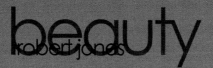

beauty
robert jones

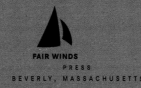

FAIR WINDS
PRESS
BEVERLY, MASSACHUSETTS

First published in the USA in 2012 by
Fair Winds Press, a member of
Quayside Publishing Group
100 Cummings Center
Suite 406-L
Beverly, MA 01915-6101
www.fairwindspress.com

16 15 14 13 12   2 3 4 5

ISBN: 978-1-59233-371-4

Digital edition published in 2012
eISBN: 978-1-610581-385-5

Library of Congress Cataloging-in-Publication Data available

Edited by Ellen Phillips
Hair and makeup by Robert Jones
Assisted by John Ball
Representation by Seaminx Artist Management, www.seaminx.com
Produced by MB Assets
Photography by Larry Travis

special thanks to all the women in my life who have and will inspire me.
www.robertjonesbeauty.com

Printed and bound in China

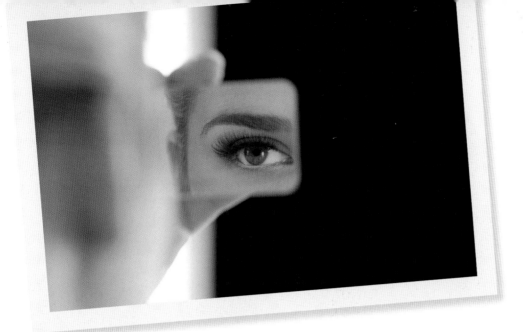

This book is dedicated to all the women out there who wake up everyday wanting and trying to look their most beautiful. Also three very important people: my grandmother Carolyn Scoville, my very first beauty inspiration; Chip McFadin, the love of my life and my rock; and Melissa Brumley, without whose support this book would not exist.

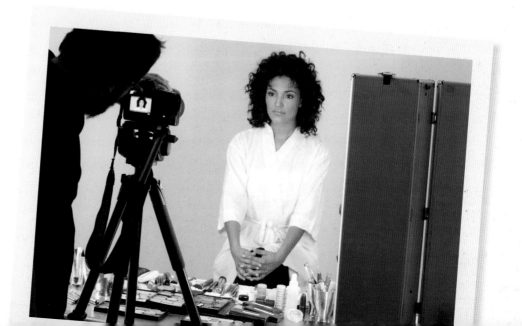

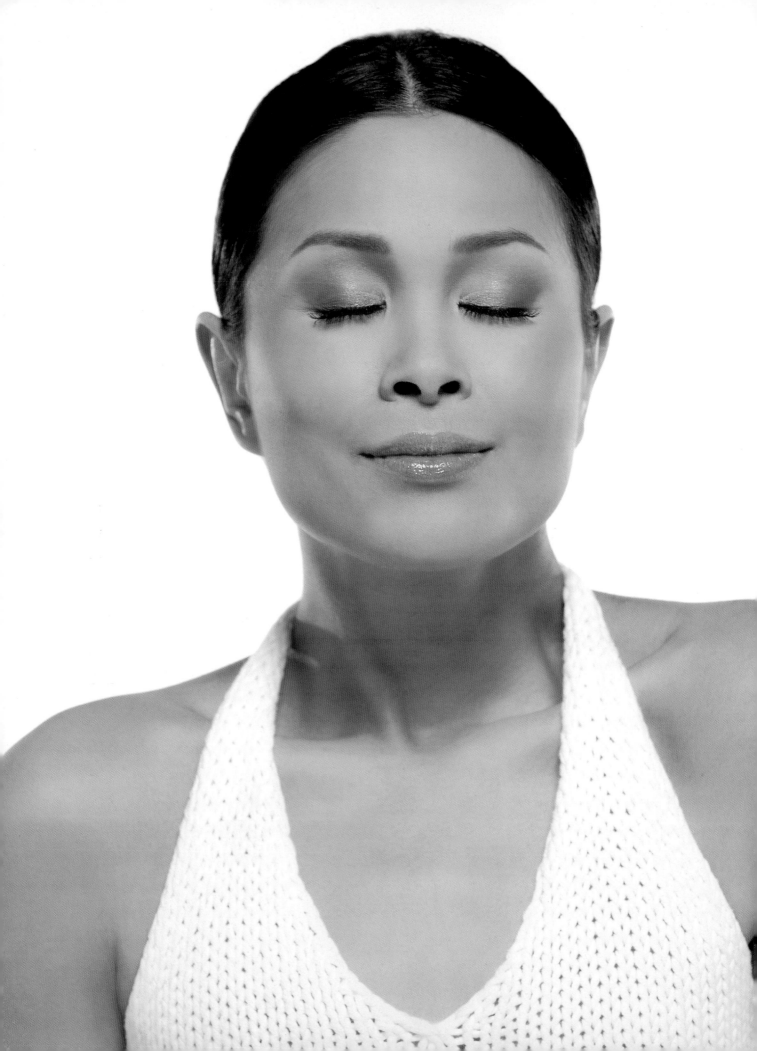

introduction: it had to be you

There is one thing I know for sure: Makeup can change your life. Not in the sense that it will put a roof over your head or cure cancer, but it can change how you look at yourself and the world. When you feel your most beautiful, it will give you confidence like nothing else can. And we all know that confidence is what true beauty is all about.

It has always been my goal to teach women to love who they actually are, not who they wish they could be. As many of you know, I have written several bestselling books that have focused on just that. Love who you are today and every day. Find what makes you special and celebrate it. Love your big baby blues; embrace that gorgeous pucker. Play and experiment to find your perfect you.

No matter how many women I've worked with, how many workshops I've led, or how many books I've written, I always find it hard to express what I want for you and what I hope you can achieve. Yes, I have an opinion about how you can achieve your own true beauty and am always willing to share it, but are you ready to receive it?

We all have preconceived notions about what is beautiful and how we look our best. Unfortunately, so often our perception is not where the truth lies. (Think of your girlfriend who's still wearing her hair the way she did in high school.) I always tell women to try new things because that's what keeps you looking your most beautiful.

I thought and thought in the process of writing this book, "How do I express what makeup and the right application can do for you?" I decided to ask a few women whom I'd worked with and see what they thought. I had changed the way they thought about beauty and the way they looked at themselves and shown them how they could change the way the world sees them. I wanted to share with you how learning the tricks and the secrets of the trade have changed it all for them.

"For beautiful eyes, look for the good in others; for beautiful lips, speak only words of kindness; and for poise, walk with the knowledge that you are never alone."

—Audrey Hepburn

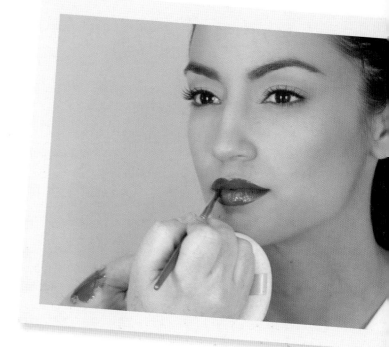

I could list celebrity after celebrity I've worked with to try to impress you, but that won't help you understand how you can change your own reality. It won't help you find *your* beauty. But I do think that women just like you—the gorgeous woman in line next to you, your beautiful next-door neighbor, the hottest mom in your child's class at school, or just the woman walking down the street who looks so good and pulled-together—are the ones who can help you see your potential. And here's what they had to say:

"One of the most important and unique traits about Robert is that he finds beauty in everyone. *He immediately can size up what features need to be highlighted and how to conceal a less-appealing trait. He's different from anyone I have ever known: Not only can he do this flawlessly, but he can also teach it . . . I've gained courage and confidence through his showing me how to change my look based on the occasion, yet still be true to my 'style' and still authentic in my skin. I have learned that I can* pull off *looks that I might not have tried, and I've learned to trust him when he tells me it's wrong for me because Robert is* always right!*"*
   —Pamela (the hottest mom in your child's class)

"Robert doesn't just teach and show you how to achieve a look, but he teaches you why you do the steps that you do to get the look. And that is when the learning really sinks in and you then become able to master the art of makeup for yourself and to share those skills with others. When people understand the 'why,' the 'how' becomes easy and second nature. Robert takes the extra steps and time to make sure you understand the 'why,' and to do that he breaks everything down into simple steps."
   —Julianne (your beautiful next-door neighbor)

"Robert Jones has the amazing ability to not only make women look beautiful but also feel beautiful. He looks at makeup not as a superficial thing, but as a tool to empower women and help them gain confidence."
   —Karen (the gorgeous woman in line next to you)

"After purchasing Robert's books, I became enthralled with the way he was able to create beauty for all types of women—real women with real beauty challenges . . . Robert taught me the really amazing tips that truly had the ability to transform. An average look became a drop-dead, over-the-top, can't-take-your-eyes-off-it look! Robert and only Robert . . . The knowledge I've gained in my wonderful association with Robert has been life-changing, as an artist and a makeup-wearing woman."
   —Christy (the stunning pro)

Hopefully, hearing from real women, you can see how makeup is going to change your life. The looks in this book are fun and easy! I show you everything step by step. No matter how much time you have or don't have, you'll see that beauty is obtainable for you *every* day. I see the beauty in you! Now *you* just need to be able to see the beauty in you. And with this book, you will. I promise!

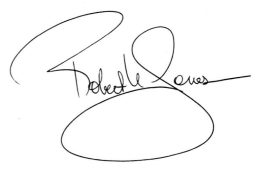

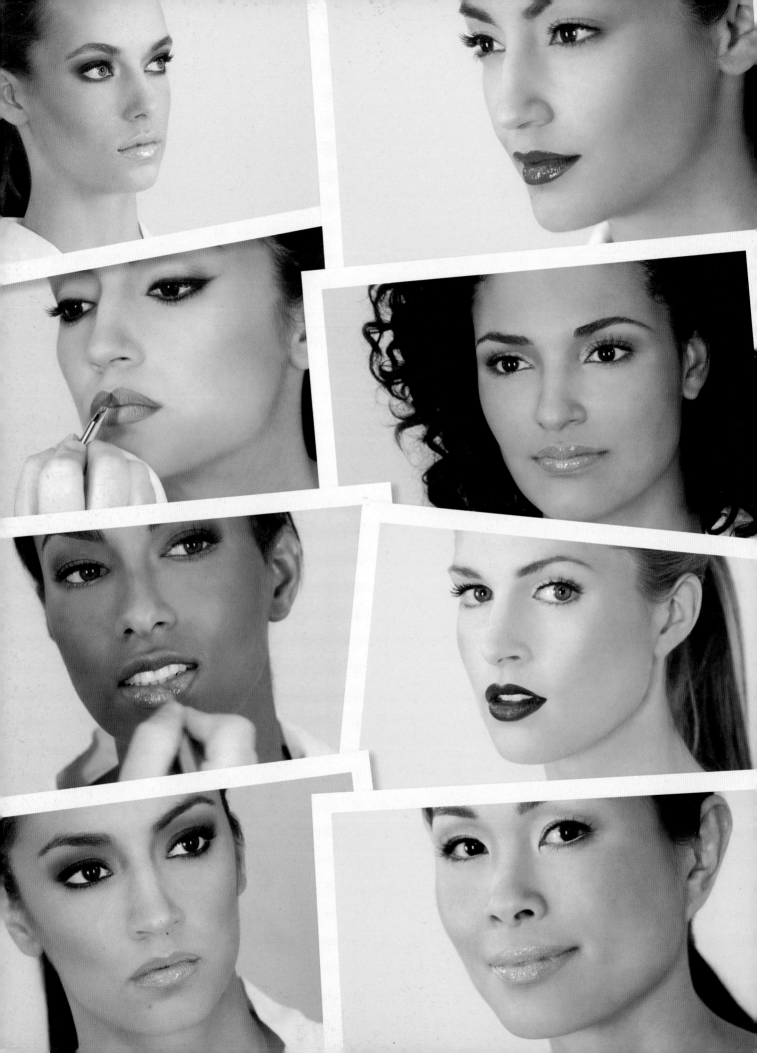

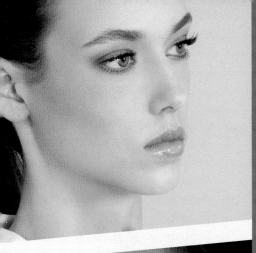

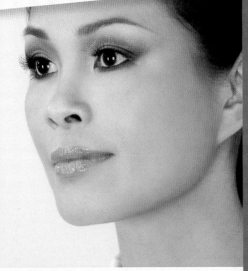

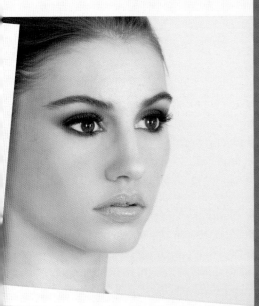

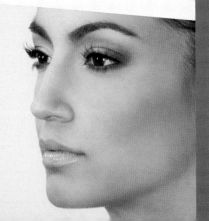

1

pretty is as pretty does

When you wake up each day, do you feel like you are just repeating yesterday, or is today a new day? For many of us, each day is a repeat of the day before. But for you, each day *can* be a new day— a beautiful day.

I know that your time can be limited, and some mornings you sleep an extra 10 minutes because you can (okay, you needed to), so you have even less time to get ready before you rush out the door. I know that some nights before you go out, you race home and only have 5 minutes to get ready. My goal with this book is to help you make the best use of whatever time you have.

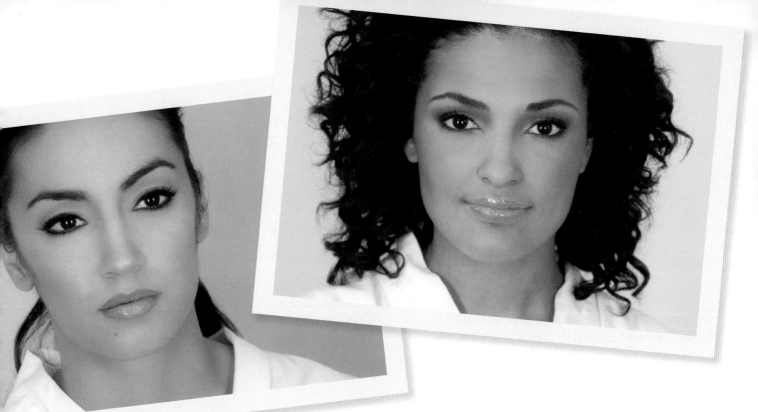

"Don't be afraid to experiment and play. Try every look. Why not?"

You have heard it your whole life: "Pretty is as pretty does." And in this case, it is so true. The looks in this book are based on how much time you have to put your look together on any given day, and it's organized so you can easily see what the results will look like. I promise you this: Whether you have 5 minutes or 15, you can always look your most beautiful. Whether you want a natural look or one with tons of color, you can always look your most beautiful. Whether you like to play or you are searching for your signature look, you can always look your most beautiful. Every day is a new chance to be the prettiest that you can be.

Makeup can transform your day and how you feel as you travel through your day. I have created look after look in this book that will take little to no time at all, as well as looks that you can take more time with when you have just a few more minutes. And trust me, they're all beautiful. With each look, there are step-by-step instructions and photos to lead you as you go about your journey. Don't be afraid to experiment and play. Try every look . . . why not, right?

"I truly believe *every* woman is beautiful."

coming soon to a mirror near you

Within these pages, we will discuss everything you need to create these looks at home. I discuss the basic types of makeup and application in chapter 2, and in chapter 3, we'll review the essential tools you will want to have on hand. As you'll see, the right makeup brush for a given application can make a big difference! You'll notice that I keep the palette of makeup shades limited to show you how little it takes to create a plethora of fast, fun, gorgeous looks.

You are going to learn how to create the perfect foundation; then you can build any of these looks on it. You'll find out exactly how to conceal what you don't want to see and how to draw attention to what you want to emphasize. You will learn tricks of the trade and secrets that make application fast and fun. Creating the illusion of perfection is always fun!

But the fun *really* starts once you've mastered the basics and start creating look after look. Wait 'til you start playing with color, experimenting with application, and—best of all—becoming the prettiest you can be.

I truly believe *every* woman is beautiful. It's simply a matter of finding what makes her special and pretty, then focusing on just that. I don't care if you have 5 minutes or all the time in the world; together we can make you look and feel your most beautiful.

There are looks for everyone in this book, whether you want a 5-minute day or evening look or you have 20 minutes to create your day look or 15 minutes for your evening look. Whatever you are looking for, it is here for you to try. And I say, try it!

With the knowledge in this book, you hold your beauty fate in your own hands. And together, we will create a unique beauty for you like no other. Gather your tools, bring your clean face, and let the fun begin!

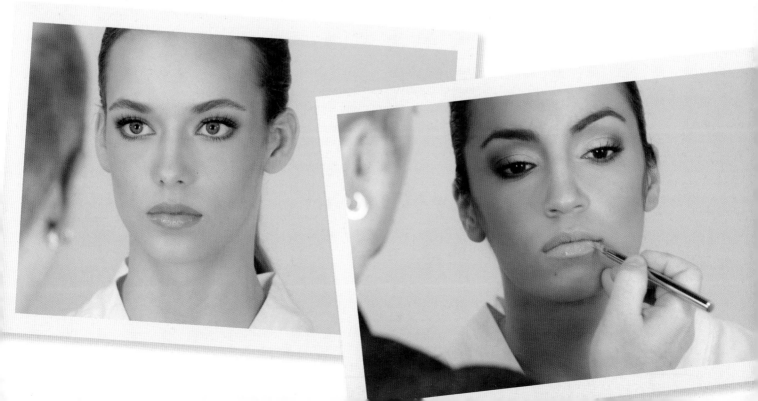

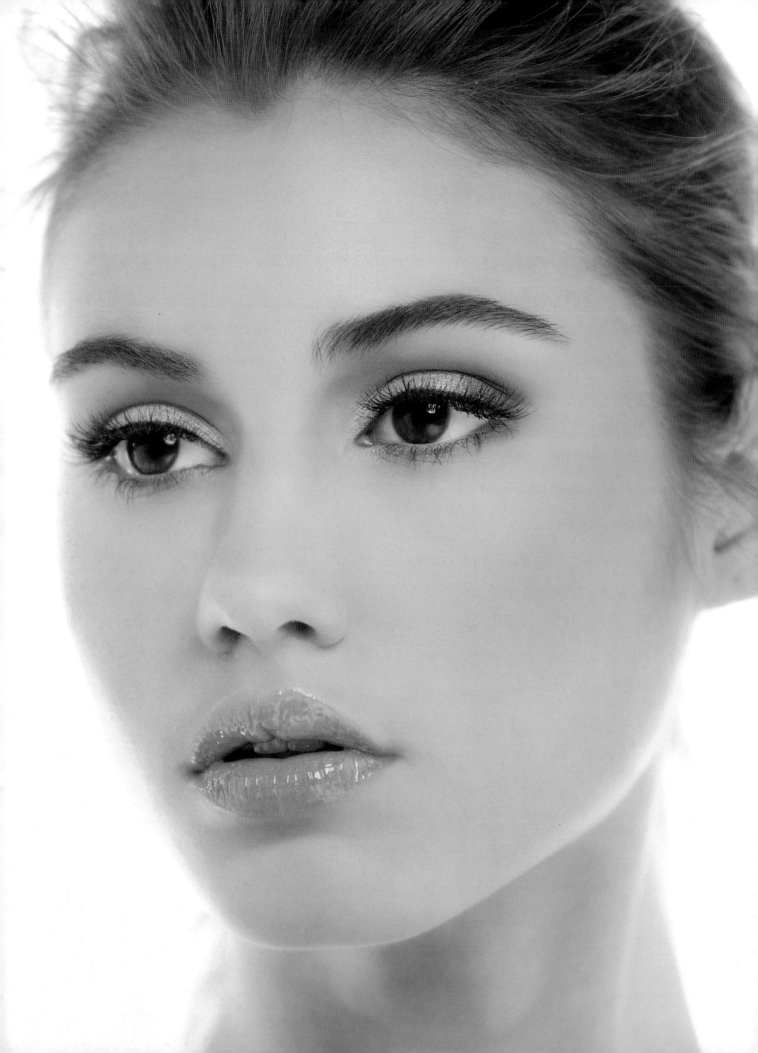

2

building the perfect foundation

foun·da·tion [foun-DAY-shuhn]

The basis or groundwork of anything; the natural or prepared ground or base on which your creation rests.

We all know that for any makeup look to appear its best, we must create a perfect canvas or foundation before we begin the transformation. In this chapter, we are going to discuss how to do just that: create the ideal palette or canvas for each and every look in this book. Without this step, none of the looks could reach perfection. You are about to see what the correct foundation application can do for someone's appearance, without adding a single finishing touch. Hang on—you might be shocked. You know what? Maybe you should sit down!

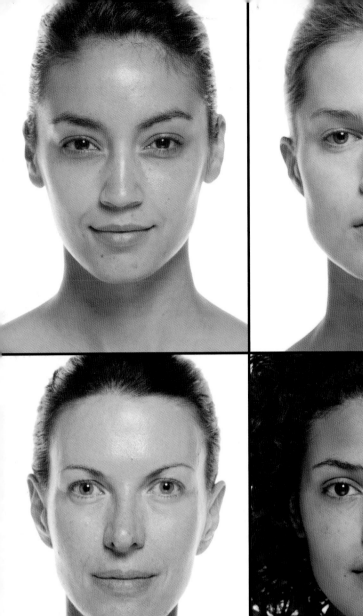
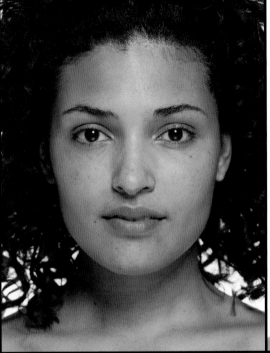
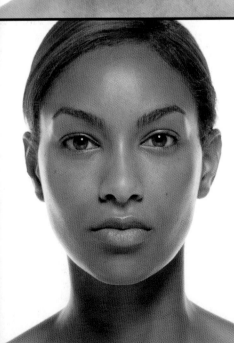
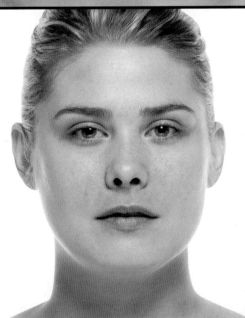
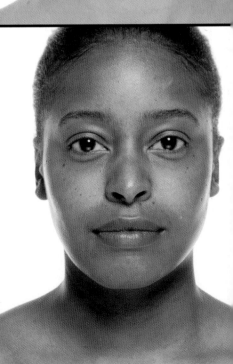

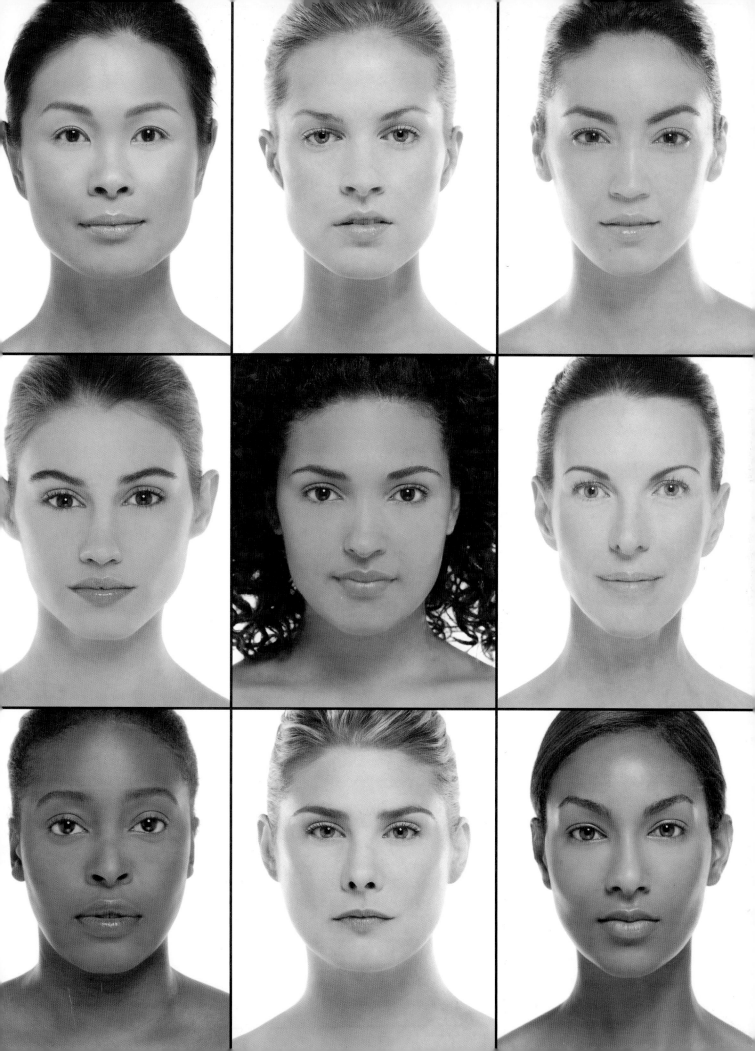

foundation

There are a few general things we need to think about here before moving on to foundation specifics: skin type, benefits, and—last but not least—coverage.

skin type: Depending on your skin type (dry, oily, combination, or normal), you will need different characteristics to your foundation. For instance, if you have dry skin, you'll need a foundation with added hydration. If you have oily skin, you will need one with oil absorbers. For combination skin, you need to decide if you need hydration or oil absorption. And for normal skin (lucky you!), the world is yours. No matter what your choice or needs, I advise you to make sure your foundation is oil-free.

benefits: Decide what benefits you want from your foundation. Options include SPF, buildable coverage, antiaging, transfer resistance, and an oil-free formula.

coverage: How much coverage do you want or need? Do you have very little to cover and want a sheer foundation, or do you have a lot to cover and need full coverage? There are so many options out there. Pick what you like best, but I always feel that you will look your most natural with the least coverage needed. I am not saying that some of you don't look your best with full coverage (you might), but only choose as much coverage as you actually *need*.

foundation formulas

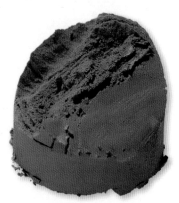

liquid foundation is the most common and comes in the most variation for all skin types. Depending on the formula, it can give you sheer to full coverage, but most formulas of this type give you medium coverage.

crème comes in both compact and stick forms. This formula most often gives you medium to full coverage. Of course, as with any formula, your application can change the coverage. If you apply it sparingly, it gives you less coverage, and if you apply it more liberally, it will give you more coverage. This formula most often will have added hydration, but doesn't always.

whipped crème (mousse) is different from its compact counterpart. This whipped version gives you a sheerer coverage than its sister in the compact (with sheer to full coverage), and it might or might not have added hydration. I love the versatility of this formula: Your application totally determines your coverage.

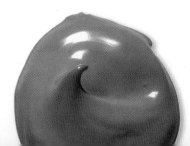

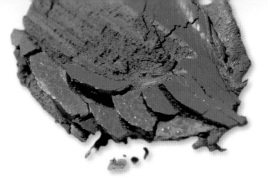

crème-to-powder gives you full coverage. Some women find this formula very convenient due to the fact that it does not have to be powdered after application to set it and it is very portable. It's best suited for normal skin.

tinted moisturizer gives you the sheerest coverage. It is moisturizer with just a hint of color. It is absolutely perfect for someone who just wants to even out her skin a bit. It's great for normal to dry skin.

mineral powder gives you sheer coverage, but it can also be built up (with multiple layers) for medium coverage. This loose powder is a very popular type of foundation right now due to its convenience and sheer coverage. Just keep in mind that if you have a lot of fine lines, it might not be your best friend. And I personally prefer a formula without sunscreen in it, because most times the ingredient used for this can cause the skin to look ashy.

compact powder is the same as mineral powder, just pressed into a compact. So it gives you sheer coverage, but can be built up for more coverage.

"you will always look most natural with the sheerest foundation coverage."

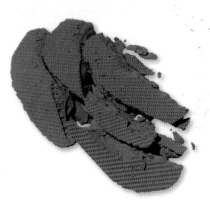

color choice

When making the correct color choice with your foundation, you must consider two very important factors: your skin's undertone and its depth level. Let's start with the easier of the two, depth level. The depth level of your foundation (and your skin) is how light or dark it appears. The lighter it is, the lighter its depth level; the darker it is, the darker it's depth level. Simple enough, right?

Now for the harder of the two, understanding your skin's undertone. To fully explain this, I need to divide all you girls into two categories: ivory/beige and bronze/ebony.

When dealing with ivory/beige skin, you are looking at three possible undertones: yellow, pink, or olive. If you have bronze/ebony skin, you have basically three undertones as well: yellow (gold), golden orange, or warm brown.

Whatever skin color you have, stripe testing is the only way to find your perfect shade match. Stripe testing is when you take multiple shades of foundation and apply them to your skin to test if they match you skin's undertone and depth level. You will want to stripe test from jaw to neck because this way, you extend your shades on to your neck to ensure a perfect match.

Many women with ivory/beige skin have pink or redness in their face and not their neck. Remember that it's your goal to match the neck. So in this case, you will need a yellow undertone to counteract the pink or red and make the face match the neck. The only time you want a pink undertone is when you have pink in both your neck and your face.

Keep in mind that undertones on bronze/ebony skin are very specific, so it is super important to get an exact match. When stripe testing bronze/ebony skin, you should apply the foundation from cheek to jaw. This is because it is more likely for this skin tone to have more color variations on your face, and you want to be able to find what you need to make your skin look flawless. But remember, you still need to try to match your neck.

timely tips

When choosing a foundation, you always want to match your neck. This way, you don't have to extend your application past your jaw line.

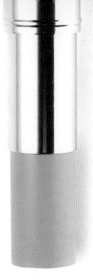

concealer

Concealer is probably the biggest factor in creating perfection (or as I prefer to look at it, the illusion of perfection). Your product formula is critical. This is especially true with concealer because different formulas give you different amounts of coverage and are created for different usages.

concealer formulas

stick concealer is probably the most common and most popular. It gives you great coverage, and the formula is usually moist enough yet dry enough to conceal just about any discoloration.

tube concealer is usually a more moisturizing formula due to the nature of the form it comes in. Very versatile due to its texture, it can give you a lot of coverage, or you can sheer it out to give a lighter amount of coverage.

pot concealer really gives you complete coverage. The formula can vary from creamier all the way to drier. So depending on your formula choice, you can find one for anything you might want to cover.

wand concealer is the sheerest of all formulas. It gives you the least coverage, but blends very easily, so it is a great choice if you are wearing minimal foundation and just want to conceal minor imperfections.

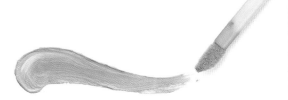

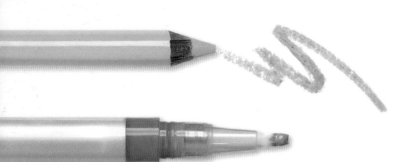

pencil concealer gives you complete, fast, easy coverage for dots, spots, and veins. Its dry texture helps it stay put all day, and because it's a pencil, getting it right where you need it is a breeze. I could not live without this.

highlighting pen is not a concealer in the sense of a cover-up, but I am putting it here because it is part of creating the illusion of perfection. If your skin is rough, uneven, pitted, or wrinkled, a highlighting pen can work wonders when used together with your concealer. That's because this product contains light-reflecting particles that help bring forward recessed areas of the face. So anywhere you have any type of indention, apply it and it will visually bring forward that recessed area, creating the appearance of smooth skin.

concealer color choices

Depth level and undertone matter. Let's talk about depth level first. When choosing a concealer, for the most part, you want a shade that is the same shade as your foundation or a shade lighter. That's the theory, anyway. I will say that I almost always choose a shade lighter because you are lightening something darker than your skin tone. Just keep in mind that the darker the discoloration, the lighter your concealer will need to be, so be open to the idea that you might need one or two shades lighter than your foundation.

Now let's talk about undertone. Once again, let's divide all of you into two categories. You can get a lot of mileage out of concealers with yellow undertones. Yellow is the best color choice for severe discoloration on ivory/beige skin because it works to counteract most skin imperfections, including the purple of under-eye circles, the brown of age spots, and any ruddiness or red in the complexion. The more severe the imperfection—such as a port-wine stain or extremely dark circles—the more yellow you will want in your concealer.

On bronze/ebony skin, a golden-orange concealer for lighter to medium skin tones works wonderfully. For really deep tones of ebony, a warm brown concealer usually covers best. The more intense the discoloration of the skin, the more intense the undertone of the concealer should be so that it can correct more.

If you're using a concealer that matches your foundation exactly, you may apply it either before or after your foundation. But if you're using one that is lighter than your foundation, it is best to apply it first.

powder

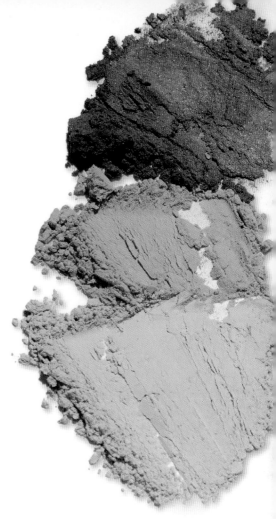

Girls, again you have a variety of choices, and as we're about to see, each has its benefits and purposes. As with foundation and concealer, we need to consider formula and shade choice. Just keep in mind that the purpose of powder is to set all crèmes and liquids and to help keep the skin looking fresh and oil-free.

powder formulas

loose powder comes in a loose form rather than a compact. This is perfect to set any and all liquids and crèmes. Keep in mind that the finer it is milled, the better it is. The more velvety a powder feels to the touch, the more finely milled it is. This formula is also the most oil absorbing, so it will give your skin a long-lasting matte finish and keep it looking fresh longer.

pressed powder is powder pressed into a compact. This formula is also great for setting liquids and crèmes and so very convenient for carrying with you for touch-ups all day.

powder color

When choosing a shade of powder, select one that matches your foundation. That way, the powder will reinforce everything you have applied (foundation, concealer, highlighting pen) before you powdered, rather than fighting it. There is also the option of using a translucent powder, which is fine for paler skin tones, but "translucent" does not mean that the powder has no color. Translucent powder is not invisible (transparent), though the two words are easy to confuse. It is less opaque than other powders, but it is not colorless, and can often appear unnatural and ashy on dark beige, olive, bronze, and ebony skin tones.

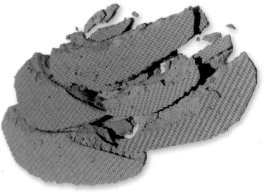

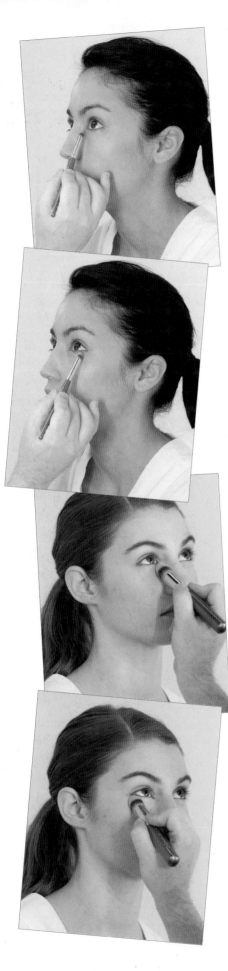

application: building your foundation

Now let's talk application because you can have the products you need, but if you don't know how to use them, they are of no benefit to you. It is all pretty basic, but I think it's essential to review application techniques.

applying concealer

I'm reviewing this first because in most cases, you are probably going to want to apply concealer before you apply foundation. I will let you know when it is best to apply it after foundation.

I have to say, the secret to concealing anything and everything is coloring within the lines, just like when you were a child and learned how to color. I repeat, you *must* color within the lines!

There are many tools and brush options to help with perfect placement. You just need to make the right choices. For even more complete and detailed concealing instructions, be sure to pick up my book *makeup makeovers: beauty bible* for all the basics you could want or need.

Let's look at the specifics of where and how you might want to apply concealer.

dark circles

1. Using a #53 concealer brush, apply concealer along the line of demarcation—where the discoloration begins on your skin. Extend the concealer up and over the entire discolored area with your brush. You never want to extend the concealer past the line of demarcation (onto the skin that you are trying to match). If you do, you will lighten skin that is already the correct color, and you'll be back to two contrasting shades of skin.

2. Now, take your finger and using a stippling (patting) motion, stipple the concealer along the line of demarcation to blend it in. This blends in the texture of the concealer, making it invisible.

3. Be sure to conceal any darkness in the inside corners of your eyes or your eyelids, if necessary.

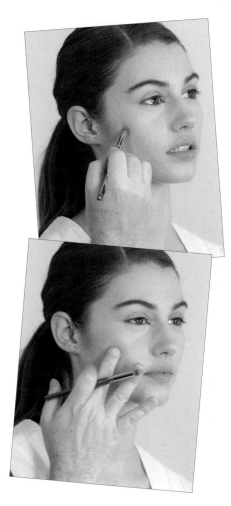

blemishes

1. Apply your foundation first. This is definitely one time when you want to apply your foundation *before* you conceal. It makes the process much easier.

2. Choose a concealer with a dry texture and one with a depth level that is not lighter than your foundation. Your concealer should match your skin exactly. A light concealer will only make the blemish seem larger. Using a #53 concealer brush, apply the concealer directly to the blemish.

3. Now with your finger, using a stippling (patting) motion, blend the edges all around the blemish into the skin. Stippling blends in the texture of the concealer, making it invisible.

timely tips

Whenever you are applying foundation over an area that you just concealed, always stipple it on with a patting motion. Never wipe it on because you could wipe off the concealer that you just applied!

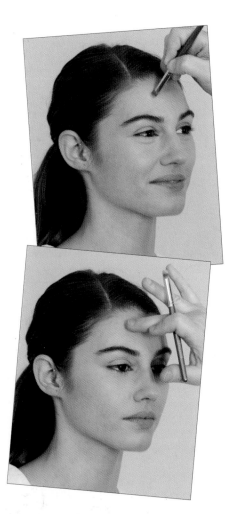

under-eye puffiness

1. First, apply your foundation. Everything you need to do to disguise the puffiness happens after you apply your foundation.

2. Next, take a highlighting pen and apply it just underneath the puffiness, right where the shadow is being created. Be sure not to extend the product up onto the puffy area because it will just make it look puffier. The highlighting pen has light-reflecting properties, making it appear as if the recessed area comes forward so it's even with the rest of the face and we do not see the indented area.

3. Now, take your finger and use a stippling (patting) motion where you applied the highlighting pen. This will blend in the color and texture, making it invisible.

hyperpigmentation (also known as melasma, age spots, and pregnancy masking)

1. Using a #53 concealer brush for precision (if you have a large spot, use your fingers or a sponge), apply your concealer only to the dark, discolored area, coloring within the lines. If there are multiple spots, cover each one separately.

2. Using your finger, stipple all around the outer edges of every spot that you concealed. This will blend in the texture, making the area look completely and perfectly natural.

broken capillaries or veins

1. Take a #50 concealer brush and draw a line of concealer right along the broken capillary or vein. You can't conceal the general area, so you must apply it only to the vein. If you extended the concealer past the edges of the vein or broken capillary, it would only lighten the skin we are trying to match, disguising nothing. This is why a concealer brush makes everything so much easier because it is so precise. Or use a concealer pencil for concealing veins—it's amazing. You simply draw it right along the vein.

2. Now, using the tip of your finger, stipple all along where you applied your concealer. This will blend in the texture of your concealer and make it look completely natural.

rosacea

1. To counteract the redness of rosacea, you will need a yellow-based concealer. Apply a thin layer of concealer to the entire area. This thin layer will get rid of the general area of redness, but you will probably be left with a few darker areas of redness still showing through. No problem—we will tackle them next.

2. Now, using the same concealer, go back and apply another layer to the darker areas that are still showing through (but only to the spots that are still visible). By covering in two steps, you do not have a thick layer of concealer over a large area of your face, so your skin looks more natural.

3. Stipple all around the outer edges of the area you concealed to blend in the texture.

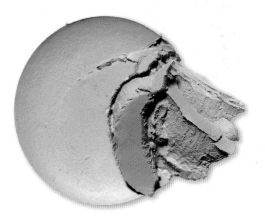

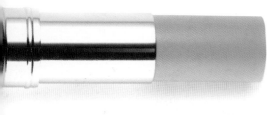

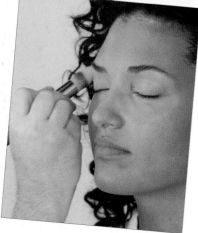

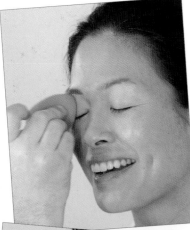

eye zone

Okay, you have one more place you need to conceal. In order to make your eye shadow and all the fun you have with your eyes look fabulous, you need to conceal your eyelid before you start your color application. Take a little concealer and apply it from lash line to brow, followed by a light dusting of powder. This creates the perfect blank canvas to paint and have fun with. Everyone has some discoloration on her eyelids, and this concealer/powder application is better than any other technique. It gives you the best start for perfect eye makeup application.

On bronze/ebony skin, especially dark depth levels, you might want to conceal your lids a bit lighter than your skin tone. It will allow all your eye shadow shades to show up better. Since you're going to be adding color over your entire lid, it won't hurt for it to be lighter to start.

timely tips

Don't be afraid to ask for samples when at beauty counters, and don't be afraid to exchange a product if you discover you've made the wrong choice!

applying foundation

Foundation is one of the hardest products for you to choose, but one of the most important you will purchase. That's why I say you should invest the most money in your foundation, concealer, and powder. They are the foundation of every look you choose to wear, and it is important for them to be the best that you can afford. Save money on all the fun color!

When applying liquid or crème foundation, you have three basic tools to work with. All three can give you great application:

A **sponge** is probably the most commonly used option. Always dampen your sponge before use; it will help it glide across your skin better and prevent it from absorbing too much product. If you stipple, your sponge will give you more coverage, and if you use your sponge to glide your foundation across your face, it will give you less coverage. You are in control!

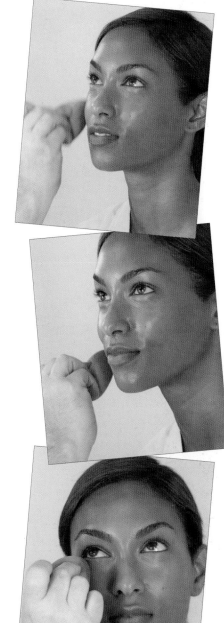

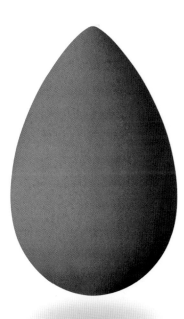

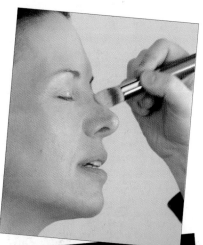

A **brush blends** well, so it gives you great coverage. The head of the most current foundation brush is tapered and pointed in its design to promote smooth, even coverage, helping your foundation blend as you apply it. Still, the only time a brush is a better choice than a sponge is when you want to touch up makeup that you have had on all day before you go out, but don't want to start over. If you stipple with your brush, it will give you more coverage, while you'll get less coverage if you swipe the brush across your face. Keep in mind that this brush always has synthetic bristles so that it won't absorb your foundation.

Don't have a brush or sponge handy? No problem, because the third tool is your **fingertips**. Just be sure to wash your hands after you've applied your moisturizer and treatment products and before you apply your foundation. The residue from the treatment products can compromise the integrity of your foundation.

Whether you use a sponge, a brush, or your fingers, the best technique for applying foundation is to begin your application at the center of your face and work your way outward. You can dip your tool in foundation and apply it directly to the skin, or you can start by dotting foundation on the cheeks, the forehead, the chin, and the nose and then blend it outward. Always remember to finish with your final strokes blending downward (no matter what your tool choice) to make sure all the small facial hairs lie flat.

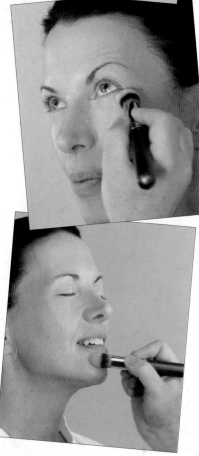

After application, give the foundation a couple of seconds to dry. Then blot with a tissue to absorb any excess moisture left from the product even though when you powder, it will absorb the excess moisture. This simple blotting step can really enhance the staying power of your foundation.

"powder is a must!"

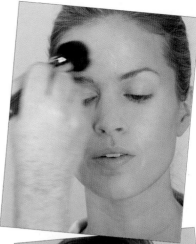

applying powder

I think that powder is a must. It sets all liquids and crèmes, while keeping your skin looking flawless all day long. So don't skip it, even if you only use it on your T-zone. There are several ways to apply both loose and compact powder:

A **brush** is the easiest and most commonly used tool. It will give you light to medium coverage. It is great for blending. To ensure smooth, even coverage, apply a little bit of powder at a time with a brush instead of applying it all at once.

A **powder puff** offers the most coverage. Press your puff into the powder, tap the excess off in the palm of your hand, and then "roll" what is left on the puff onto your skin. To finish, lightly sweep your face with a brush, using gentle downward strokes to remove any excess powder.

A **fingertip** works well for a light powder application. It's a great way to powder underneath the eyes or any area where you don't want to draw attention to fine lines. Just dip your finger in loose powder. Rub your finger in the palm of your hand to brush off the excess. Then trace your finger over the area you are trying to set.

A **sponge** works well for tight areas and is great for "spot" powdering.

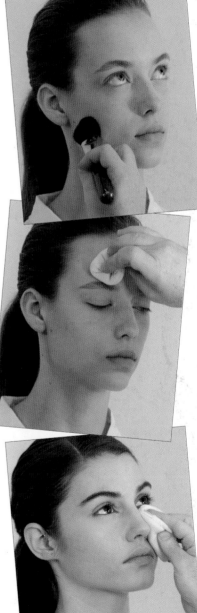

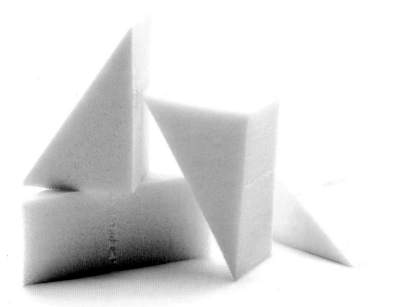

"any face can look more oval with nothing more exotic than foundation and powder."

highlight and contour

Here's a technique that can really make a huge difference in giving your face a glow and defined shape. This is definitely an optional step, but I have to say, once you see the benefits you can create with this technique, you'll know why you are going to love doing it.

I'm talking about highlighting and contouring your face. It's the makeup artist's equivalent of an optical illusion. That's because everything you highlight (or lighten) comes forward visually, and everything you contour (or darken) goes away from you.

The face shape that's considered to be the most perfect is oval, so by highlighting and contouring, we can make your face look more oval. Let's put it this way: We can make your face look thinner and more sculpted. (Does that sound more exciting?) You'll be amazed how simply highlighting and contouring your face really creates shape. You pull forward the area of your face you want to see (the oval area) and push back the areas you don't want to see. So you will minimize that fullness around the outer edges of your face that is making you feel like your face looks too round.

Not only will this technique shape the face, but it will also add color, warmth, and life to every face. You will be thrilled by how this subtle effect can add the most incredible glow to your skin.

And guess what? Any face can look more oval with nothing more exotic than foundation and powder!

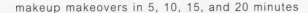

choose the right shades

Before you start, you will need to select three shades of foundation or powder in three different depth levels.

1. The first color should match your skin exactly. It is your true foundation color.

2. The second color, your highlight color, should be one level lighter than the first, preferably with the same undertone.

3. The third shade, your contour color, should be one level darker than your first, preferably with the same undertone.

4. The more dramatic you want your final result to be, the more dramatic the contrast between the three shades' depth levels should be. For example, if you want your contouring to be more noticeable, you could use a shade that is two or three levels darker than your natural shade. This will create a much more dramatic result. To create contrast if you have dark ebony skin, you could choose a highlight shade that is two or three levels lighter than your natural shade to get even more impact out of your sculpting. Just keep in mind that the more dramatic your choices, the more thoroughly and carefully you will have to blend the shades together.

timely tips

Don't forget my simple rule: With ivory/beige skin, contour more than you highlight, and with bronze/ebony skin, highlight more than you contour.

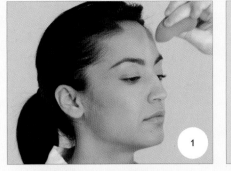
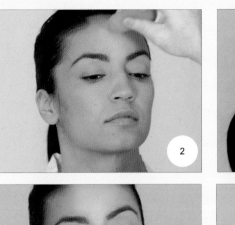
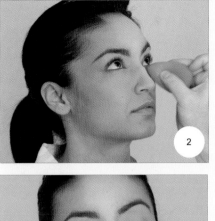
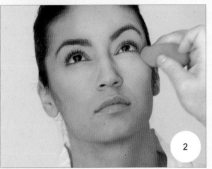

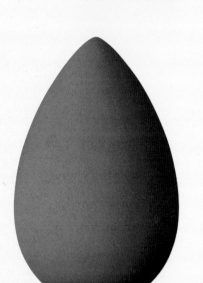

how to sculpt your face

Application takes just four simple steps:

1. Apply your first or true foundation color over your entire face. Then visualize an oval on your face. The width of the oval is your eye sockets; the height and length of your oval extends from the tip of your forehead to the tip of your chin. The reason you do this is that it helps you see where to highlight and where to contour.

2. Apply your second or highlight foundation color to the high points inside the oval, including your forehead, under the eyes at the top of the cheekbones, and the tip of your chin. The features that you highlight will be what the eye will focus on first. So if your face is too full, you'll be drawing attention to the narrow area in the middle of your face and away from the fuller sides.

"by highlighting and contouring,
we can make your face look thinner
and more sculpted."

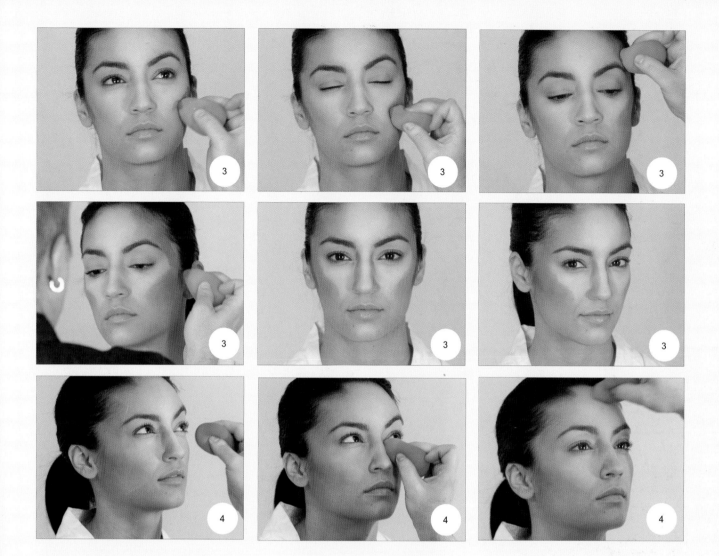

3. Finally, use your contour or darkest shade and apply it to the areas outside the oval, including the temples, along your hairline, and the sides of your cheeks down to the jaw. By deepening the outside areas, you are visually helping those areas recede, making your face appear more narrow and oval.

4. Blend everything really well. The secret to this technique appearing natural is all in the blending.

If you have ivory/beige skin, you will contour your face more than you highlight. Especially if you have really pale skin, the last thing you want to do is wash out your skin tone even more! So contouring is going to give you the most dramatic change. On bronze/ebony skin, you will highlight your skin more than contour. Especially if you have darker bronze/ebony skin tones, God gave you beautiful dark pigment in your skin, and contouring will not really show. But what *will* make a huge difference is what you highlight because it will brighten your skin and add life.

When you've finished applying your three foundation shades, simply powder with a shade that matches your natural skin tone. It will not negate all the work you have just finished, but it will set everything beautifully.

If you want your results to be even more dramatic, you can finish with three shades of powder: one that matches your true foundation shade, one that matches your highlight shade, and a darker or matte bronzing powder to match your contour shade. This will reinforce all of your work and give you a beautifully sculpted, three-dimensional effect that will make any face shape appear more oval and add that ever-so-important glow.

highlight powder

1. I prefer to use a sheer translucent highlight powder with no shimmer.

2. Apply it with your #76 powder brush underneath your eye on top of the cheek bone.

3. Now apply your highlight powder to the center of your forehead.

4. Apply your powder to the tip of your chin.

5. Here you can see proper placement.

6. Using your #73 powder brush, blend off the excess highlight powder.

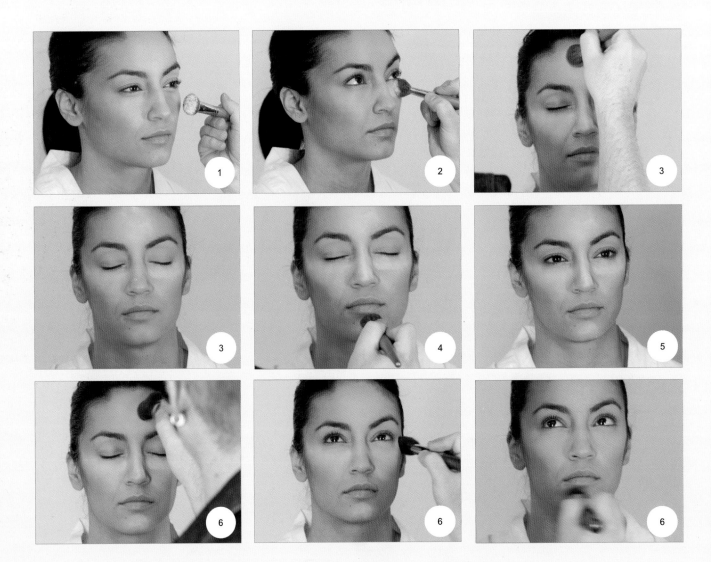

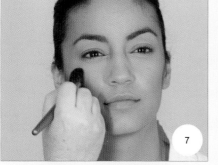
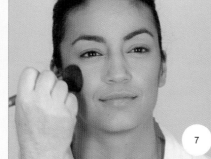
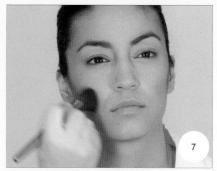

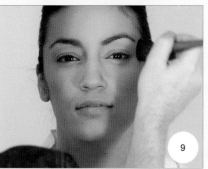
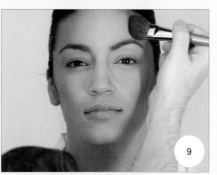
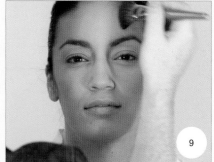

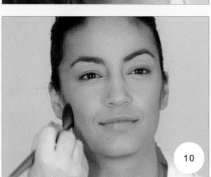
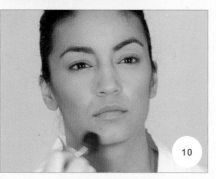

contouring powder

You can use either a matte bronzer or a darker shade of powder.

7. Using your #73 bronzer/blush brush, apply your matte bronzer beginning at the back of your cheekbone and sweep it forward toward the apple of your cheek. Then take the brush back towards your ear. This lays your color in place.

8. Now take your brush and use it in the opposite direction (up and down) to blend. Be sure to blend well, or it will not look natural.

9. Don't forget to add a little at the temples to help shape your face. Sweep the bronzing powder up around the temples and eye sockets.

10. Now apply your bronzer along your jawbone to help create shape.

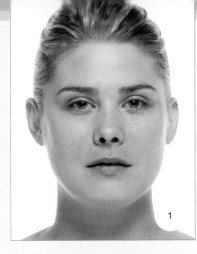

before

seeing is believing

The photos on pages 38-41 will help you understand the purpose and placement of your three shades. Keep in mind that, in these photos, I have **exaggerated** my highlight and contour so that you can truly see where to place your shades. Blend the three shades well because it is the blending process that makes the sculpting method work.

1. My goal is to warm up her skin and narrow her face.

2. This is an example of highlighting and contouring with foundation.

3. I have layered powder over the foundation to exaggerate the effects, but it also shows you where your highlight and contour shades go. Remember: blend, blend, blend! If you layer multiple powder shades over your foundation shades, it will make your highlighting and contouring more dramatic.

4. I know, it's okay for you to be shocked. Maybe you should sit down.

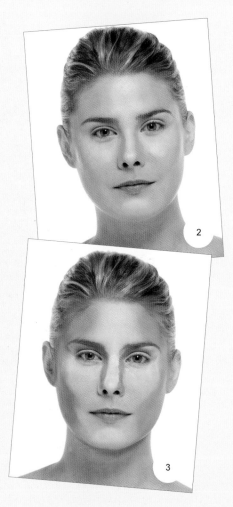

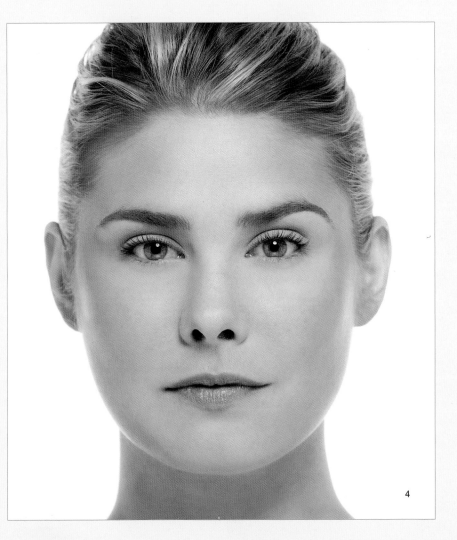

after

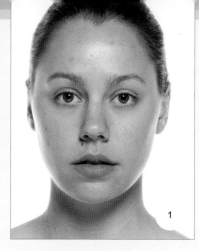

1. My goal is to bring out her cheekbones by contouring, which will also create a glow.

2. Once again, I've exaggerated the effects here with foundation. Also remember that with ivory/beige skin, you get more bang for your buck when you apply foundation like this.

3. Now I've reinforced the effects with powder and shown how to really chisel the cheekbones.

4. You can see how it really brings out her cheekbones.

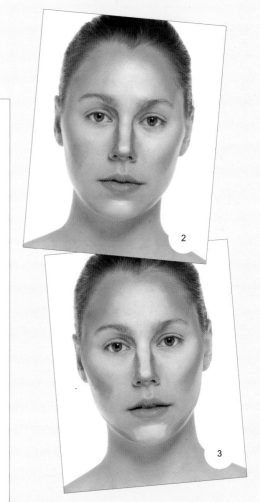

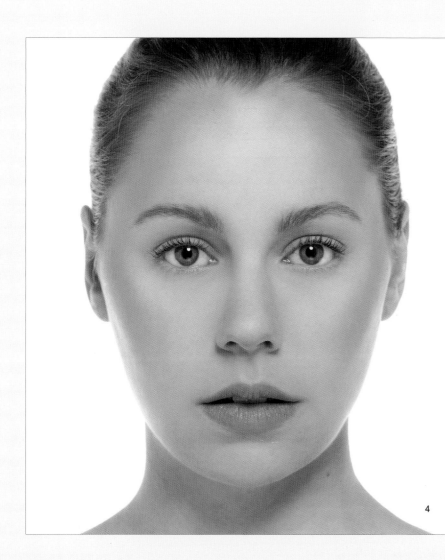

after

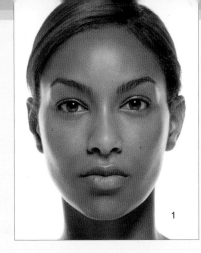

before

1. Here I am not trying to narrow her face; I am trying to brighten her face and give it a glow.

2. The foundation is showing you proper highlight placement. It's exaggerated, but because it is bronze/ebony skin, I highlighted like this because you get more impact. The darker the skin, the less contouring you will do, so highlighting gives you the most wow.

3. I followed with powder to exaggerate even more and show you where to contour as well.

4. You can see that it looks as if we turned the lights on. Her skin is glowing!

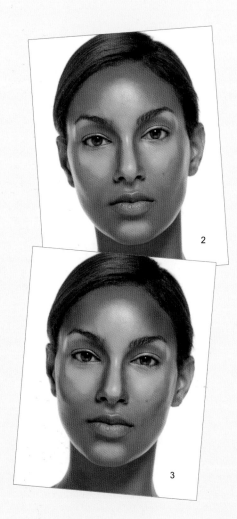

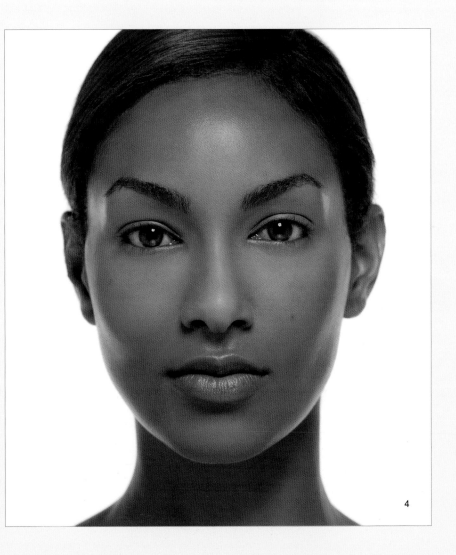

after

1. Here I want to draw attention to the center of her face (her highlight area) to give the illusion of narrowing the face.

2. The foundation is showing you proper highlight placement. It is exaggerated, but notice the effects on her bronze/ebony skin. I highlighted because it's an easy way to get a great effect on dark skin. Most of the time, I only highlight on bronze/ebony skin.

3. The foundation is showing you exaggerated, but proper, highlight and contour placement. Notice that because her skin tone is so dark, the contour does not do as much, which is why her highlight is more important than her contour.

4. I followed with multiple powder shades. Notice that her highlight powder has a golden-orange undertone.

5. You can see how this gives her face shape and a gorgeous glow.

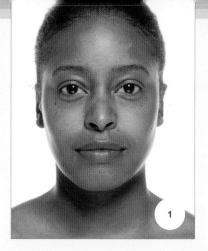

before

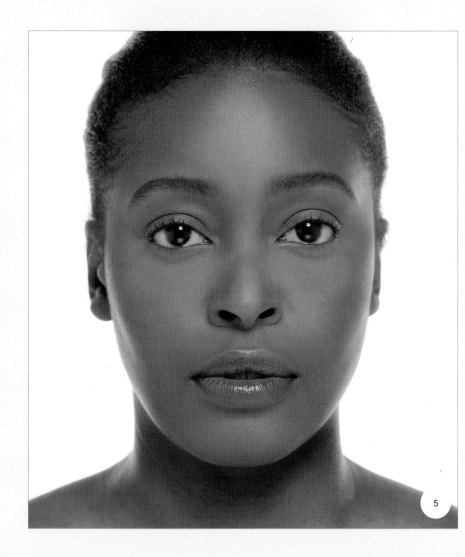

after

"there is *no* quicker, cheaper, faster facelift than curling your eyelashes!"

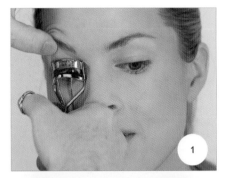

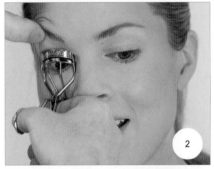

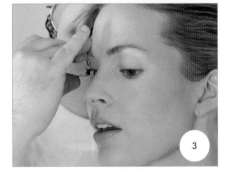

luscious lashes

I have five words to say about eyelashes: curl, curl, curl, curl, and curl. There is no quicker, cheaper, faster facelift than curling your eyelashes. It opens your eyes up and lifts your lids. Yes, you *have* to curl your lashes!

Nowadays, you have many curling options and multiple tools to get the job done. You have choices that range from the classic crimp curler to a precision eyelash curler or one of my favorites, the heated eyelash curler. No matter what your choice is, just remember to curl!

If your choice is a classic **crimp curler**, you can only use it before applying mascara, never after. The trick to curling your eyelashes correctly using a crimp curler is to crimp them more than just once at the lash line. So, "walk" the eyelash curler up the length of your lashes, taking care to close, open, and move the eyelash curler up several times until you reach the end of your lashes. Some women can crimp once, some three times (see images 1 and 2).

A **precision eyelash curler** works the same way a classic crimp curler works: You crimp it down on the lash, and it curls. The big difference is the size: It is only about one-fourth the width of the classic version, making it easier to get right at the base of the eyelashes (see image 3).

There is now an alternative eyelash-curling tool for those who are afraid of crimp-style eyelash curlers: a **heated eyelash curler**. This tool is used after you've applied mascara. I love this feature because many times when you apply your mascara, it can slightly uncurl your lashes. Starting at the base of your lashes, work the heated curler back and forth from side to side so that your lashes can fit into the grooves of the curler. Now push up and roll the curler in toward your lid, and your lashes will be curled to perfection—no crimping needed!

"mascara is the most important makeup you can own! Curled, thick, dark, long lashes are 80 percent of the battle."

mascara

Mascara is probably the most important piece of makeup you can own. It is the first step in defining your eyes. Personally, I think that curled, thick, dark, long lashes are 80 percent of the battle—your lashes are *that* important.

I think every woman should want long, thick lashes. But ultimately, you'll control whether or not your lashes appear longer and thicker by the application technique you choose.

for thicker lashes: Start at the base of the lashes and hold your mascara wand in a horizontal position, working it from side to side as you work your way up to the end of the lashes. This makes the mascara particles attach to the sides of your lashes, making them appear thicker.

for longer lashes: Hold your mascara wand in a vertical position. Starting at the base of the lash line, pull the wand up and out to the end of your lashes. The mascara particles will attach to the ends of your lashes, making them appear much longer.

If you want both—and you *deserve* both!—simply apply multiple layers each way. For example, apply your first coat thick (horizontally) and then let it dry. Apply your next coat so that it lengthens (vertically), let it dry, and so on. Don't forget: If you want to waterproof your lashes, just make your final layer waterproof.

With that said, I think every one of you needs more than one coat of mascara. You should always apply at least a couple of layers to your top lashes. (I personally prefer at least three to your top lashes, but just one on the lower lashes.) There is definitely a method to your madness in getting the perfect multiple-coat application!

timely tip

The trick to mastering multiple-coat mascara applications that look natural is making sure you apply very thin coats, letting each dry completely between coats.

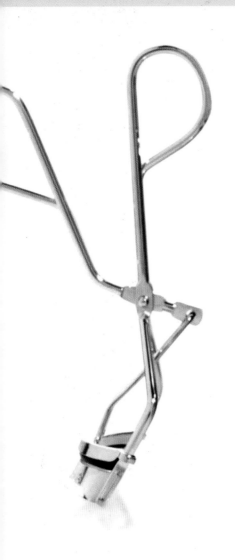

lashes that last

Here's the best way to layer several coats of mascara to "build" lashes that last:

1. Curl your eyelashes with a crimp-style eyelash curler because it opens up the eyes and makes them appear larger. (If you opt to use a heated curler, do so once you've applied your mascara and it's thoroughly dried.)

2. Pull the mascara wand out of the tube and wipe the brush against the opening of the tube or on a paper towel to remove any excess product. Don't be afraid of cleaning too much product off—there is plenty on there!

3. Apply the small amount that is left on the brush to your eyelashes.

4. Using an eyelash comb, comb your lashes before the mascara dries. This will help keep your lashes well separated and prevent them from clumping.

5. Let each coat of mascara dry between applications. This could take a couple of minutes, so be patient, but each coat must be completely dry. If you do not wait for each layer to dry, your lashes will clump.

6. After one coat is dry, pull your wand out, clean it off, and apply your next coat. And so on and so on and so on—you get the picture!

The trick to mastering multiple-coat applications is making sure you apply very thin coats, letting each dry completely between coats.

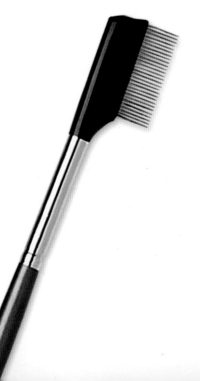

beautiful brows

Your brows are the frame of your face. Beautiful brows are a finishing touch that completes and polishes any look you choose to try and play with. I am often asked if everyone needs brow color, and I would say 95 percent of women need at least some brow color. But before you can color, you need to trim and shape your brows.

trimming

Often, brow hairs are actually longer than they appear because the tips of the hairs are lighter in color, and when they reach a certain length, they tend to curl. By trimming them, you trim away some of the density and that slight curl so that the hairs lie flat.

To trim your brow hairs, simply brush them up and snip any stray hairs that extend past the upper brow line. Next, brush them down and snip any unruly hairs that extend past the lower brow line. Now brush them back into place. Notice how much better they lie and how much softer they look on your face.

It's important to remember that if you need to trim your brows, it should be done before you start to tweeze. Otherwise, you might ruin your brow line by tweezing away hairs that should have stayed but were simply too long.

shaping

How do you determine where to start? By locating three key points of reference, we will know where and what to tweeze. Simply locate these three critical points and follow these directions, and you'll have perfect brows!

point A: Hold a pencil or the handle of a brush vertically against the side of your nose, noticing where it meets the brow. That is where your brow should begin.

point B: Hold the pencil against your nostril and move it diagonally across the outer half of the iris of your eye. Notice where the pencil meets the brow: This is the best place for the peak of your arch. If you tweeze from point A to point B, tapering the line slightly thinner toward the peak, you will create the ideal shape for your brow. It is a gentle taper, using the natural width at the beginning of your brow (point A) and slowly tapering it thinner as you get to the arch (point B).

point C: Again, place the pencil against your nostril, but this time, extend it diagonally to the outer corner of your eye. Where it meets the brow is the best place for your brow to end. If you tweeze from point B to point C, tapering the line even thinner, you will create the best brow shape for your face.

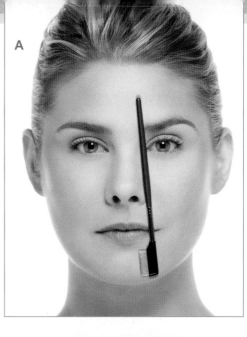

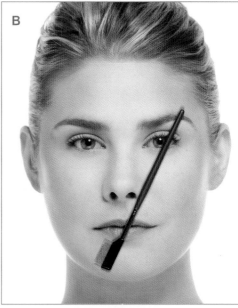

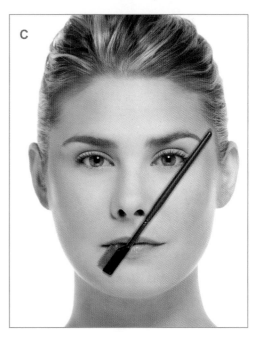

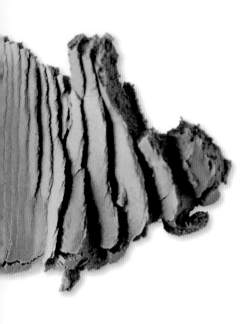

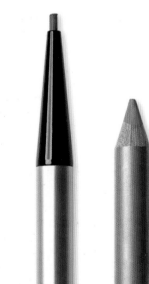

choosing brow color

Did you know that you can choose a brow color as easily as a hair color? It's true, and you should take advantage of it, especially when you're trying to look younger. When selecting a brow color, the basic rule of thumb is that it should pretty closely match your hair color (whether natural or chosen). Let's elaborate a little bit, though, because it isn't really as simple as that. Here are the perfect brow colors for each hair color:

light blonde: same color as hair or one shade darker

medium to dark blonde: same color as hair

auburn: same color as hair

light brown: same color as hair or one shade lighter

medium to dark brown: same color as hair or one shade lighter

very dark brown to black: one shade lighter than your hair color

silver or gray: use a blonde or soft taupe color for ivory/beige skin tones and use a light golden brown for bronze/ebony skin tones (a silver or gray brow color to match your hair would just wash you out and make you look older)

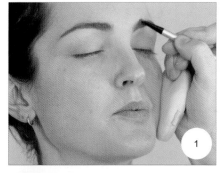
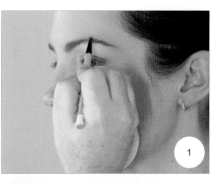

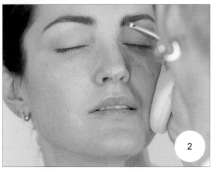
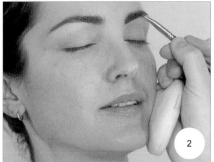

application

Now it's time to add some color!

1. Apply your pencil using short, feathery, hairlike strokes angled in the same direction as the hairs' growth. Your strokes are meant to mimic natural brow hairs; never draw a solid straight line!

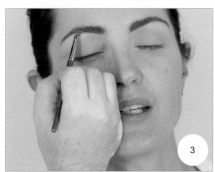
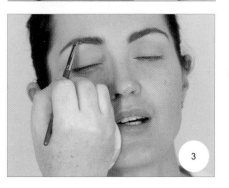

2. Using a small stiff-angled brush, go over the pencil you just applied, using the same short strokes. This will blend your color even more, making it look extremely natural.

3. Take your brush and dip it into your brow powder. Once again, apply the powder using short, feathery, hairlike strokes angled in the same direction as the hairs' growth. Make sure you cover the entire brow. The powder and pencil layered together like this will give you more complete coverage, help the color last longer, and look more natural.

4. When grooming your brows, always finish by using a brow brush (my favorite is shaped like a toothbrush) to brush all your brow hairs upward and outward. This will ensure that your brow hairs are lying in place and blend your color beautifully to give you an absolutely natural effect.

Now you have all the techniques you need to create a perfect foundation. It's time to look at your essential tools in the next chapter!

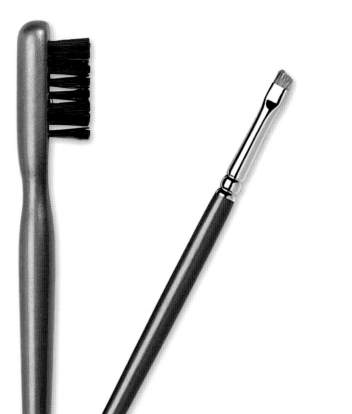

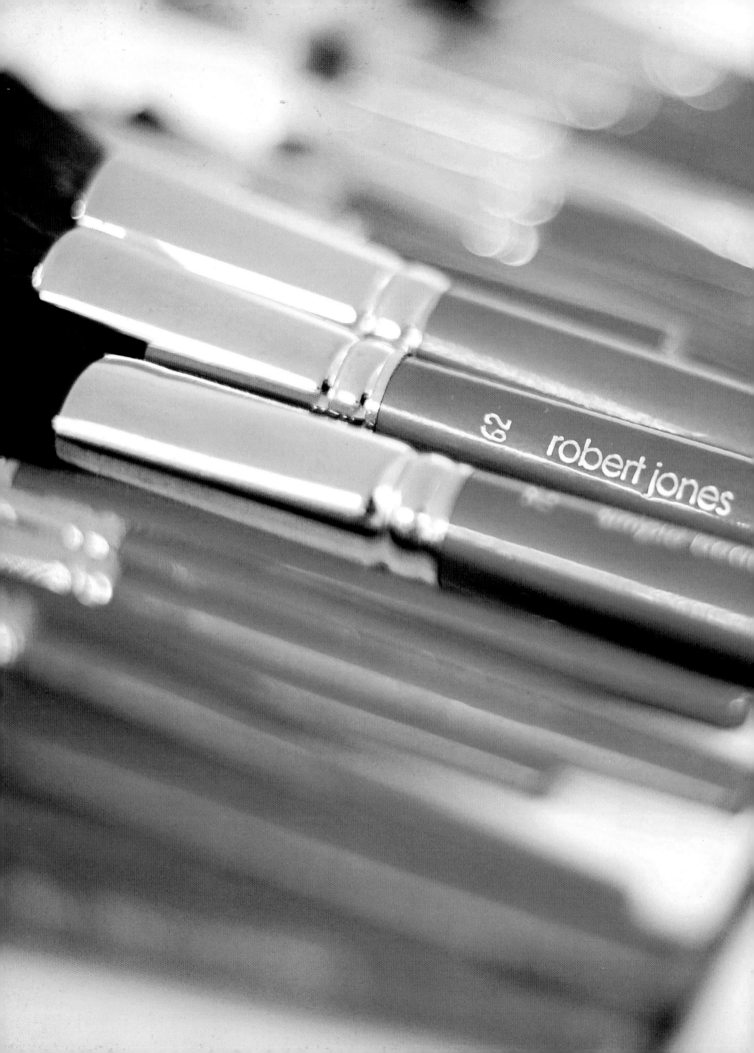

3

must-have tools

It's time to gather your tools to create a look you will love. In this chapter, I am going to help you put together the makeup shades you need as well as the brushes that help create every look. I tried to keep the palette of shades simple, so you can see that it just takes a small number of items to create an amazing number of looks. There is no need to own every eye shadow under the sun. You can create so many looks with a collection of just a few perfect shades.

Keep in mind as you go through the book and study all the different looks and application techniques that you can always substitute other shades and still use the same application to customize a look.

the eyes have it

Let's talk about eye makeup first. It takes three shades to shape an eye: a highlight (everything you highlight comes forward), a midtone (a natural shade that is an extension of your skin), and a contour (the dramatic fun color). So I have divided up the shades accordingly.

eye shadow powder

You can create every look in this book with a combination of these shades.

shimmer peachy gold

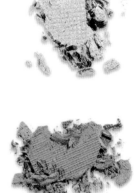

highlight

matte beige

shimmer acid green

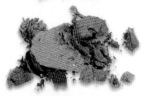

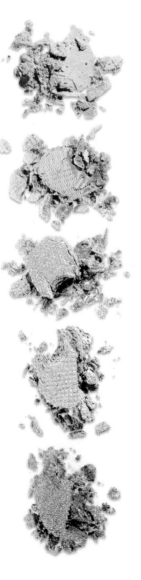

midtone

matte flesh

matte taupe

shimmer champagne

matte dark taupe

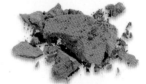

shimmer white

matte caramel

shimmer gold

matte ginger

"it takes three shades to shape an eye: a highlight, a midtone, and a contour."

contour

shimmer iridescent purple

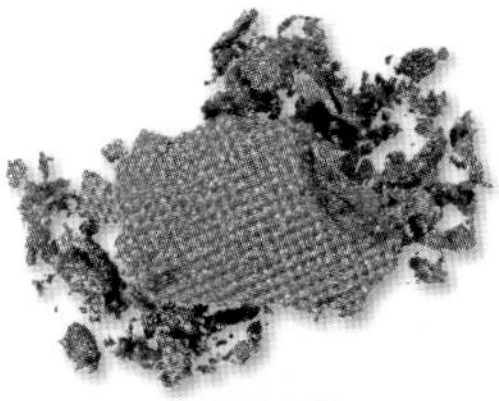

shimmer purple

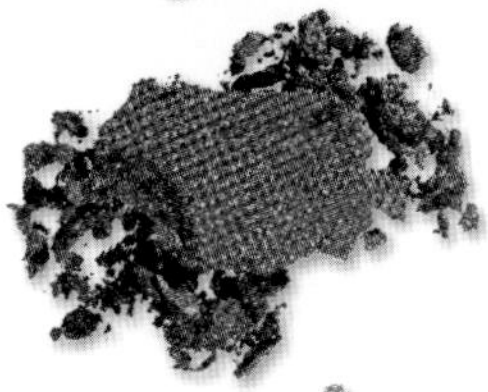

shimmer teal

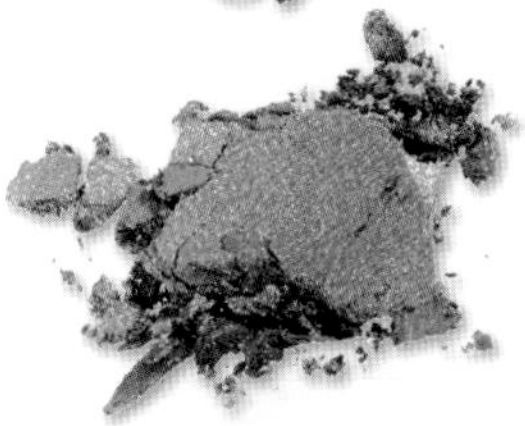

shimmer dark blue

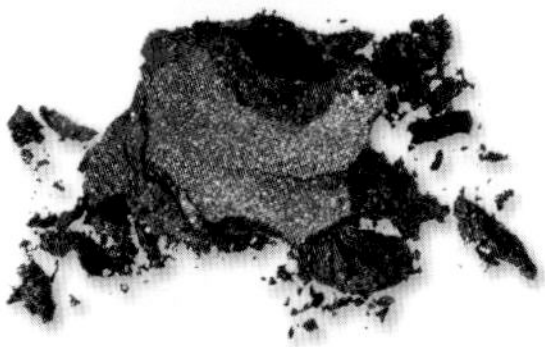

shimmer dark green

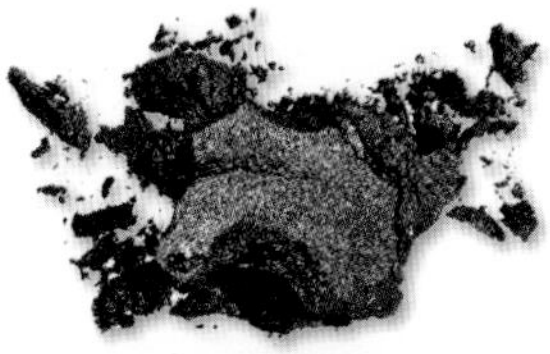

shimmer burgundy

shimmer copper

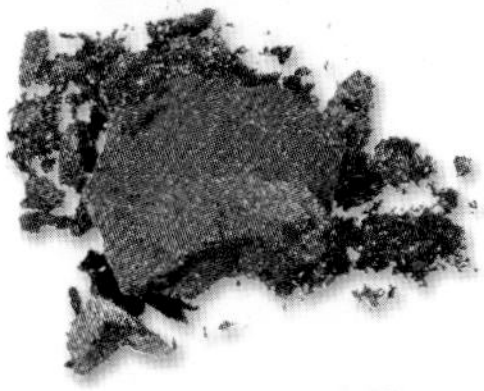

shimmer terra-cotta

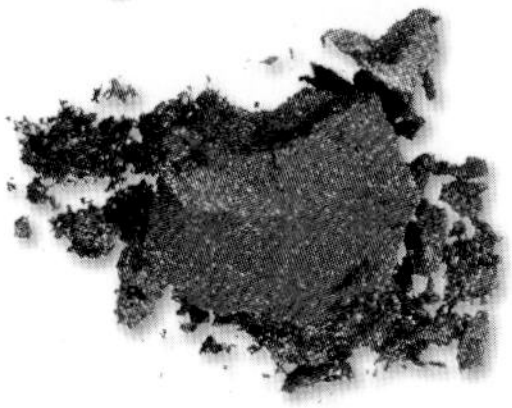

shimmer bronze

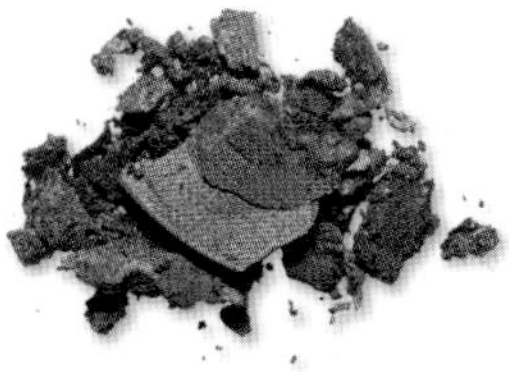

shimmer pinky gray

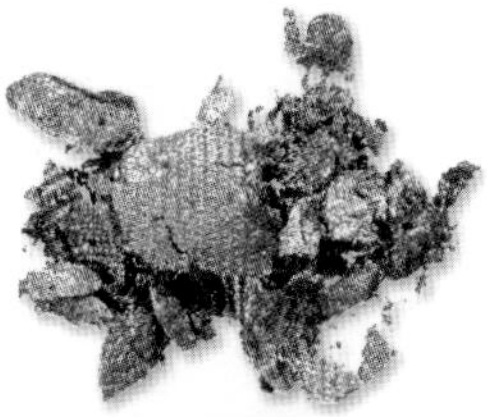

shimmer golden brown

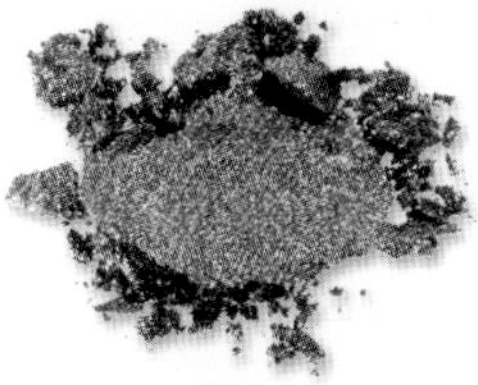

matte dark brown

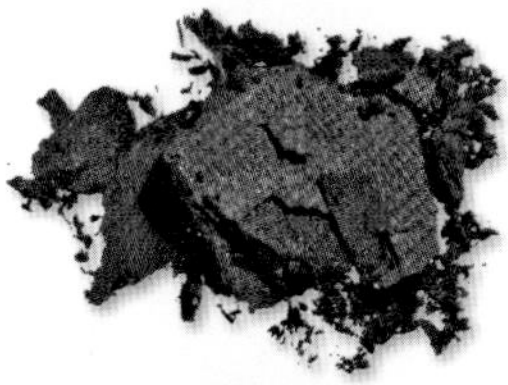

shimmer dark brown

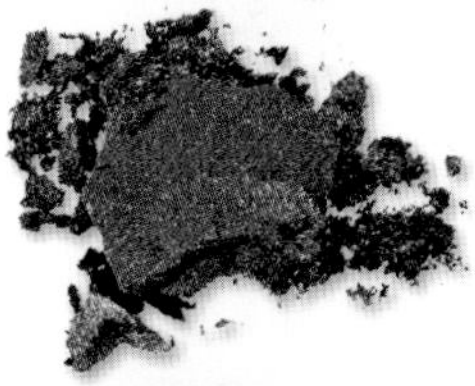

shimmer dark gray

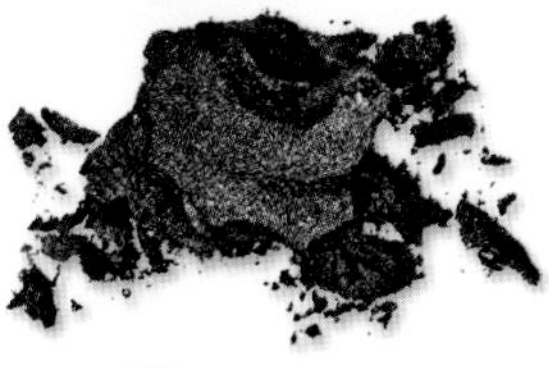

matte black

"I'm a big believer in brown and black because basic shades work the best."

eye shadow crème-to-powder

The purpose of using a crème (the majority of the time) is to intensify your color and your payoff. So layer your crème on first. Then follow it with your powder.

eyeliner

You'll notice that I use very few eyeliner colors. I have to say, I'm a big believer in brown and black, simply because the purpose of eyeliner is defining the eye, and so basic shades work the best. I only use color when doing a colorful eye.

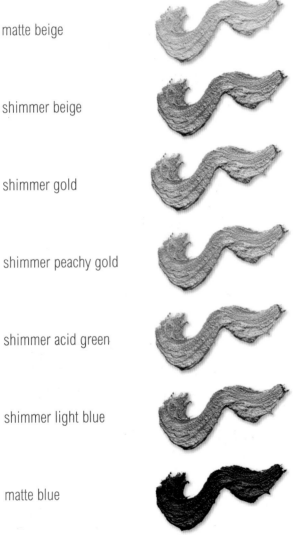

matte beige

shimmer beige

shimmer gold

shimmer peachy gold

shimmer acid green

shimmer light blue

matte blue

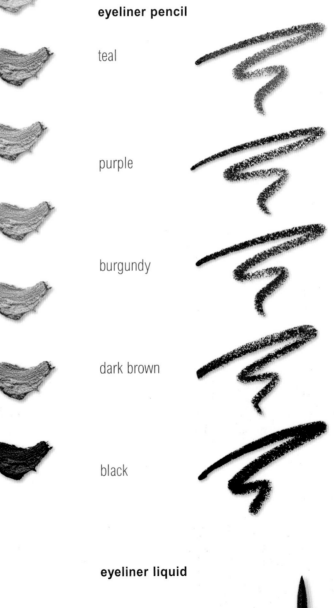

eyeliner pencil

teal

purple

burgundy

dark brown

black

eyeliner liquid

black

blushing beauty

My blush palette is so basic! That's because your blush is supposed to create a very natural flush. You do not need a crazy number of shades, just what looks natural. Then, depending on how strong or soft you want the look, you simply add more or less or layer crème and powder together for more flush.

blush powder

I find that three blush shades are enough to bring out the beauty in every woman's skin tone! Wondering what happened to pink and red? Trust me, girls: These are *not* the colors God gave you! Go with these blush tones instead for a beautiful, natural flush.

peach

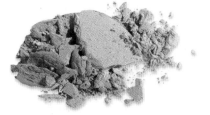

apricot

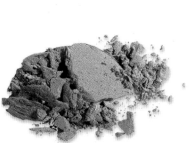

raisin

blush crème-to-powder

For a richer color, choose one of these natural looking crème-to-powder shades.

peach

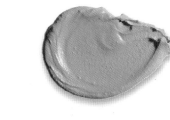

apricot

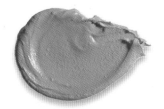

"the purpose of blush is to create a natural-looking flush."

luscious lips

For the looks in this book, I've chosen to use a very pared-down palette. As you'll see, you don't need a million shades to create a ton of looks. Play, experiment, and have fun!

lip liner

Lip liner defines your lip outline. But as with blush, you want a natural liner, not a bold, harsh color that draws attention to itself instead of to your beautiful lips!

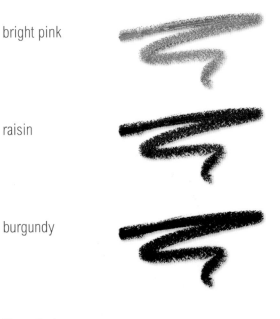

bright pink

raisin

burgundy

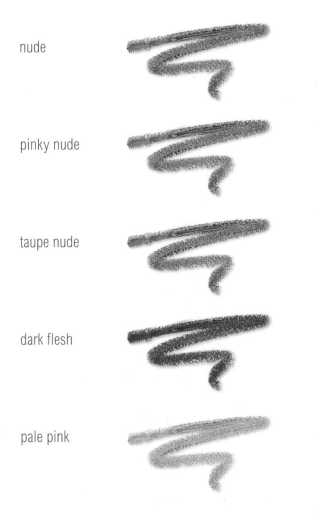

nude

pinky nude

taupe nude

dark flesh

pale pink

lipstick

Lipstick is your chance to play with color, from subtle nudes to bold red, fuchsia, and deep berry. Check out the looks in chapters 4 to 7 to see how I match lip colors to each look!

nude

pink nude

peach nude

pale pink

"you don't need a million shades to create a ton of looks."

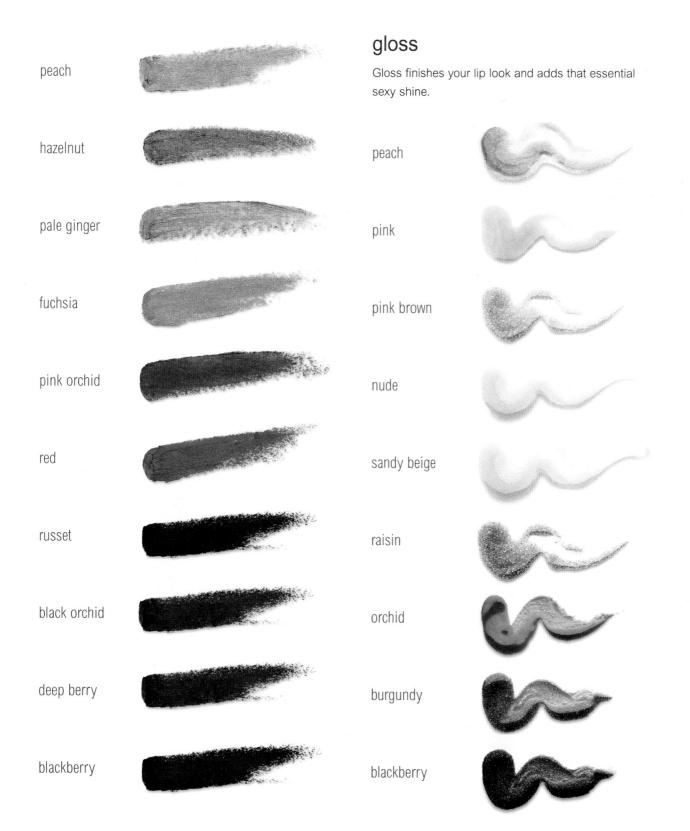

peach

hazelnut

pale ginger

fuchsia

pink orchid

red

russet

black orchid

deep berry

blackberry

gloss

Gloss finishes your lip look and adds that essential sexy shine.

peach

pink

pink brown

nude

sandy beige

raisin

orchid

burgundy

blackberry

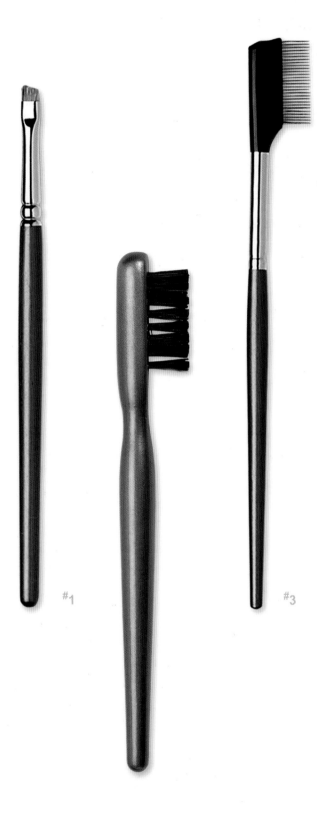

#1

#3

brushes

There are so many choices, shapes, sizes, and types of brushes out there that I can completely understand how it can become very confusing when making your choices. Believe it or not, the different brush head shapes make a huge difference in the effect they create. So I have designed brushes for every purpose or effect you need to create. I am going to describe each shape so that between the picture and the description, you will know which brushes to buy.

In this book, I've used brushes from my own signature collection of *robert jones beauty* makeup tools (www.robert-jonesbeauty.com), where you can find every shape you could ever need.

eyebrow/eyelash brushes

#1: This is the perfect brush for applying color and shaping your brows. Its short, stiff, natural bristles and narrow angle will give you an exact application. The firmness of this brush is so important to its ability to give precise placement of color. The edges of the angle are also tapered for softness of color and to help blend.

brow brush: I know it may look like a toothbrush, but it's not. This brush is the perfect shape for grooming and shaping your brows. It is perfect for trimming brows because of its ability to brush the entire brow. It's also great for blending everything after every color application.

eyelash comb #3: An eyelash comb is a must for perfect lashes. After applying mascara, combing your lashes will help separate every lash while removing any clumps. The fine metal teeth allow for exact precision.

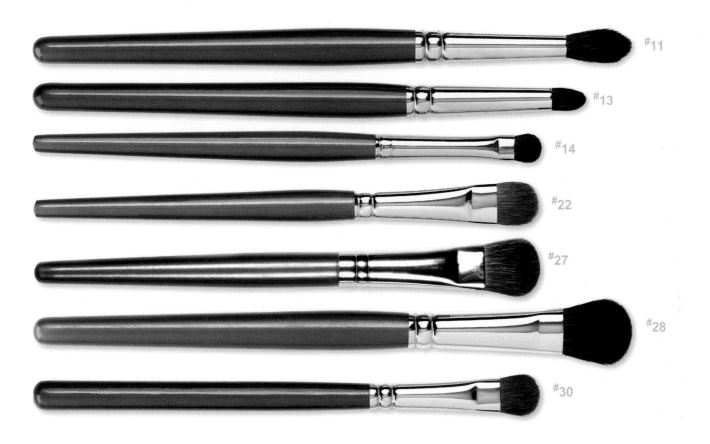

eye shadow brushes

#11: This tapered natural-bristle brush expertly applies your favorite midtone shade in the crease with precision, from the outer corner of the eye to the inside corner. The shape helps apply your color right where you want it while helping blend your color.

#13: This precision-shaped natural-bristle brush is perfect for applying your favorite shade of eye shadow along the lower lash line while giving you a smudged and blended effect with no harsh lines. It's also perfect for creating a very defined line of color in the crease of the eye.

#14: This natural-bristle brush is perfect for applying your highlight shade at the inside corner of the eye and along the lower lash line (which, as you'll discover, opens the eyes for a wide-eyed, youthful look). It's also perfect for smudging liner and detailed color application.

#22: Use this professional-quality natural-bristle eye shadow brush to precisely apply your highlight shade to your brow bone and lid. It's also perfect for applying color anywhere to your eye whenever you want a brush with a slightly stiffer feel. The stiffness can make it easier to control placement.

#27: This natural-bristle brush is the perfect size and shape for applying color over a large area of your lid. Its soft flexibility makes it the must-have tool for creating the perfect smoky eye.

#28: This soft, natural-bristle brush is perfect for all-over blending. It's a must when you're wearing more than one eye color. Keep this brush free of color so you can use it to blend multiple shades of eye shadow flawlessly. Use it to blend over and across the lid after you have applied all your eye shadow; this will blend all your shades together without making the colors on your lid look muddy.

#30: This precision brush, made of natural bristles with the edges tapered for blending, is perfect for applying your most intense shade of eye shadow along the lash line and into the outer corner of the crease of the eye. Its shape is ideal for creating a wide variety of looks and effects.

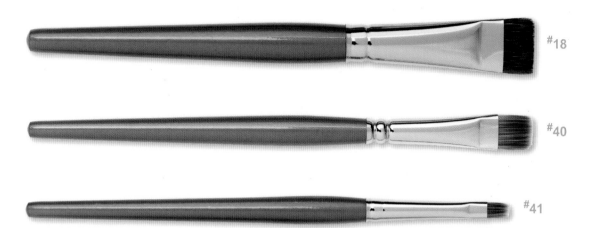

#18

#40

#41

eyeliner brushes

#18: Use this wide, flat natural-bristle brush to precisely apply a line of bold or soft eye color along the lash line and blend up onto the lid. It makes your application so easy because of its shape: Simply lay the brush flat on your lid along your lash line and brush up. It's great for helping you create intensity at your lash line for a smoky eye.

#40: This flat, synthetic brush is used to line and define eyes with eye shadow or to apply powder over your pencil liner to create a more subtle effect. It is also great for blending your pencil without adding color: Simply brush across the pencil you applied to smooth and perfect the line. It's perfect for wet or dry use.

#41: My secret weapon for eyes that grab attention with subtle perfection is a tiny brush with big results. Use this brush to push color into your lash line, which makes your eye color really pop and your lashes look so thick. It's also perfect for very detailed lining.

timely tip

Keep in mind when applying a powder product that you want a brush with natural bristles, and when applying crème products, for the most part you want a brush with synthetic bristles, but if you are applying a crème-to-powder product, you can use either.

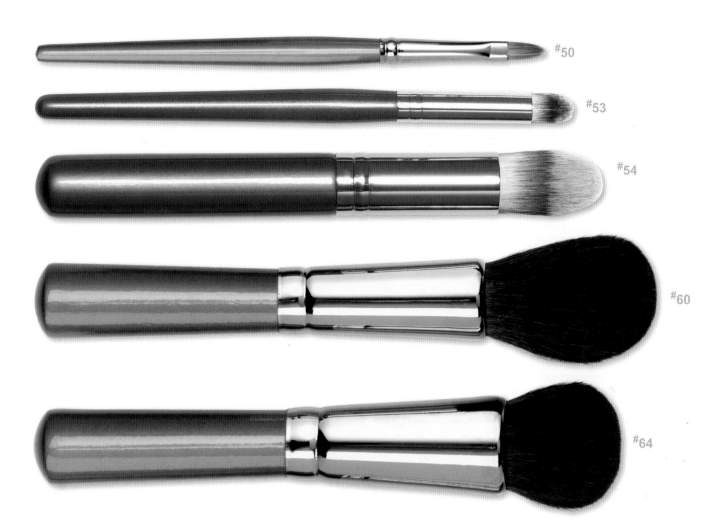

#50

#53

#54

#60

#64

complexion/face-perfecting brushes

#50: Use this synthetic brush to apply concealer with exact precision. Its pointed, tapered shape allows you to cover very detailed areas of the face without overblending or over-working your concealer. A concealer brush is an absolute must-have.

#53: This new updated pointed shape is amazing for con-cealing. This synthetic brush is perfection for concealing larger areas or for use on curved areas of the face. Talk about fast, perfect application!

#54: Use this perfectly tapered, pointed, synthetic-bristle brush to apply crème or liquid foundation evenly and flaw-lessly onto the skin. It's the best tool for end-of-the-day touch-ups, when you don't want to start over but need to touch up.

#60: This is the ultimate blush and bronzer brush. It's made with the softest natural bristles, the best for applying blush or bronzer. Its full, round shape and expert tapering blend your blush or bronzer for the most professional application.

#64: This is the perfect blush brush made of the softest, highest-quality natural bristles. The round, full, tapered shape is perfect for applying color to the "apples of the cheeks" without creating any hard or definite edges. I created it to work perfectly with crème-to-powder blush.

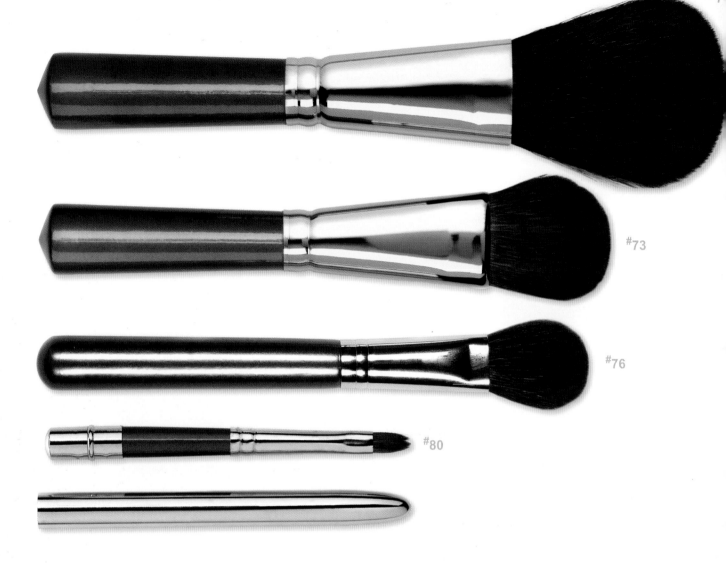

#7

#73

#76

#80

lip brushes

#70: This is a big and fluffy natural-bristle brush that is perfect for brushing on loose powder smoothly, giving you sheer, even application. The slightly tapered head shape really assists with your application.

#73: This natural-bristle brush is so versatile and irreplaceable! So many uses, so little time. It's perfect for loose and pressed powder application, unbelievable for removing excess loose powder after powder-puff application, and priceless for detailed blush and face contour application.

#76: This natural-bristle brush is the ultimate for detailed powdering. Due to its shape and size, it can't be beat for powdering in small areas, like under eyes and eyelids. There is no better brush for applying powder highlights and face shimmers with precision.

lip brush #80: This lip brush with a fine, tapered point is perfect for applying lipstick and lip gloss with precision. And we all know that if you apply lipstick with a brush, it will last longer, and if you apply lip gloss with a brush, it will look shinier.

timely tip

The right brush is the true secret to great application. It is one of the key things that make a pro's work look professional.

good brush hygiene

You have to clean your brushes regularly, or you won't get the application and clarity of color that you want and need. The cleaner the tool, the better the application. You have a couple of cleaning options:

brush cleanser: This option is certainly simplest: There are professional brush cleansers available that work beautifully. One great benefit is that most of them are fast-drying, which makes them even more convenient. You dip your brush in the cleanser and wipe it off on a towel, and it's cleaned to perfection.

shampoo: Your other option is to shampoo your brushes. Because brushes are made from hair (natural or synthetic), shampoo works great, but it will take longer for them to dry. Just dampen your brush and then, with a bit of shampoo in the palm of your hand (a gentle baby shampoo works best and will not be too harsh), work the brush into the shampoo and rinse. I find it best to lightly condition the brushes after washing (a light leave-in hair conditioner works best because it will be very lightweight, but be sure you rinse it out afterward), then rinse them. Finally, squeeze out all the excess moisture (being sure to reshape the brushes, so that when they dry the shape will be correct) and lay them flat on a towel to dry.

"The cleaner the tool, the better the application."

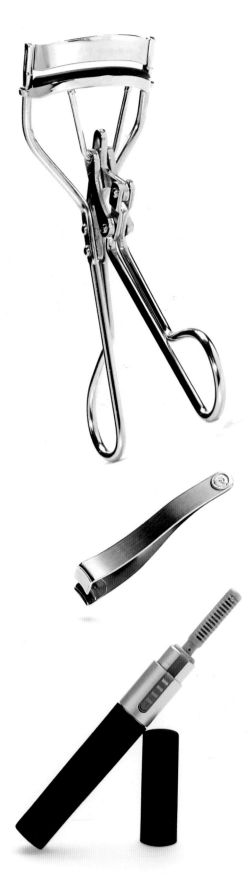

"eyelash curlers make you look younger, so use them!"

eyelash curlers

No woman should be without a good eyelash curler. Because of modern technology, there are several good choices available. No matter which you choose, the goal is still the same: to curl your lashes and make yourself look younger.

There are basically three versions: a crimp curler, a precision eyelash curler, and the can't-live-without heated eyelash curler:

crimp curler: The most common (usually metal) and most widely used, this version is used only before applying mascara, never after. Make sure the rubber pad or pads have curved edges to create a better curl, not a crimp. You must also make sure that you replace your curler at least once a year and the rubber piece at least once every six months. Turn to page 42 to learn proper curling technique.

precision eyelash curler: This curler works just like a crimp curler, but its width makes it easier to get right at the root. I love it because I can use it to curl the far inside and outside corner lashes that most crimp curlers miss. It is also easier to use on lashes that are extremely short.

heated eyelash curler: This miracle product is a must-have! The beauty of this curler is that it works *after* you apply your mascara. (I am sure many of you have experienced for yourselves that applying mascara can start to uncurl the lashes you have just curled.) If you try to use a crimp or precision curler after applying mascara, they could rip lashes out. The heated curler actually uses the mascara as a curling catalyst, which helps the curl last all day. This curler will curl even the most stubborn lashes that no other curler will. See page 42 for usage instructions.

sponges

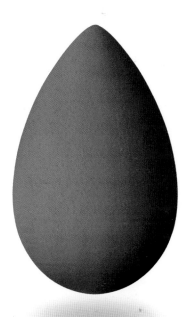

There are a couple of things to consider when choosing a sponge. First, look at the texture and quality. The better the quality, the better looking the application will be. So price can definitely matter. The shape can effect how a sponge performs as well, depending on what you're using it for; different shapes make it easier to get makeup where you want it. The material a sponge is made from will also have a huge effect on how flawless the application is.

In today's world of beauty, you have many choices, including your traditional triangular wedge, oval, and round sponges. One of my latest favorite tools is a new egg-shaped sponge called the Beauty Blender. What makes it so amazing is the texture and shape, allowing you to create an airbrushed finish to your foundation. Also, it is latex-free, so if you are allergic to latex, it is a great option.

Ready to get your tools and go? Great! In the next chapter, you'll see how to put the tools and techniques you've just learned about to work to give yourself a fabulous new look in just 5 minutes. Did I say 5? You bet I did!

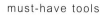

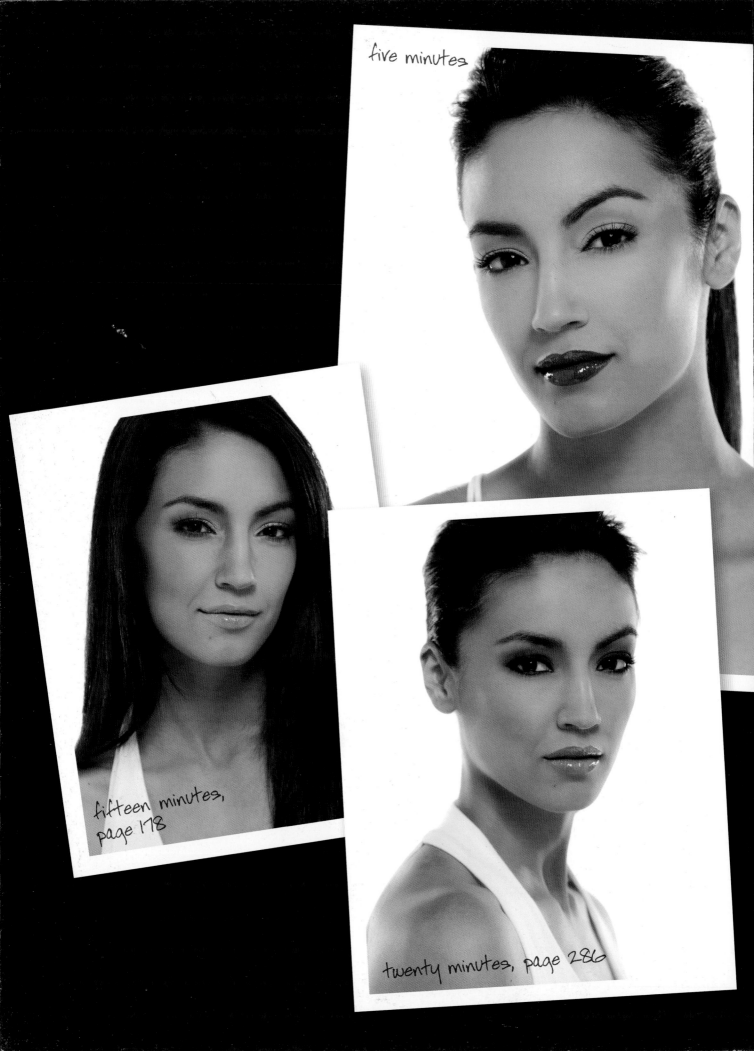

five minutes

fifteen minutes,
page 178

twenty minutes, page 286

5 minutes to gorgeous

Are you ever walking down the street, at the mall, or just sitting at a traffic light when you see a woman who looks so gorgeous and pulled together? Do you get jealous and think, "I would never have time to get myself that flawless looking?" Guess what: It doesn't take forever to get gorgeous. It could take as little as 5 minutes!

Check out the looks I've created for this chapter, try them out for yourself, and you'll know I'm right. Imagine the thrill of looking beautiful in just 5 minutes. What are you waiting for?!

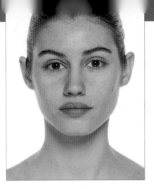

color wash

I love this look because it's fun and colorful, yet quick and simple. This look is so easy because it just requires a quick wash of color, but the results are fabulous! Remember, when doing a simple wash of color like this, choosing the right shade can go a long way toward bringing out your eye color. You'll get soft definition, but as you can see with Alex, your eyes will really pop.

Here's how to get this look:

eyes

1. Start by defining your crease. Using your #11 midtone brush and starting from the outside corner of your crease, glide your brush across to the inside corner. Use a soft matte taupe eye shadow—a shade just a bit darker than your skin tone—so that you get soft definition.

2. Always follow with your #28 blending brush (remember, this is the one that you always keep clean and ready to blend with) and blend your midtone so there are no hard edges.

3. Next, grab your #30 contour brush and some of your midtone eye shadow and define the outer third of your eyelid.

4. Again, follow with your #28 brush to blend. This step starts your lid definition.

5. Now, with your #27 eye shadow brush, use a soft iridescent purple and starting at the base of your lash line, bring the color all the way across the lid and up into the crease. Once again, start from the outside corner and work toward the inside, so the deepest color is on the outside of the lid.

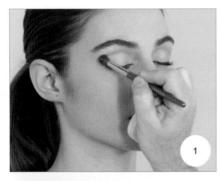

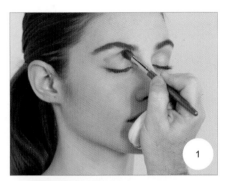

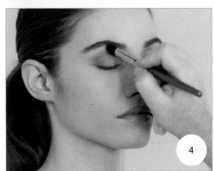

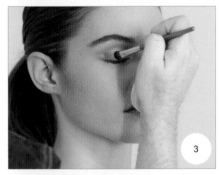

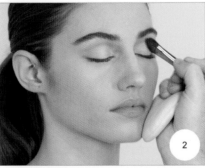

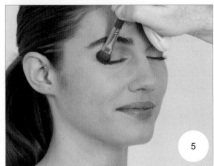

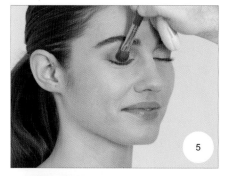

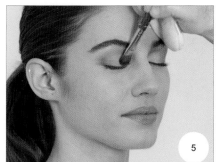

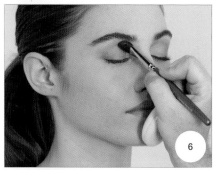

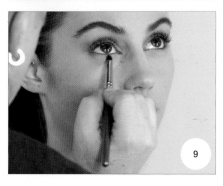

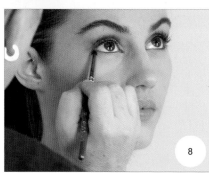

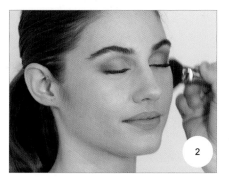

6. Pick up your #28 blending brush again and blend the area where your contour shade meets your midtone shade.

7. This is a perfect time to apply your first layer of mascara to your upper lash line. Of course, by now you know you have to curl first! (See page 42 to review how to curl properly.)

8. Now, grab your #13 detail eye shadow brush and apply your midtone eye shadow all along your lower lash line. Once again, start your application from the outside corner, sweeping it across to the inside corner.

9. Follow this with your soft purple shadow and layer it right on top of the midtone eye shadow that you just applied to your lower lash line.

10. Finish by adding another layer of mascara to your top lashes and then define your lower lashes with mascara. (See page 44 to review how to layer your mascara properly.)

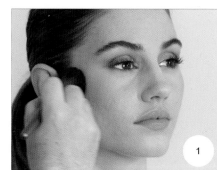

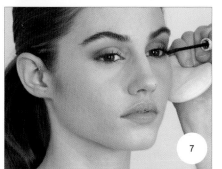

cheeks

To make this simple and fast, we are only going to use a matte bronzer to define the cheek and add color. Bronzer often provides the perfect amount of color all by itself, especially when paired with a colorful eye.

1. Grab your #73 bronzer/blush brush and let's get your glow on! Beginning at the back of your cheekbone, sweep it forward toward the apple of your cheek. Then take the brush back toward your ear. This lays your color in place.

2. Next, take your brush and use it in the opposite direction (up and down) to blend. Be sure to blend well, or it will not look natural.

3. Don't forget to add a little bronzer at the temples to help shape your face. Sweep the bronzing powder up around your temples and eye sockets. This always gives the face more color and gives you a healthy glow.

4. Feel free to blend some bronzer along your jawbone. This also helps create that glow and define your face.

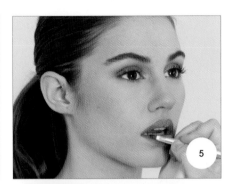

lips

Here the cheeks are minimally enhanced and the eyes are brought out with a soft wash of color, so you can focus on creating very defined lips.

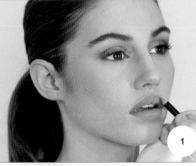

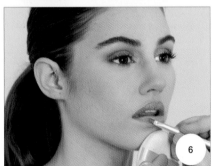

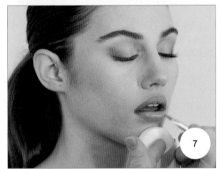

1. First, using a nude lip liner, line your lips. Begin with a V in the "cupid's bow," or center curve of the lips. Bring the liner up and around the curves of your bow.

2. Next, starting at the outer corners, move toward the center bow with your pencil.

3. On the lower lip, first accentuate the lower curve of the lip. Then begin from the outer corners, moving toward the center. Outline your entire lip: Take the color to the almost invisible line just at the edge of the colored part of your lips.

4. Now, using the same pencil, fill in halfway toward the center of your lips. This will help your lip color last longer and make it easier to blend your liner.

5. Using a #80 lip brush, blend your liner before you apply your lipstick. Use this lip brush to apply your lipstick because it gives you better application and helps the color last longer.

6. With your brush, fill in your entire lip with the perfect peach lipstick. Blend the lipstick really well over your lip liner.

7. As always, I like to finish with a coat of sheer peach lip gloss to add shine. And I love that sexy shine! Make sure you apply your gloss with your #80 lip brush because if you apply gloss with a brush, it will appear shinier.

"the trick to creating a look that's fast and easy is using fewer products."

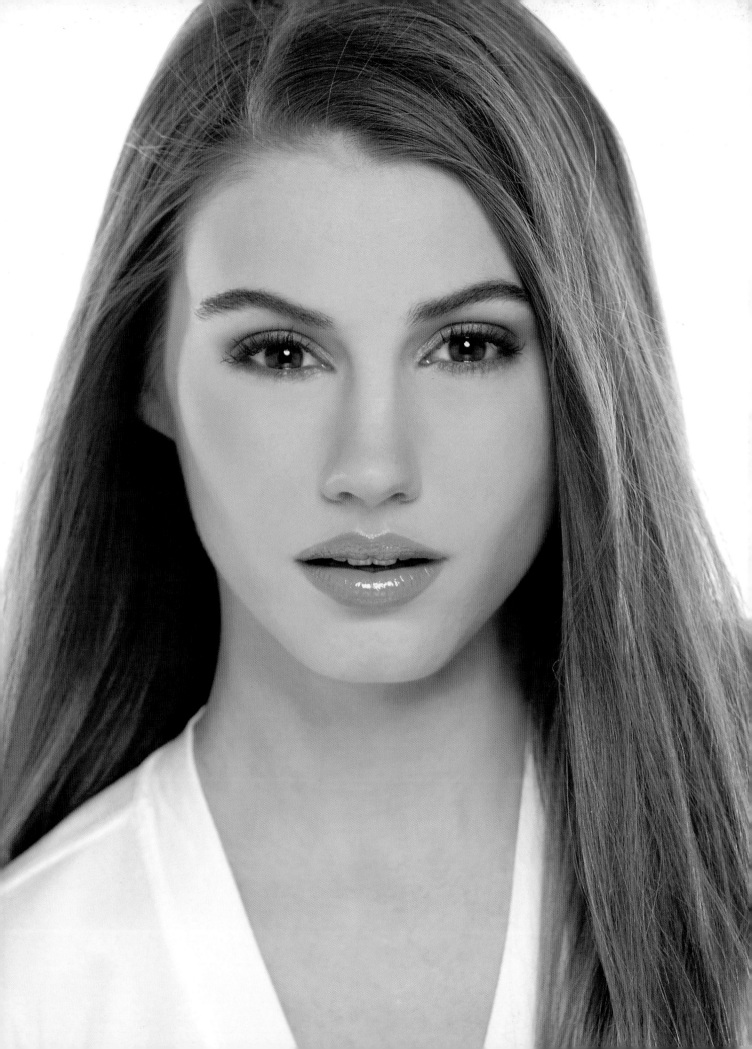

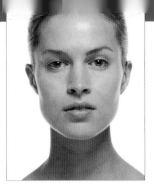

sun-bleached beauty

I call this look sun-bleached because it looks like your makeup was applied, then bleached out from being in the sun. What I love about this look is the beautiful glow it gives to the skin.

Obviously, your skin is the focus of this look. But as always, your eyes still have the perfect amount of definition so they don't disappear! This look is perfect for whenever you want a summer beach glow, no matter what time of year it is.

Here's how to get this look:

eyes

1. One of the most important aspects of creating this look is highlighting the eye. Using your #22 highlighting brush and a pale matte beige eye shadow, highlight your lid and brow bone. When I say brow bone, I mean the area just under the arch of your brow.

2. Follow your matte beige shadow with a shimmer white, layering it right on top of your matte shade, but only on your lid, not your brow bone. I almost always prefer the lid to be a bit more high-lighted than the brow bone. This shimmer over your matte will give you a more dramatic highlight.

3. For very subtle lash line definition, use your #41 detail eyeliner brush and push black eye shadow into the base of your lash line.

4. Now, taking a little matte bronzer, define your crease. Using your #11 midtone brush, start from the outside corner of your crease and glide your brush across to the inside corner. This softly defines your crease.

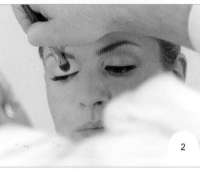
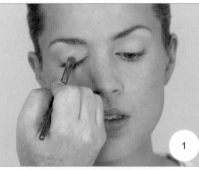
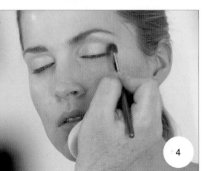
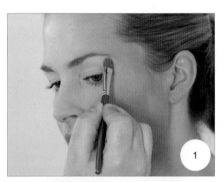
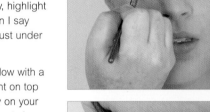
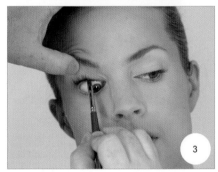
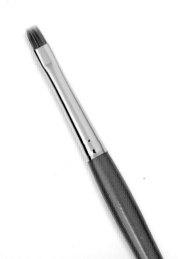

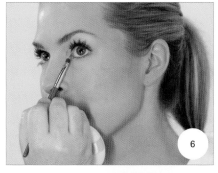

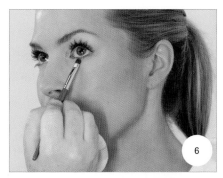

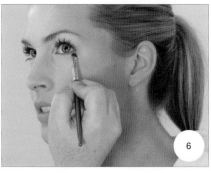

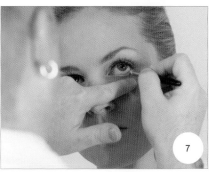

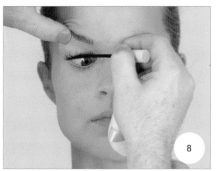

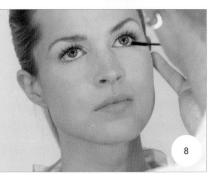

5. It's time to curl your eyelashes and apply your first layer of mascara to your top lashes. (See page 42 to review how to curl properly.)

6. Here comes more highlight. With your #14 detail highlighting brush, apply your shimmer white shadow all along your lower lash line from the inside corner to the outside corner, along the lash line.

7. Using a concealer pencil, line your water-line. (Remember, the waterline is the inner rim above the lower lash line.) I do not do this often, but for this look it is so part of creating that sun-bleached style.

8. Now it's time for mascara on your lower lashes and another coat to your upper lashes. (See page 44 to review how to layer your mascara properly.)

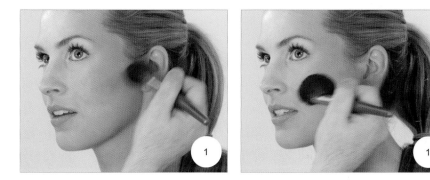

cheeks

1. This look is all about bronzer, so we want a lot of bronzer used in the cheek area. Now grab your #73 bronzer/blush brush and your matte bronzer. Apply the bronzer beginning at the back of your cheekbone and sweep it forward toward the apple of your cheek. Then take the brush back toward your ear. This lays your color in place.

"this look is perfect whenever you want a summer beach glow."

2. Now take your brush and use it in the opposite direction (up and down) to blend. Be sure to blend well, or it will not look natural.

3. Don't forget to add a little at the temples to help shape your face. Sweep the bronzing powder up around the temples and eye sockets. This always gives the face more color and gives you a glow, and that is what this look is all about.

4. Also, feel free to blend some bronzer along your jawbone. This also helps create that glow and softens your face shape.

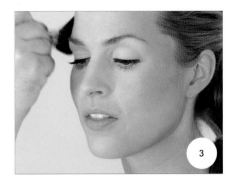

lips

1. To finish off this look, it is so important for the lips to look sun-bleached as well. With that in mind, the first thing you should do is conceal your natural lip line. This helps create a super-natural nude lip.

2. Now, using a barely-there nude lip pencil, line your lips. Begin with a V in the "cupid's bow," or center curve, of the lips. Bring the liner up and around the curves of your bow.

3. Starting at the outer corners, move toward the center with your pencil.

4. On the lower lip, first accentuate the lower curve of the lip. Then begin from the outer corners, moving toward the center. Remember to use your entire lip: Take the color to the almost invisible line just at the edge of the colored part of your lips.

5. Be sure to fill in at least halfway toward the center of your lip. This will help your lip liner look more natural and your lip color last longer.

6. Now blend with your #80 lip brush to make it look more natural.

7. Using your lip brush (because it gives you better application and helps color last longer), fill in your entire lip with the perfect pale nude lipstick. Make sure you blend really well over your lip liner.

8. End with a quick sweep of the perfect nude lip gloss to make your lips shiny, fuller looking, and sexy. Apply your gloss with your #80 lip brush, because if you apply gloss with a brush it will appear shinier. Hello, summer!

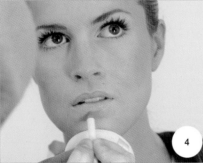

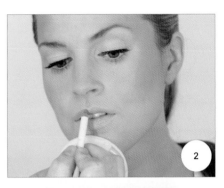

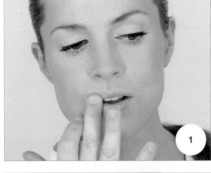

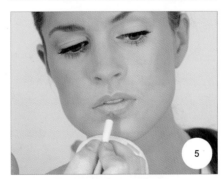

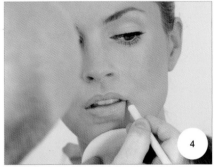

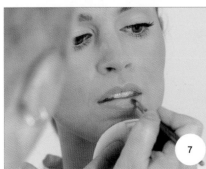

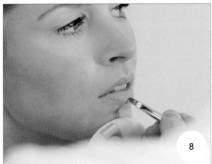

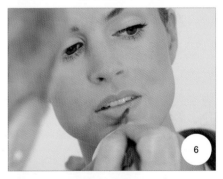

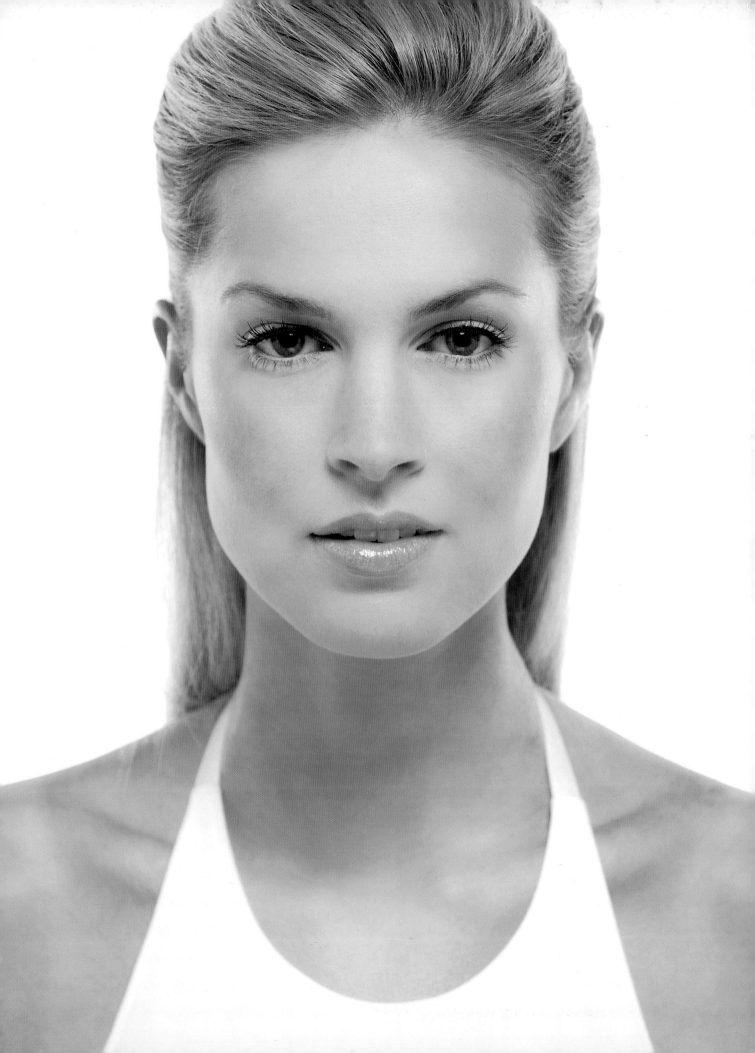

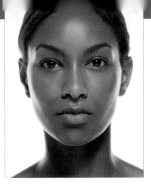

bronze and beautiful

Even bronze/ebony girls sometimes want that natural bronzed glow. It is all about beautiful glowing skin, softly defined eyes, and glossy, nude lips. For this look, you will choose the perfect, barely-there colors and apply them to the perfect intensity. Remember, natural doesn't mean naked: It's about your color choices. It's time to learn tricks to define your eyes while making it look like there's almost nothing there. And don't forget your naked glossy lip. Girl, let's get your glow on!

Here's how to get this look:

eyes

1. Using your #22 highlighting brush, apply a shimmery gold highlight to your lid and brow bone. When I say brow bone, I mean the area just under the arch of your brow.

2. Now it's time to curl your eyelashes and apply the first layer of mascara to your top lashes. (See page 42 to review how to curl properly.)

3. Next, using your #11 midtone brush and a matte midtone eye shadow and starting from the outside corner of your crease, glide your brush across to the inside corner. Use a matte ginger shadow (a shade just a bit darker than your skin tone) so that you get nice, soft definition.

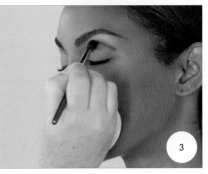

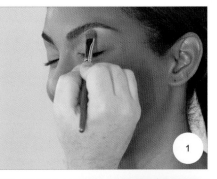

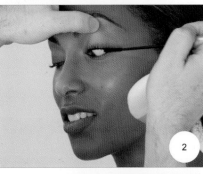

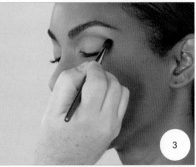

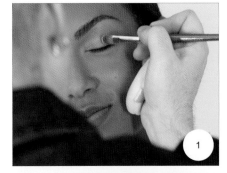

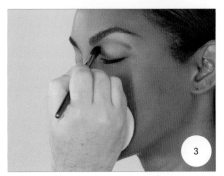

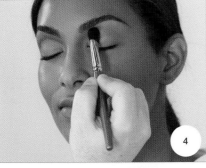

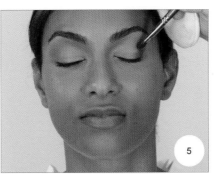

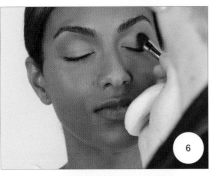

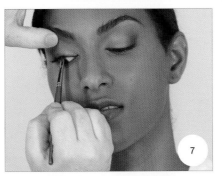

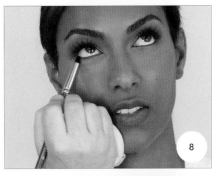

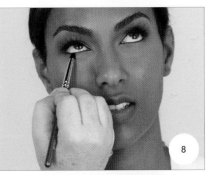

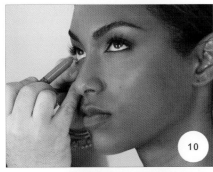

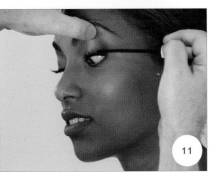

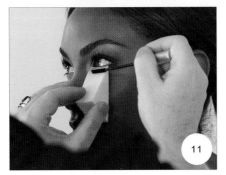

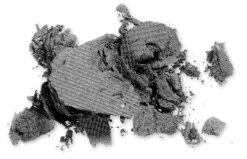

4. Use your #28 blending brush (the one that is always clean and ready to blend with) and blend your midtone so that there are no hard edges.

5. Grab your #30 contour brush and some of your midtone eye shadow and define the outer third of your eyelid.

6. Follow with your #28 brush to blend. This just starts your lid definition.

7. For very subtle lash line definition, use your #41 detail eyeliner brush and push black eye shadow into the base of your lash line.

8. Grab your #13 detail eye shadow brush and apply your midtone eye shadow all along your lower lash line. Start your application from the outside corner, sweeping it across to the inside corner.

9. Using your #14 detail highlighting brush, highlight the inside corner of the lower lash line. Because there is so little color to this look, this step really brightens the eye and opens it up to give you a wide-eyed effect.

10. Now it's time for another little trick: Using a concealer pencil, line the waterline of your lower lid. (Remember, the waterline is the inner rim above the lower lash line.) This really gives you a great, open-eyed effect.

11. Time for another layer of mascara on your top lashes and a layer on your lower lashes. After you finish the rest of your makeup, add yet another layer to the top lashes. Remember, with this look, lush lashes are very important, so you want to really layer your mascara on your top lashes. (See page 44 to review how to layer your mascara properly.)

5 minutes to gorgeous

cheeks

1. The secret to this look is a perfectly flushed cheek. You are going to achieve this by layering your blush, starting with a great crème-to-powder blush. Using your #64 crème blush brush, apply a bright apricot blush to the apple of the cheek, starting at the front of the apple and working toward the back.

2. Follow with a light dusting of loose or pressed powder.

3. Now to reinforce that flush, smile and apply your powder blush (the perfect bright sheer apricot color) with your #74 bronzer/blush brush on the apple of your cheek, starting at the front of your apple and working toward the back.

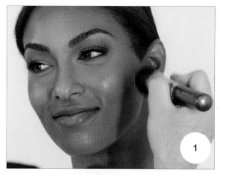
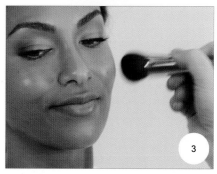
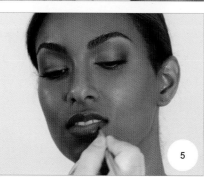
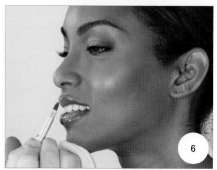

lips

1. I chose to use lip liner with this look to even out your natural lip color and help it last longer. Grab your pencil and begin with a V in the "cupid's bow," or center curve, of the lips. Bring the liner up and around the curves of your bow.

2. Next, starting at the outer corners, move toward the center with your pencil.

3. On the lower lip, first accentuate the lower curve of the lip. Then begin from the outer corners, moving toward the center. Remember to use your entire lip: Take the color to the almost invisible line just at the edge of the colored part of your lips.

4. Be sure to fill in at least halfway toward the center of your lip. This will help your lip liner look more natural and your lip color last longer.

5. Now blend with your #80 lip brush to make it look more natural.

6. Simply finish with a coat of the perfect sheer peach lip gloss. Apply it with your lip brush. Remember, if you apply gloss with a brush, it will appear shinier.

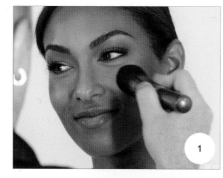
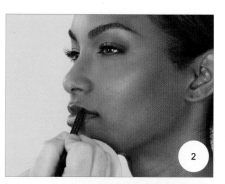
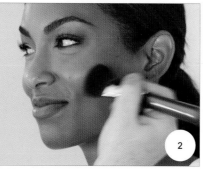
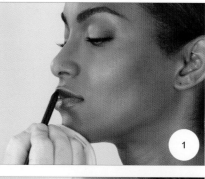
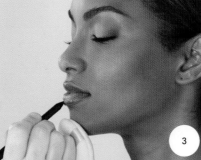
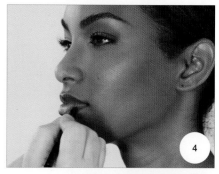

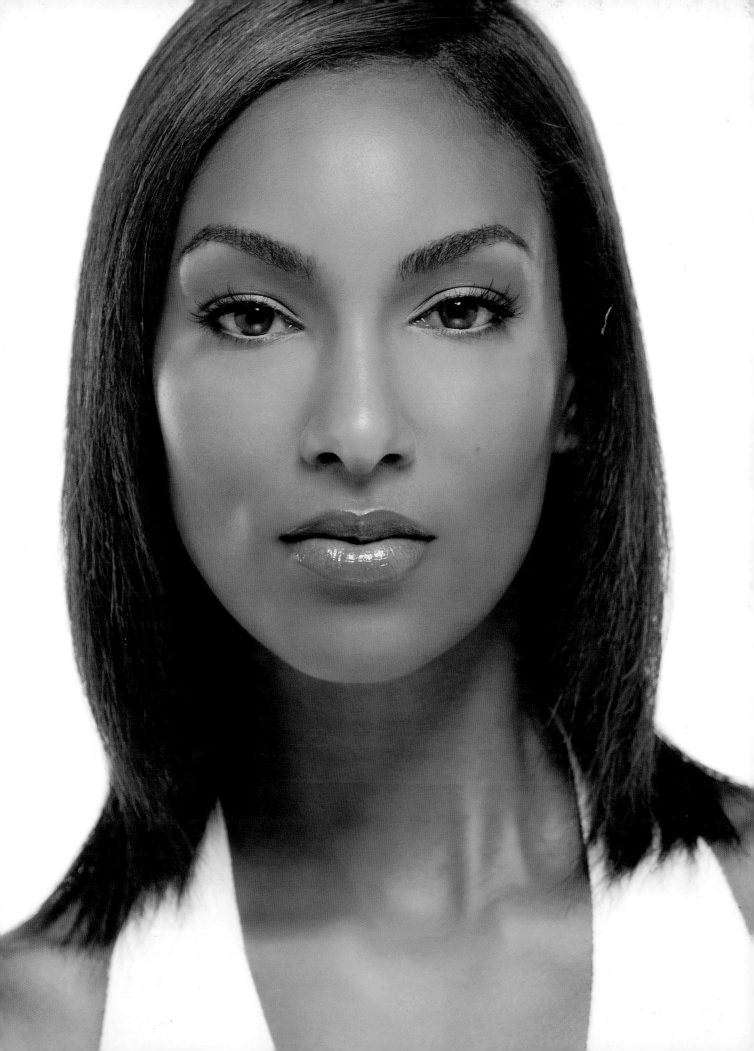

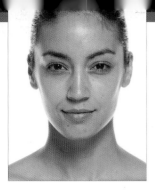

perse pout

There is nothing that says "evening" better than a barely-there eye and a fabulous lip color. A look like this is the fastest way to create an evening face that can take you anywhere. It's perfect for taking your little black dress to new heights. It's also a go-to look for days when you want to look super-polished, yet with minimal effort. Play and learn how to create this lip and make it last.

Here's how to get this look:

eyes

1. Because this look is all about the lips, you want your eyes to be understated. First, apply a matte flesh-colored eye shadow to your lid and your brow bone with your #22 highlighting brush. We do not want your eyes to look made up, but we *do* want them to have definition, and by using highlight and midtone eye shadow, you'll create contrast that will give your eyelid shape.

2. Using your #11 midtone brush and a matte midtone eye shadow and starting from the outside corner of your crease, glide your brush across to the inside corner. Use a soft matte caramel shadow (a shade a bit darker than your skin tone) to get soft definition.

3. Use your #28 blending brush (the one that is always clean and ready to blend with) and blend your midtone so that there are no hard edges.

4. Also, before you move on, curl your eyelashes and apply the first layer of mascara to your top lashes. (See page 42 to review how to curl properly.)

We'll let your mascara dry and put on another coat at the end of the look.

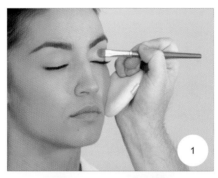
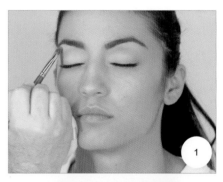

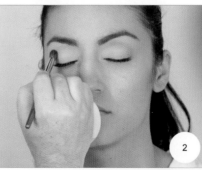
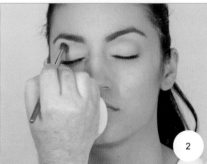

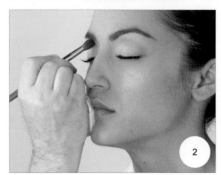
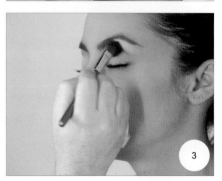

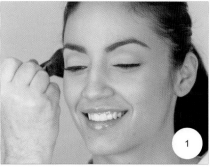
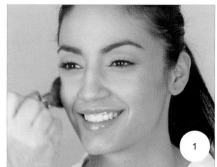

cheeks

1. Using your #73 bronzer/blush brush, apply matte bronzer, beginning at the back of your cheekbone and sweeping forward toward the apple of your cheek. Then take the brush back toward your ear. This lays your color in place.

2. Now, take your brush and use it in the opposite direction (up and down) to blend. Be sure to blend well, or it won't look natural.

3. Don't forget to add a little at the temples to help shape your face.

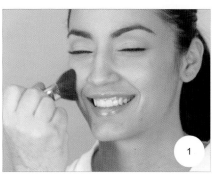
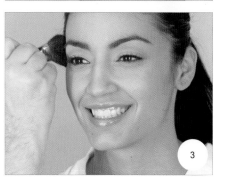

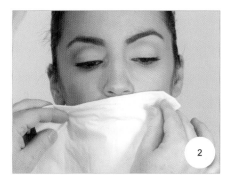
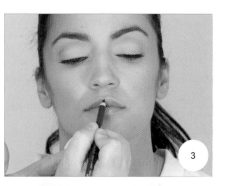

lips

1. Because this look is all about the lips, you really want them to look sumptuous and smooth, so before you start your color application, moisturize them with lip balm. This will help the color go on smoothly and evenly.

2. After the balm has had a bit of time to soak in, blot the excess off with a tissue so that it won't shorten the staying power of your lipstick.

3. Whenever you choose to wear intense lip colors, always ground your color with a slightly deeper shade of lip liner. This will help create a better edge to your lip. Grab your burgundy lip pencil and begin with a V in the "cupid's bow," or center curve, of the lips. Bring the liner up and around the curves of your bow.

4. Next, starting at the outer corners, move toward the center with your pencil.

5. On the lower lip, first accentuate the lower curve of the lip. Then begin from the outer corners, moving toward the center. Remember to use your entire lip: Take the color to the almost invisible line just at the edge of the colored part of your lips.

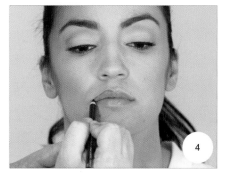
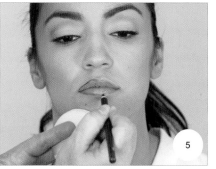

6. Next, fill in your entire lip, except for the center of the top and bottom lips. This will ground your color and help it last much longer.

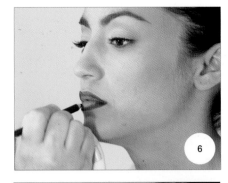

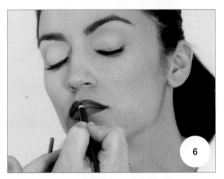

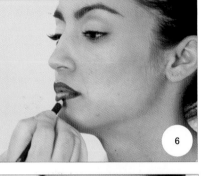

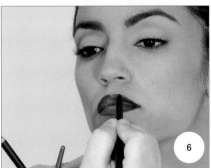

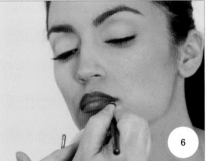

"A look like this is perfect for taking your little black dress to new heights."

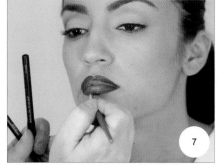

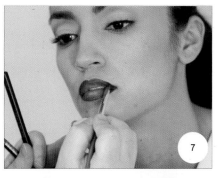

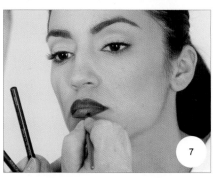

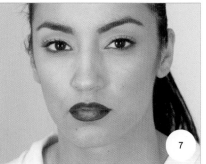

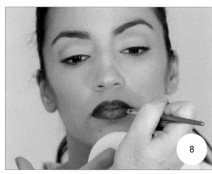

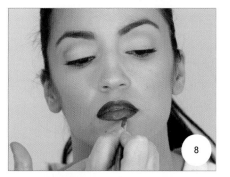

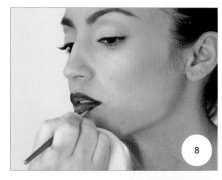

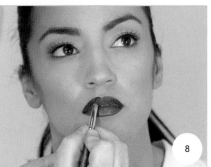

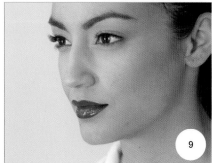

7. Now blend with your #80 lip brush to make it look more natural.

8. Using your lip brush (because it gives you better application and helps color last longer), fill in your entire lip with the perfect pink orchid lipstick. Make sure you blend really well over your lip liner.

9. Using your lip brush, end with a quick sweep of a sheer orchid lip gloss, being sure to concentrate it in the center of your lip. This will give you a great shine without causing bleeding.

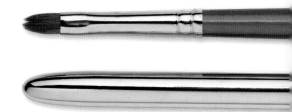

eyes

Here are the final step for your eyes.

5. Add another layer of mascara on your top lashes and a layer on your lower lashes. After you finish the rest of your makeup, add yet another layer to the top lashes. Remember, with this look, lush lashes are very important, so you want to really layer your mascara on your top lashes. (See page 44 to review how to layer your mascara properly.)

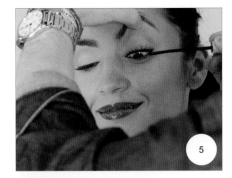

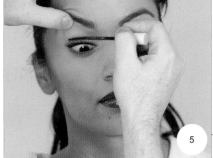

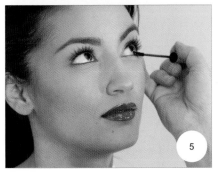

"nothing says 'evening' better than a barely-there eye and fabulous lip color."

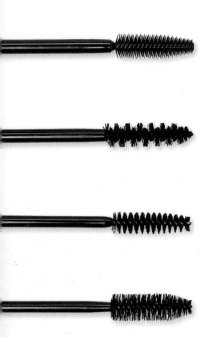

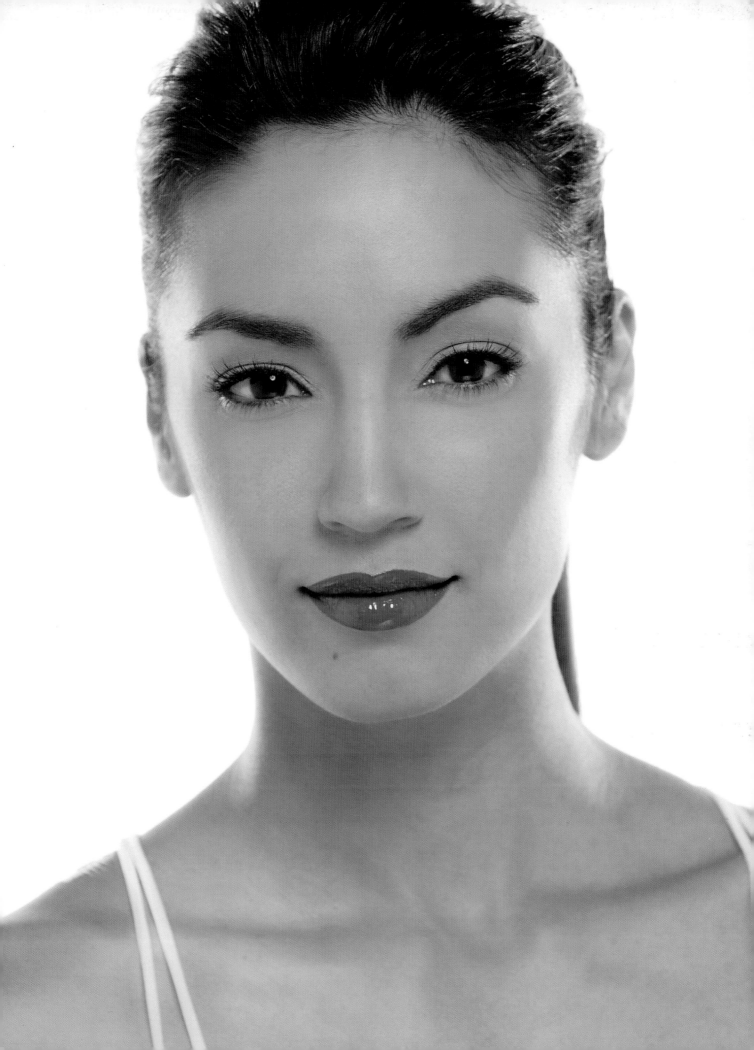

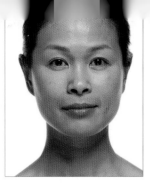

ready, set, shimmer

Some mornings, you wake up and just want to look soft and shimmery. A shimmery lid and lots of lashes can be such a fun and easy look to create and wear. This is such a fast, easy look because your shades are low contrast, making them super-easy to blend. Remember, with this look, it's important not to overpower your soft eye, so keep your lips soft and pastel.

　　Here's how to get this look:

eyes

This eye look is all about shimmer. Because there's low contrast between shades, it is fast and easy to achieve, without a lot of blending.

1.　To make the highlight shimmer more dramatic, you need to layer your color. First, using your #22 highlighting brush, apply a pale beige matte eye shadow to your lid and brow bone. When I say brow bone, I mean the area just under the arch of your brow.

2.　Using the same brush, layer a shimmery white eye shadow directly on top of the matte beige.

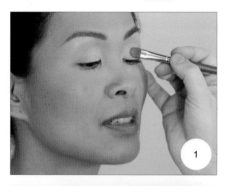

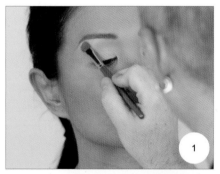

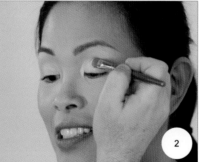

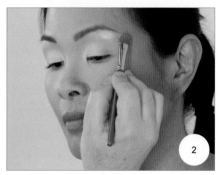

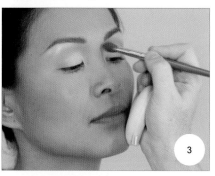

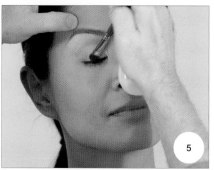

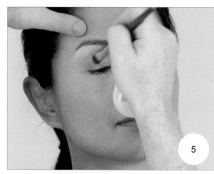

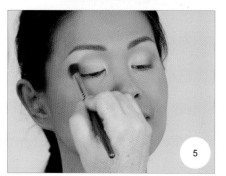

3. Using your #11 midtone brush and a matte midtone eye shadow and starting from the outside corner of your crease, glide your brush across to the inside corner. Use a matte dark taupe shadow (a shade just a bit darker than your skin tone) so that you get soft definition.

4. Use your #28 blending brush (the one that is always clean and ready to blend with) and blend your midtone so that there are no hard edges.

5. With your #30 contour brush, apply a shimmery pinky gray eye shadow to the outer third of your lid. Follow this step by blending the color with your #28 blending brush.

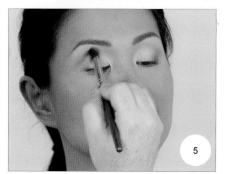

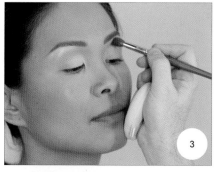

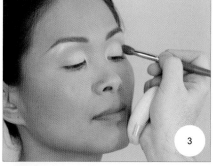

6. It's time to curl your eyelashes and apply the first layer of mascara to your top lashes. (See page 42 to review how to curl properly.)

7. Now, grab your #13 detail eye shadow brush and apply your midtone eye shadow all along your lower lash line. Once again, start your application from the outside corner, sweeping it across to the inside corner.

8. Using your #14 detail highlighting brush, highlight the inside corner of the lower lash line.

9. Next, using a white eyeliner, line the waterline along your lower lash line. (Remember, the waterline is the inner rim above the lower lash line.) This helps create that pastel watercolor look that we want for your eyes.

10. Now it's time for another layer of mascara on your top lashes and a layer on your lower lashes. After you finish the rest of your makeup, add yet another layer to the top lashes. Remember, with this look, lush lashes are very important, so you want to really layer your mascara on your top lashes. (See page 44 to review how to layer your mascara.)

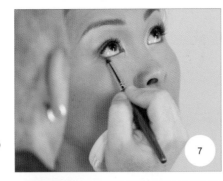

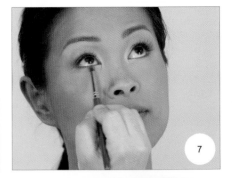

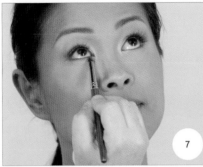

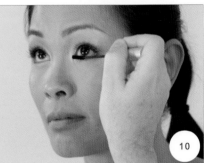

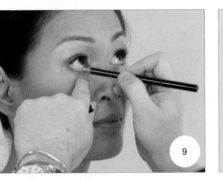

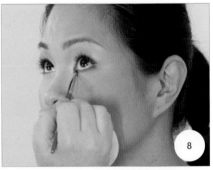

"sometimes, you just want to look soft and shimmery."

cheeks

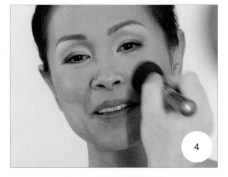

1. Using your #73 bronzer/blush brush, apply your matte bronzer, beginning at the back of your cheekbone. Sweep it forward toward the apple of your cheek and then take the brush back toward your ear. This lays your color in place.

2. Now take your brush and use it in the opposite direction (up and down) to blend. Be sure to blend well, or it will not look natural.

3. Don't forget to add a little at the temples to help shape your face. Sweep the bronzing powder up around the temples and eye sockets. This always gives the face more color and gives you a glow.

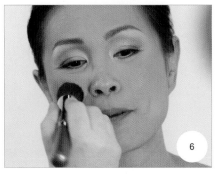

4. It's time to put a soft flush on your cheeks, which adds to this shimmery look. You are going to achieve this by layering your blush. Start with a great crème-to-powder blush. Using your #64 crème blush brush, apply a bright peach blush to the apple of the cheek, starting at the front of the apple and working toward the back.

5. Follow with a light dusting of loose or pressed powder.

6. To reinforce that flush, smile and apply your powder blush (the perfect bright sheer peach color) with your #74 bronzer/blush brush on the apple of your cheek, starting at the front of your apple and working toward the back.

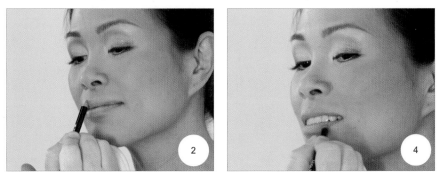

lips

1. To not compete with the eye, you want a pale lip with this look. To get those perfect pale lips, start by concealing your natural lip and lip line.

2. Now, grab a pale pink natural-tone lip pencil and define your lips. Begin with a V in the "cupid's bow," or center curve, of the lips. Bring the liner up and around the curves of your bow.

3. Next, starting at the outer corners, move toward the center with your pencil.

4. On the lower lip, first accentuate the lower curve of the lip. Then begin from the outer corners, moving toward the center. Remember to use your entire lip: Take the color to the almost invisible line just at the edge of the colored part of your lips.

5. Be sure to fill in at least halfway toward the center of your lip. This will help your lip liner look more natural and your lip color last longer.

6. Now blend with your #80 lip brush to make it look more natural.

7. Using your lip brush (because it gives you better application and helps color last longer), fill in your entire lip with the perfect pale pink lipstick. Make sure you blend really well over your lip liner.

8. End with a quick sweep of the perfect sheer pink lip gloss to make your lips shiny, fuller looking, and sexy. Be sure to apply your gloss with your #80 lip brush because if you apply gloss with a brush, it will appear shinier.

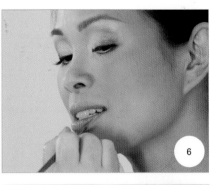

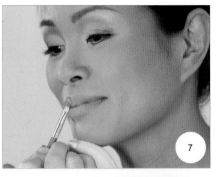

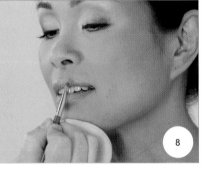

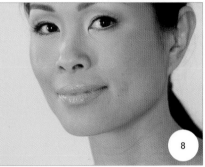

face

1. To complete your shimmery glow, apply a subtle shimmer to strategic areas of the face with your #76 detail powder brush. Apply a shimmer highlight powder to the centers of your forehead and chin and along the top of your cheekbones. This will help give your face dimension and create that glow.

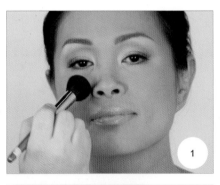

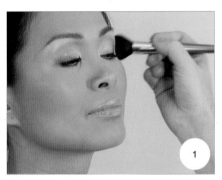

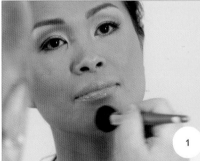

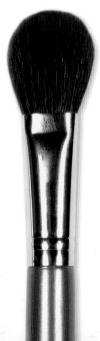

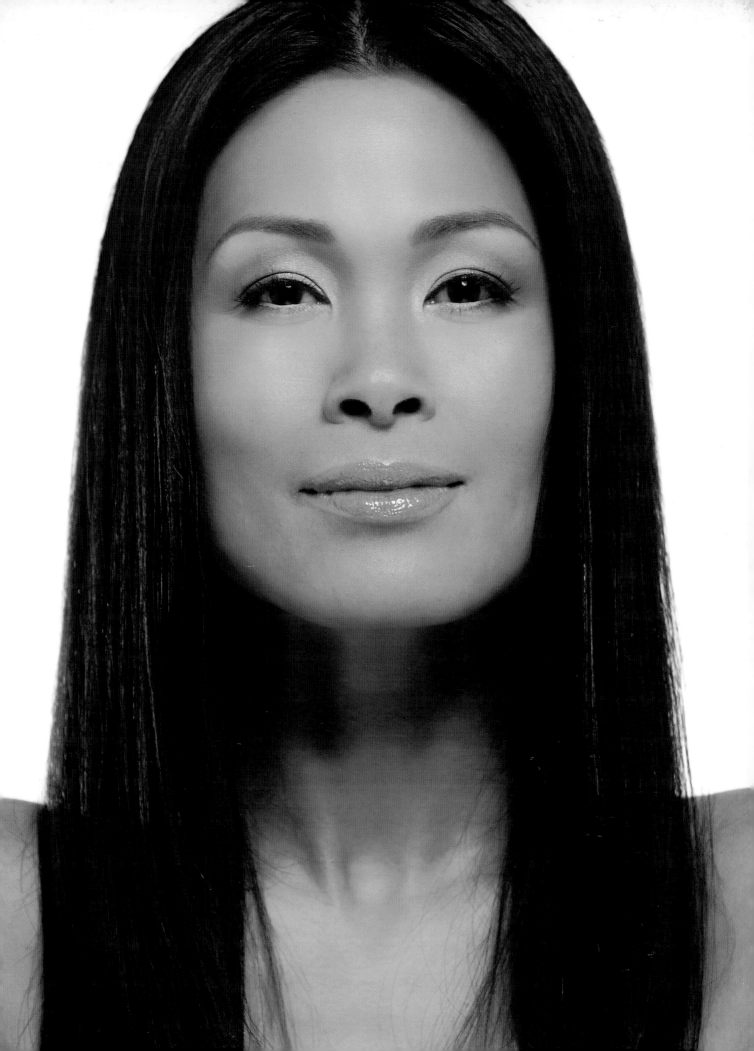

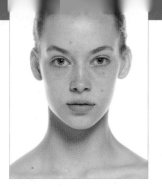

natural beauty

It doesn't take a lot of makeup to make a difference and look beautiful. This look is proof! The beauty of this look is its simplicity and super-natural glow. Notice that with this look, you are focusing on the product and application that make the most difference. This look demonstrates that, *sometimes*, less is more.

Here's how to get this look:

eyes

1. Using your #22 highlighting brush and the perfect champagne eye shadow with shimmer, highlight your lid.

2. Now, using your #11 midtone brush and your matte bronzer as your midtone (remember, the less product, the faster the application, and bronzer doubles as the perfect midtone), start from the outside corner of your crease and glide your brush across to the inside corner. This softly defines your crease.

3. Grab your #30 contour brush and apply additional bronzer to the outside third of your eyelid.

4. With your #28 blending brush, blend everywhere your midtone meets your highlight. This will give you the perfect blend and create a super-natural look.

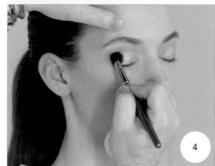
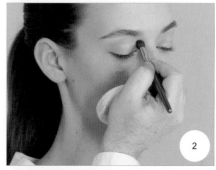
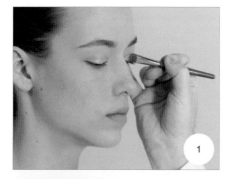
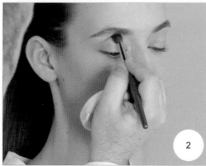
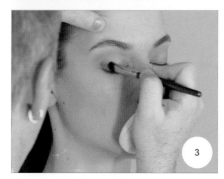
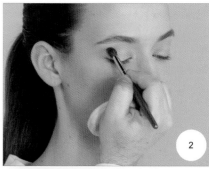

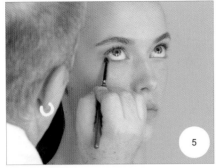

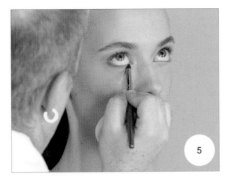

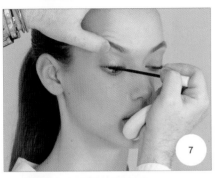

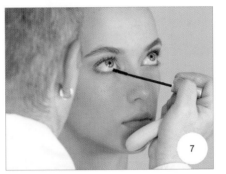

5. Using your #13 detail eye shadow brush and your bronzer (midtone for this look), define along your lower lash line. Start from the outside corner and work in toward the inner corner.

6. Using your #14 detail highlighting brush, apply your highlight shade to the inside corner of the lower lash line. This helps open the eye up and really brightens your eyes.

7. It's now time to curl your eyelashes and put your first layer of mascara on your top lashes. (See page 42 to review how to curl properly.)

8. I've decided that we need a bit more definition. To achieve this, you are going to simply use a dark brown shadow and your #18 brush, applying it right along the upper lash line. This is perfect for soft, natural definition and pops the eyes without making you look made up at all.

9. Now it's time for mascara on your lower lashes and another coat to your upper lashes. (See page 44 to review how to layer your mascara properly.)

10. Lastly, here's a little trick: Using a concealer pencil, line the waterline of your lower lid. (Remember, the waterline is the inner rim above the lower lash line.) This really gives you a great open-eyed effect.

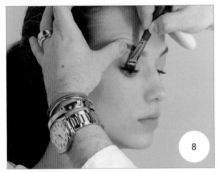

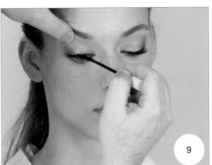

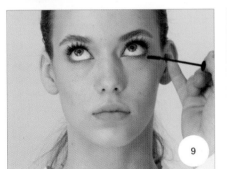

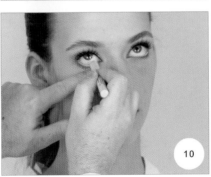

"*sometimes*, less is more."

cheeks

This look definitely requires a beautiful flushed cheek. I call it "popping your apples." This is a two-step process with a little secret.

1. The first thing you want to do is take a soft peach crème-to-powder blush, and with your #64 blush brush, apply it to the apple of your cheek. Remember to start from the front of each apple and brush it toward the back. Keep the color right on your apple.

2. Follow this with a little loose powder to help set the blush.

3. Now, grab your #73 cheek brush and bronzer (the same shade you used on your eyes) and apply it, beginning at the back of your cheekbone. Then sweep it forward toward the apple of your cheek. Finally, take the brush back toward your ear. This lays your color in place.

4. Next, take your brush and use it in the opposite direction (up and down) to blend. Be sure to blend well, or it won't look natural.

5. Don't forget to add a little at the temples to help shape your face. Sweep the bronzing powder up around the temples and eye sockets. This always gives the face more color and gives you a glow.

6. Also, feel free to blend some bronzer along your jawbone. This also helps create that glow and softens the shape of your face.

7. Lastly, using your #73 brush and a powder blush that matches your crème, apply the blush just to the apple of your cheek. Start at the front of the apple and brush toward the back. Layering powder on top of a crème will make it last longer and really gives you the perfect flush.

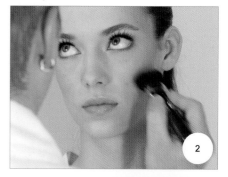

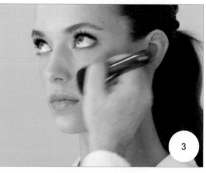

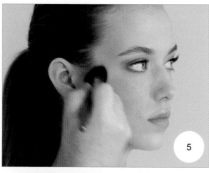

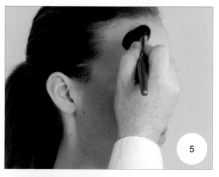

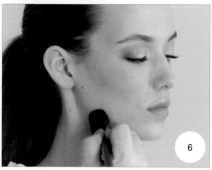

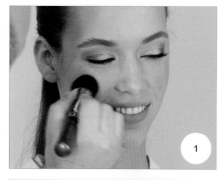

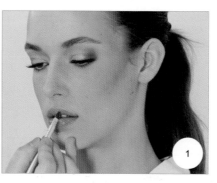

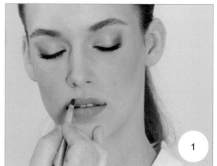

lips

1. For this look the lips are simple—just a sheer wash of a gorgeous, shiny sheer peach lip gloss with your #80 lip brush.

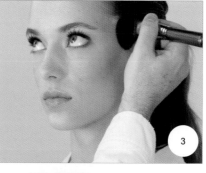

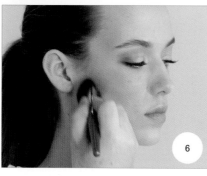

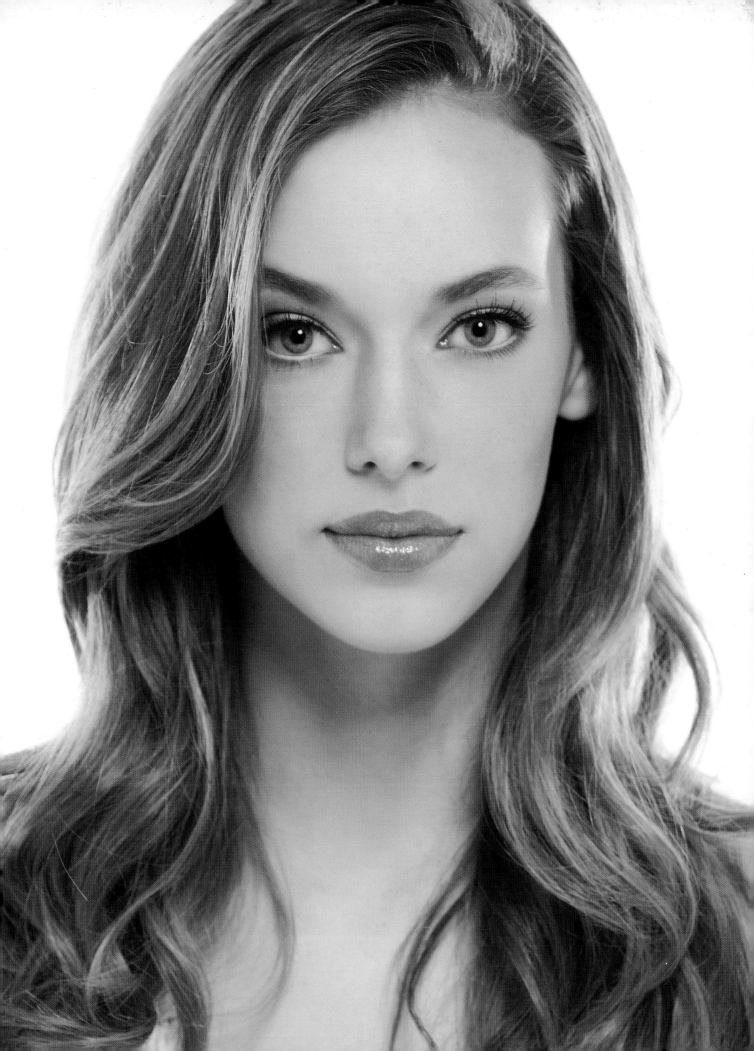

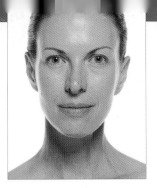

pretty in peach

We all know that peach is a very youthful color, but it definitely works on girls of every age. Beautiful peach lips, a softly defined eye, and freshly flushed peach cheeks = gorgeous. You can see how this look with the perfect color choices takes years off. I don't care what age you are, pretty is pretty, and this look is the perfect example of getting your pretty on.

Here's how to get this look:

eyes

1. Often, I highlight the lid with a shimmer and the brow bone with a matte so that the lid will be more dramatic, as with this look. Starting with your #22 highlighting brush, use a shimmer champagne eye shadow to highlight just your lid. Now, grab a matte beige shadow and highlight your brow bone. When I say brow bone, I mean the area just under the arch of your brow.

2. Using your #11 midtone brush with a matte midtone eye shadow and starting from the outside corner of your crease, glide your brush across to the inside corner. This starts to define your crease. Use a soft matte taupe shadow (a shade just a bit darker than your skin tone) so that you get soft definition.

3. Use your #28 blending brush (the one that is always clean and ready to blend with) and blend your midtone so that there are no hard edges.

4. It's time to curl your eyelashes and apply the first layer of mascara to your top lashes. (See page 42 to review how to curl properly.)

5. For very subtle lash line definition, use your #41 detail eyeliner brush and push black eye shadow into the base of your lash line.

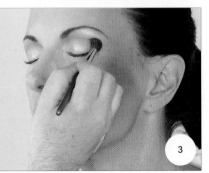

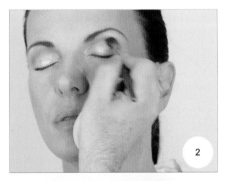

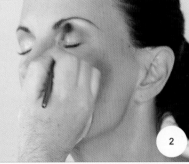

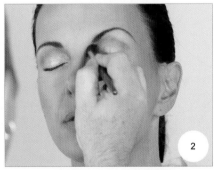

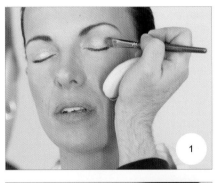

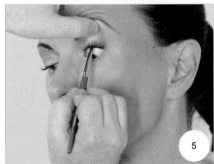

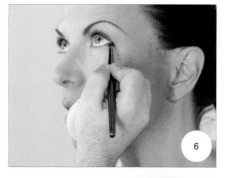

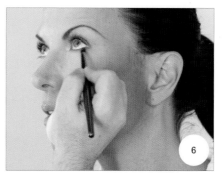

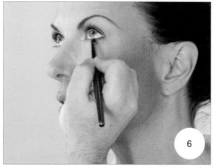

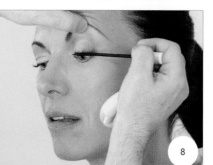

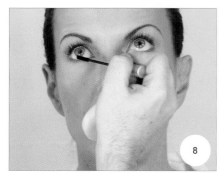

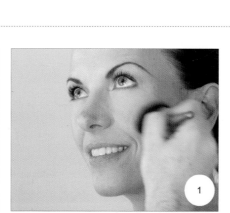

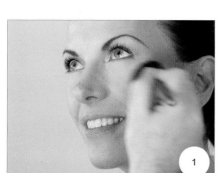

6. Using your #13 detail shadow brush, apply your midtone all along your lower lash line. Start from the outside corner and work in toward the inner corner.

7. Using your #14 detail highlighting brush, apply your highlight shade to the inside corner of the lower lash line. This helps open the eye up and really brightens your eyes.

8. Now, add another layer of mascara on your top lashes and a layer on your lower lashes. (See page 44 to review how to layer your mascara properly.)

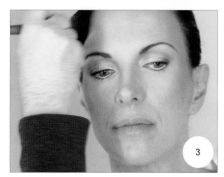

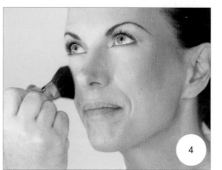

cheeks

1. Using your #73 bronzer/blush brush, apply your matte bronzer, beginning at the back of your cheekbone. Sweep it forward toward the apple of your cheek and then take the brush back toward your ear. This lays your color in place.

2. Use your brush in the opposite direction (up and down) to blend.

3. Don't forget to add a little at the temples to help shape your face. Sweep the bronzing powder up around the temples and eye sockets.

4. It's time for a little extra color! Grab your #73 bronzer/blush brush and smile. Now apply your powder blush on the apple of your cheek, blending back toward the area that you bronzed. This technique really gives your face that fresh flush.

lips

1. I have chosen to use lip liner with this look because I want a very defined lip. Grabbing your nude pencil, begin with a V in the "cupid's bow," or center curve, of the lips. Bring the liner up and around the curves of your bow.

2. Next, starting at the outer corners, move toward the center with your pencil.

3. On the lower lip, first accentuate the lower curve of the lip. Then begin from the outer corners, moving toward the center. Remember to use your entire lip: Take the color to the almost invisible line just at the edge of the colored part of your lips.

4. Be sure to fill in at least halfway toward the center of your lip. This will help your lip liner look more natural and your lip color last longer.

5. Now blend with your #80 lip brush to make it look more natural.

6. Using your lip brush (because it gives you better application and helps the color last longer), fill in your entire lip with the perfect peach lipstick. Make sure you blend well over your lip liner.

7. End with a quick sweep of the perfect sheer peach lip gloss to make your lips shiny, fuller looking, and sexy. Be sure to apply your gloss with your #80 lip brush because if you apply gloss with a brush, it will appear shinier.

"this look is the perfect example of getting your pretty on."

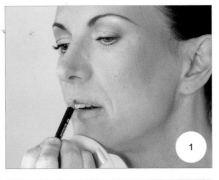
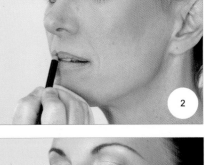

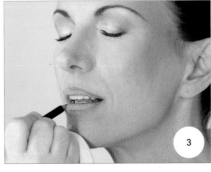
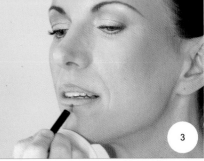

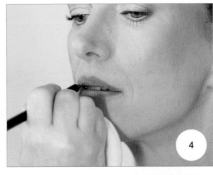
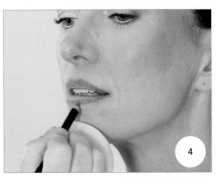

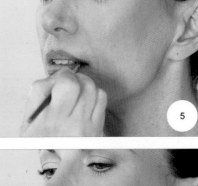
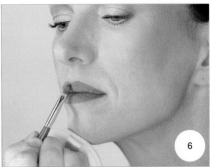

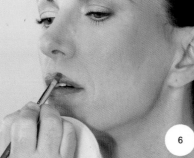
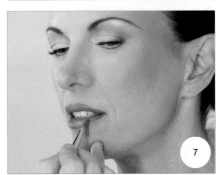

makeup makeovers in 5, 10, 15, and 20 minutes

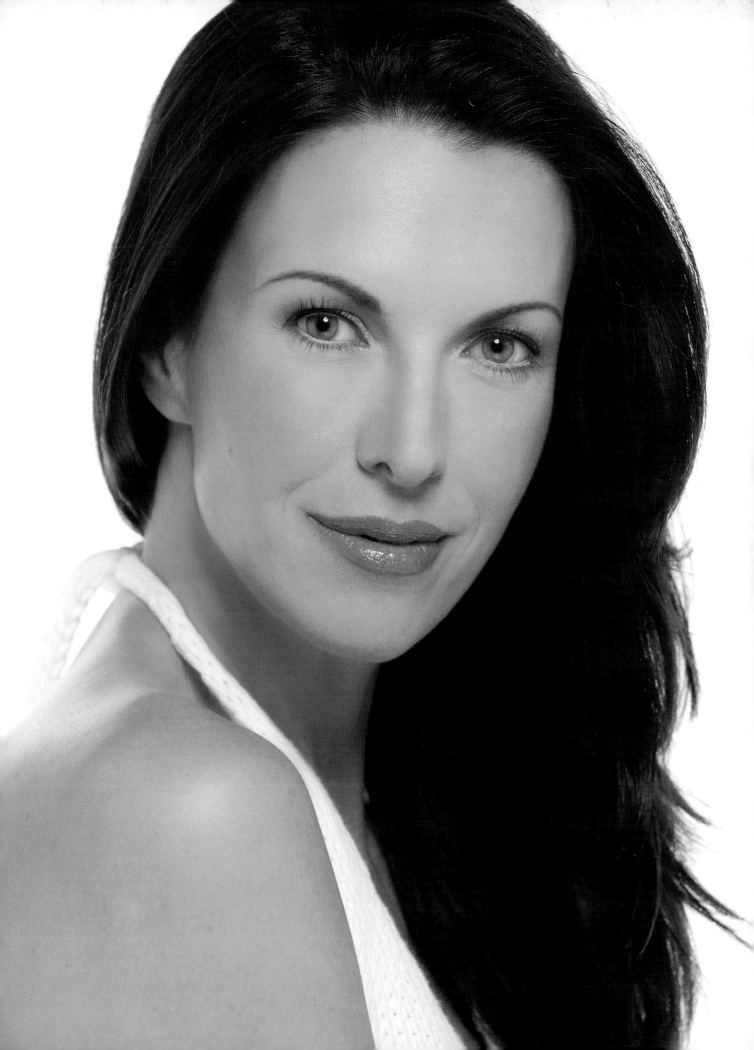

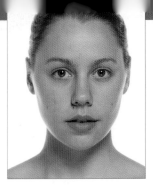

goldfinger

You could not find a simpler look to achieve than this one. It is all about gold shimmer and thick, dark lashes. Application is even easier, because you actually do some of your application with nothing more than your fingers. Perfect for those days when you want to look great, but want to wear next to nothing.

Here's how to get this look:

eyes

1. Using a shimmery gold crème-to-powder eye shadow, apply it on your lid with your finger. Make sure you apply it only from the lash line to the crease. Once again using your finger, apply a little of a shimmery powder gold eye shadow directly over the crème to set it.

2. Now it's time for a little extra definition. With your #18 brush, apply the faintest bit of dark brown eye shadow, pushing it down into the lashes.

We'll return to your eyes in a moment.

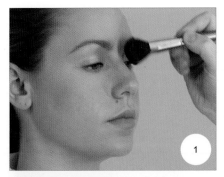

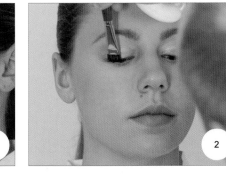

face

1. To replicate the glow that the sun would give you, the first thing we want to do is apply a subtle shimmer to strategic areas of the face with your #76 detail powder brush. Apply a shimmer high-light powder to the center of your fore-head, along the top of your cheekbones, and to the center of your chin. This will help give your face dimension and create that glow.

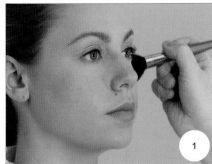

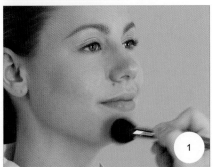

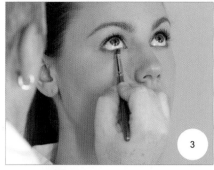
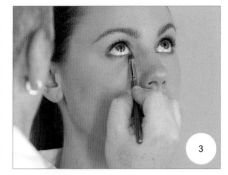

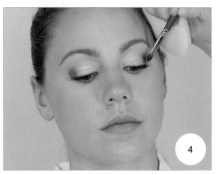
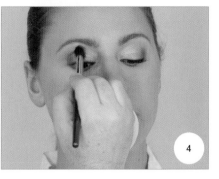

eyes

3. Using your #13 detail shadow brush, apply bronzer all along your lower lash line. Start from the outside corner and work in toward the inner corner.

4. Grab your #30 contour brush and a bit of bronzer and define the outer third of your eyelid. We are only using bronzer because we want very subtle definition. Follow with your #28 brush to blend.

5. Remember, this look is all about the shimmer and lots of lashes. Now it's time to curl your eyelashes and apply the first layer of mascara to your top lashes. (See page 42 to review how to curl properly.)

We'll let your mascara dry and put on another coat at the end of the look.

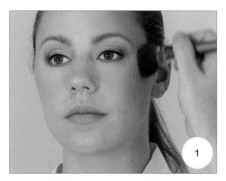
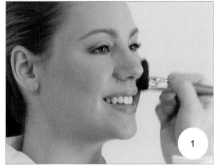

cheeks

1. Now use your #73 bronzer/blush brush to apply your matte bronzer, beginning at the back of your cheekbone. Sweep it forward toward the apple of your cheek and then take the brush back toward your ear. This lays your color in place.

2. Now, take your brush and use it in the opposite direction (up and down) to blend. Be sure to blend well, or it won't look natural.

3. Don't forget to add a little at the temples to help shape your face. Sweep the bronzing powder up around the temples and eye sockets. This always gives the face more color and gives you a glow, and that is what this look is all about.

4. Feel free to blend some bronzer along your jawbone. This also helps create that glow and defines your face.

"the perfect, easy look when you want to look great."

eyes

Here are the final steps for your eyes.

6. Now it's time for another layer of mascara on your top lashes and a layer on your lower lashes. After you finish the rest of your makeup, add yet another layer to the top lashes. Remember, with this look, lush lashes are very important, so you want to really layer your mascara on your top lashes. (See page 44 to review how to layer your mascara properly.)

7. Using your #14 detail highlighting brush, highlight the inside corner of the lower lash line and reinforce the highlight on the inner corner of your top lid.

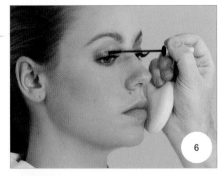

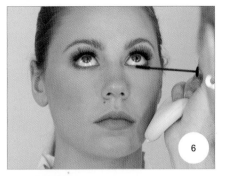

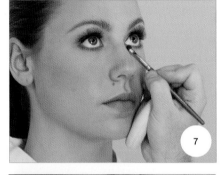

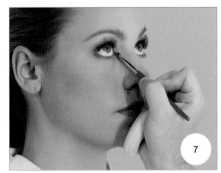

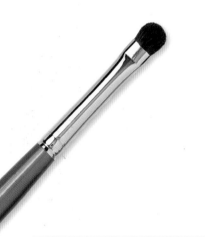

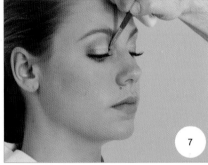

lips

1. So simple! With your #80 lip brush, apply nothing but a sheer pink-brown lip gloss. Remember, if you apply your gloss with a brush, it will appear shinier.

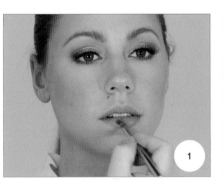

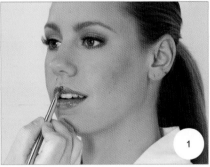

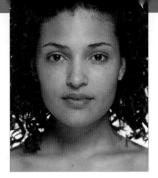

bohemian glow

This is the "I didn't try, I was just born this fabulous" look. Talk about ultra-natural, this look will make you appear flawless and fresh, as if you were wearing nothing at all. For me, this look says, "I don't care, yet I look flawless." Luminous skin, flushed cheeks, and naked, glossy lips—what is more bohemian than that?

Here's how to get this look:

eyes

1. For this look, your eye makeup is barely there, yet well defined. Using a shimmery gold crème-to-powder eye shadow, apply it to your lid with your #22 highlighting brush. Apply it only from the lash line to the crease.

2. Now, with the same brush, apply a shimmery gold eye shadow powder directly over the crème. This sets it and really intensifies the shimmer and the shine, which gives this look more definition because it increases the contrast.

3. Using your #11 midtone brush and a matte midtone eye shadow and starting from the outside corner of your crease, glide your brush across to the inside corner. Use a matte caramel shadow (a shade just a bit darker than your skin tone) so that you get soft definition.

4. Use your #28 blending brush (the one that is always clean and ready to blend with) and blend your midtone so that there are no hard edges.

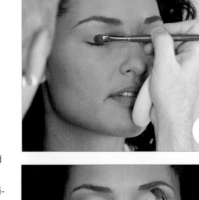
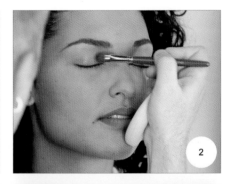
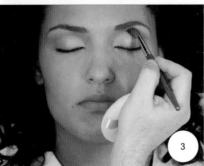
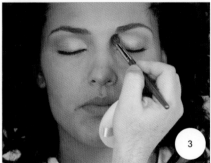

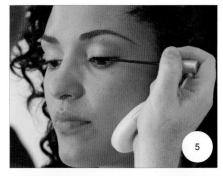

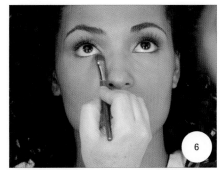

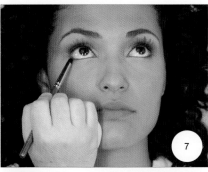

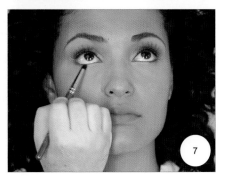

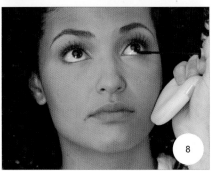

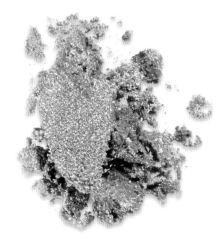

5. Now it's time to curl your eyelashes and apply the first layer of mascara to your top lashes. (See page 42 to review how to curl properly.)

6. Using your #14 detail highlighting brush, highlight the inside corner and a third of the way across your lower lash line.

7. Using your #13 detail shadow brush, apply your midtone all along your lower lash line. Start from the outside corner and work in toward the inner corner.

8. It's time for another layer of mascara on your top lashes and a layer on your lower lashes. After you finish the rest of your makeup, add yet another layer to the top lashes. Remember, with this look, lush lashes are very important, so you want to really layer your mascara on your top lashes. (See page 44 to review how to layer your mascara properly.)

"this look says, 'I didn't try, I was just born this fabulous.'"

cheeks

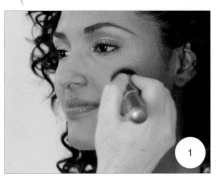

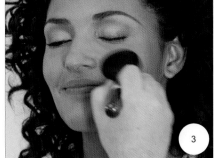

1. The secret to this look is a perfectly flushed cheek. You are going to achieve this by layering your blush. Start with a great crème-to-powder blush. Using your #64 crème blush brush, apply a bright apricot blush to the apple of the cheek, starting at the front of your apple and working toward the back.

2. Follow with a light dusting of loose or pressed powder.

3. Now to reinforce that flush, smile and apply your powder blush (the perfect bright sheer apricot color) with your #73 bronzer/blush brush on the apple of your cheek, starting at the front of your apple and working toward the back.

lips

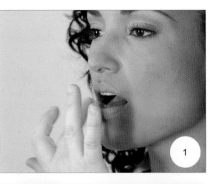

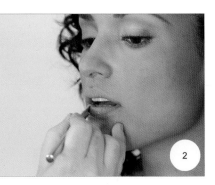

1. You want just soft, sheer lips. First, so the color will be barely there, conceal your natural lips to create a blank canvas. This way, whatever you put on top will show its true color.

2. All that is left is to give your lips a wash of the perfect sheer peach lip gloss with your #80 lip brush.

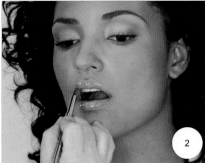

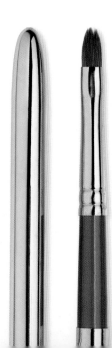

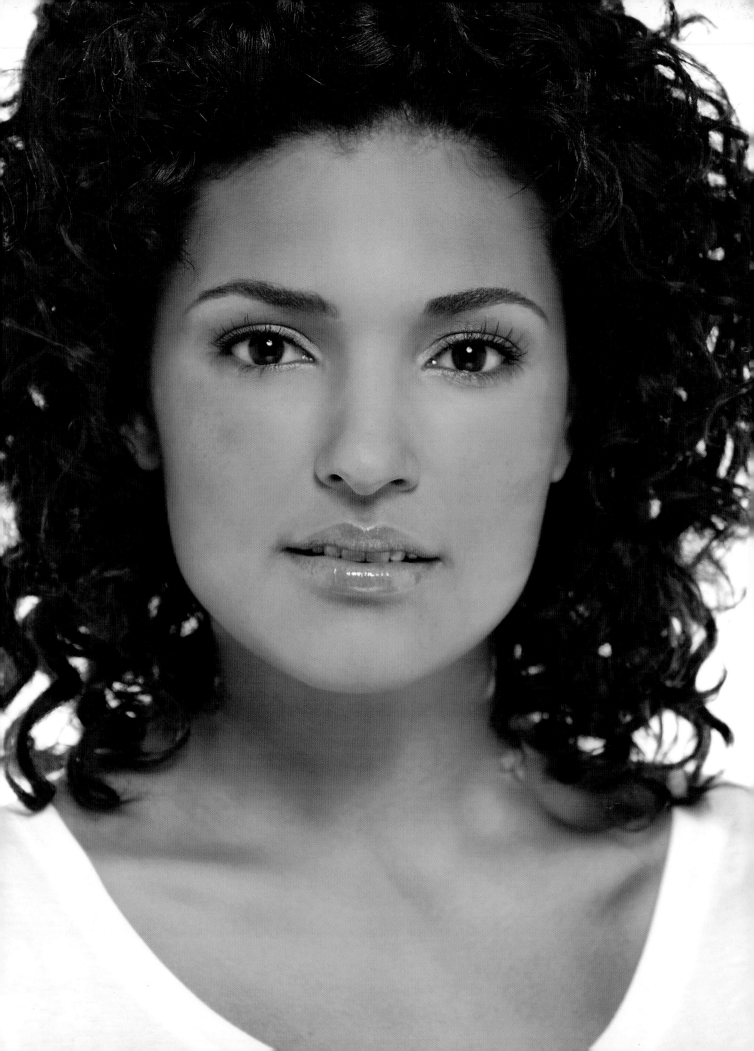

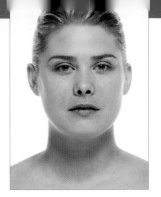

naked beauty

I call this look naked because there is so little color to this makeover. So many people think naked and natural means no makeup, but what it really means is the right (natural) color choices. I love the fact that everything looks so minimal yet defined, not to mention the soft, flushed glow to the cheek. This is a look that would work no matter what the occasion.

Here's how to get this look:

eyes

1. Using your #22 highlighting brush and a pale matte beige eye shadow, highlight your lid and brow bone. When I say brow bone, I mean the area just under the arch of your brow.

2. With the same brush, follow your matte beige shadow with a shimmer champagne eye shadow, layering it right on top of your matte shade, but only on your lid, not your brow bone. I almost always prefer the lid to be a bit more highlighted than the brow bone. This shimmer over your matte will give you a more dramatic highlight.

3. Next, taking a medium matte taupe eye shadow and your #13 eye shadow brush, define your crease. Starting from the outside corner of your crease, glide your brush across to the inside corner, creating a distinct line along your crease.

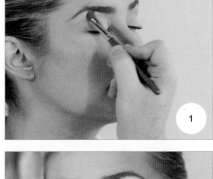

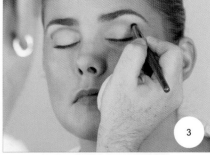

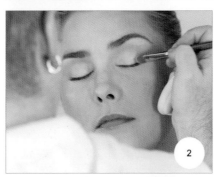

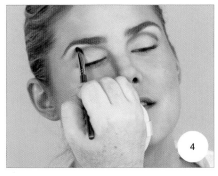

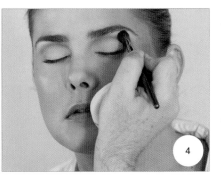

4. Follow that with a #28 blending brush, using it to blend that line. You want to start with the line before you blend so that you have a tight, well-defined crease that does not overtake your highlighted areas and creates contrast.

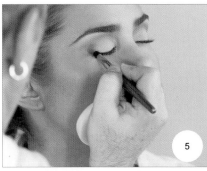

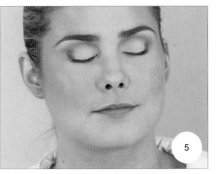

5. Using your #13 detail eye shadow brush, apply a matte brown eye shadow at the very outer corner of the eyelid. You just want to softly define the very outside edge of your eyelid.

6. Blend this area again with your #28 blending brush.

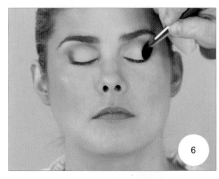

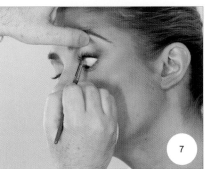

7. For very subtle lash line definition, use your #41 detail eyeliner brush and push black eye shadow into the base of your lash line.

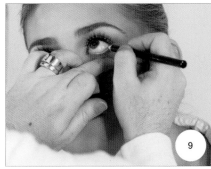

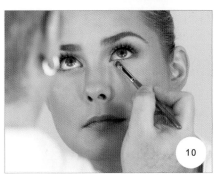

8. It's time to curl your lashes and apply your first layer of mascara to your top lashes. (See page 42 to review how to curl your lashes properly.)

9. Using a concealer pencil, line your waterline. (Remember, the waterline is the inner rim above the lower lash line.) I don't do this often, but for this look, it creates the effect of having no color on the lower lash line. For this look, the only definition we want is mascara.

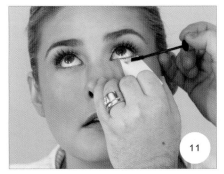

10. Using your #14 detail highlighting brush, apply your highlight shade to the inside corner of the lower lash line. This trick opens up the eye.

11. And now it's time for mascara on your lower lashes and another coat to your upper lashes.

We'll add another layer of mascara at the end of the look.

cheeks

1. Grab your #73 bronzer/blush brush and a matte bronzer. Apply the bronzer beginning at the back of your cheekbone and sweep it forward toward the apple of your cheek. Then take the brush back toward your ear. This lays your color in place.

2. Now take your brush and use it in the opposite direction (up and down) to blend. Be sure to blend well, or it won't look natural.

3. Don't forget to add a little at the temples to help shape your face. Sweep the bronzing powder up around the temples and eye sockets. This always gives the face more color and gives you a glow, and that is what this look is all about.

4. Feel free to blend some bronzer along your jawbone. This also helps create that glow, and if your face is fuller, it will narrow your face and soften your jaw.

5. Follow all this fabulous bronzing with a soft wash of a bright, sheer peach blush applied just to the apple of the cheek with your #73 brush.

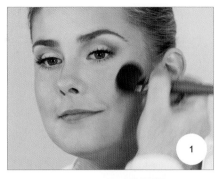

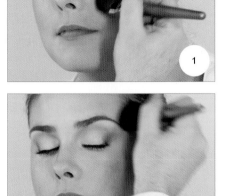

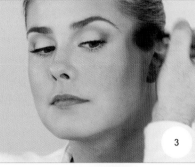

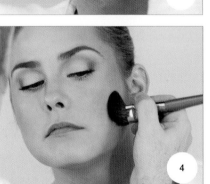

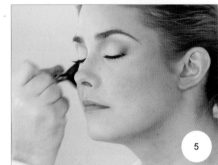

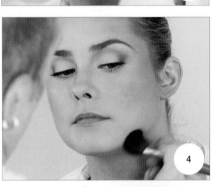

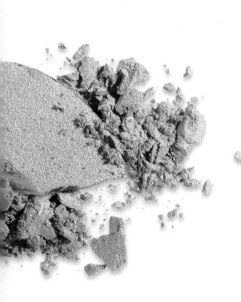

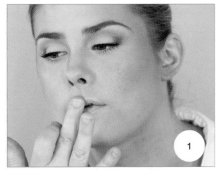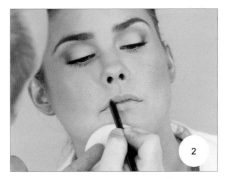

lips

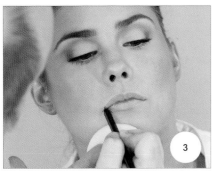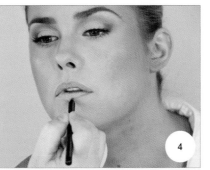

1. We want a soft taupe nude lip for this look. So the first thing you need to do is conceal your lips.

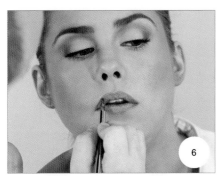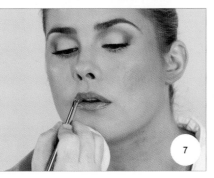

2. Line with a soft taupe nude lip liner. Begin with a V in the "cupid's bow," or center curve, of the lips. Bring the liner up and around the curves of your bow.

3. Next, starting at the outer corners, move toward the center with your pencil.

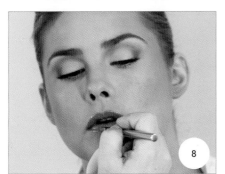

4. On the lower lip, first accentuate the lower curve of the lip. Then begin from the outer corners, moving toward the center. Remember to use your entire lip: Take the color to the almost invisible line just at the edge of the colored part of your lips.

5. Be sure to fill in at least halfway toward the center of your lip. This will help your lip liner look more natural and your lip color last longer.

6. Now blend with your #80 lip brush to make it look more natural.

7. Using your lip brush (because it gives you better application and helps the color last longer), fill in your entire lip with the perfect neutral nude lipstick. Be sure to blend really well over your lip liner.

8. End with a quick sweep of the perfect nude lip gloss to make your lips shiny, fuller looking, and sexy. Apply the gloss with your #80 lip brush—if you apply gloss with a brush, it will appear shinier.

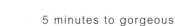

eyes

Here is the finishing touch for your eyes.

12. When you finish the rest of your makeup, add yet another layer of mascara to the top lashes. Remember, with this look, lush lashes are very important, so you want to really layer your mascara on your top lashes. (See page 44 to review how to layer your mascara properly.)

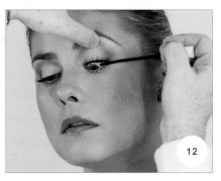
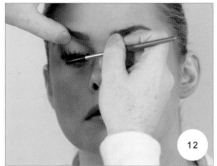

Thrilled with these stunning 5-minute makeovers? Just wait until you see what you can do in only 10 minutes!

"this look will work for every occasion."

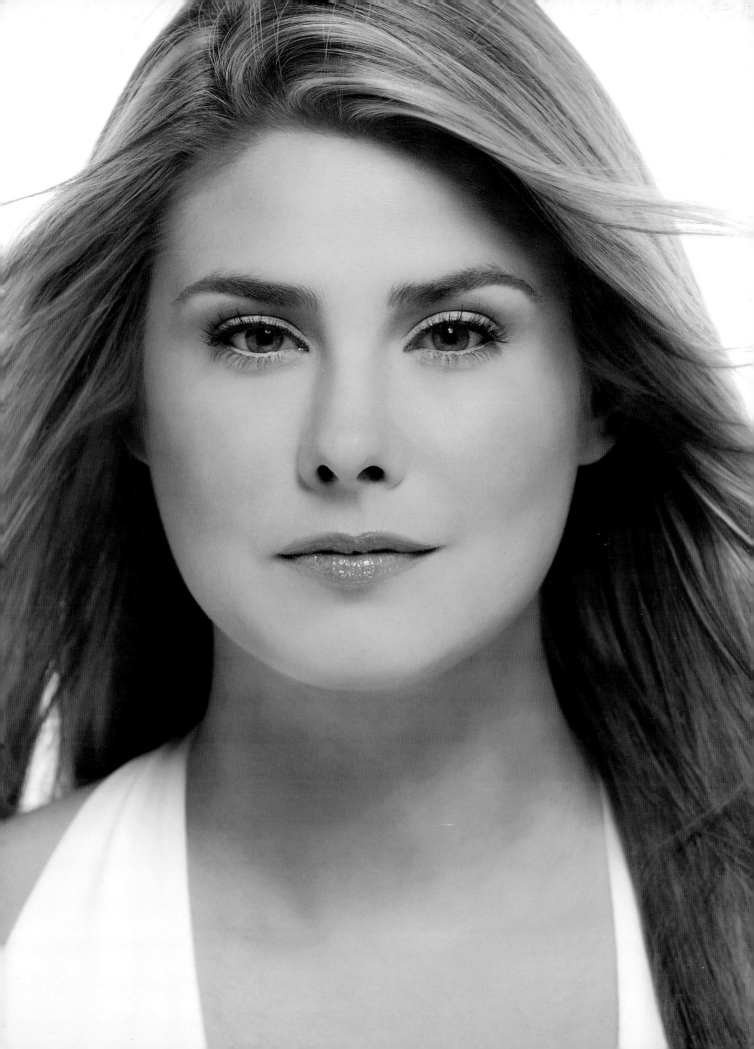

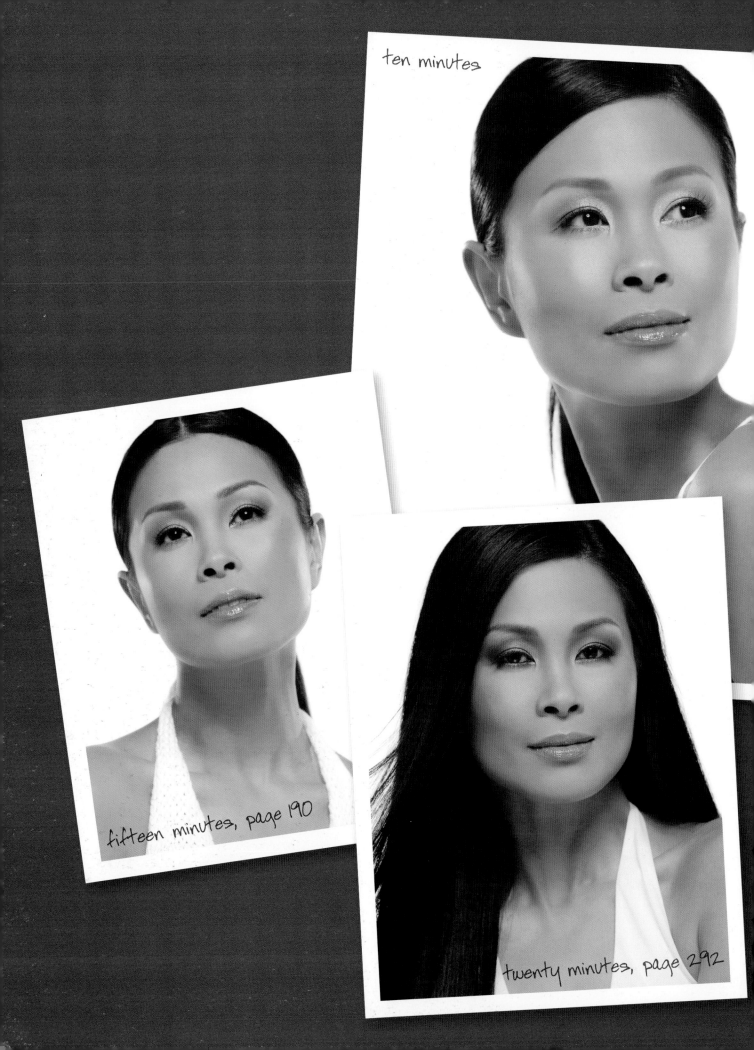

ten minutes

fifteen minutes, page 190

twenty minutes, page 292

10 minutes that could change your life

Let's say you find yourself with a little more time this morning (or evening) than you had in the last chapter. Now you have 10 minutes to give yourself a makeup makeover. Ten minutes? Doesn't sound like much. That's not even enough time to buy the perfect pair of new shoes. But, as you're about to see, it's plenty of time to make yourself beautiful! Of course, what you're *really* doing is making sure the rest of the world sees what I do—and that's how beautiful you already are. That's what makeup is really for.

What are we waiting for? Let's play!

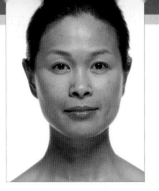

candy-coated

Shimmery bright color—is there anything more fun to play with? This look is about using fun color in a very sophisticated way. Remember, whenever using bright color, you have to ground it with a neutral. Notice the play with opposing colors, mixing complementary opposites (the green and purple shades) together. I point this out because if you want to mix colors, in order for them to pop, they have to be complementary opposites; otherwise, they blend together and look like one color. Be brave and play!

Here's how to get this look:

eyes

1. With your #22 highlighting brush, high-light your brow bone with a shimmery white eye shadow. When I say brow bone, I mean the area just under the arch of your brow.

2. Even though this eye look is all about color, we still need to ground it and add crease definition. Using your #11 midtone brush and a matte midtone eye shadow and starting from the outside corner of your crease, glide your brush across to the inside corner. Use a dark matte taupe shadow (a shade just a bit darker than your skin tone) to get soft definition. Use your #28 blending brush (the one that is always clean and ready to blend with) and blend your midtone so that there are no hard edges.

3. Using your #22 highlighting brush, apply a crème-to-powder shimmery acid green eye shadow to your lid (but only from your lash line to your crease). You are going to layer crème and powder to make your lid more dramatic.

4. With the same brush, apply a shimmery acid green eye shadow powder on top of the crème you applied to your lid.

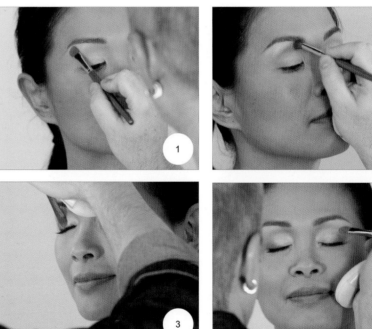

"be brave and play with your look!"

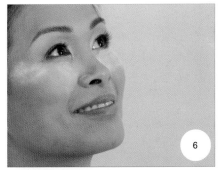

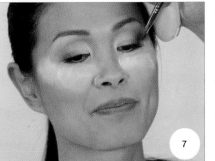

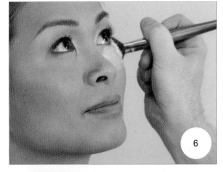

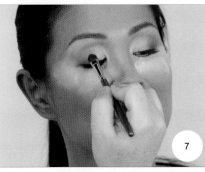

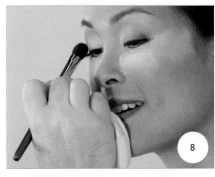

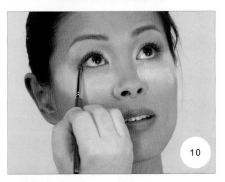

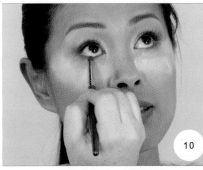

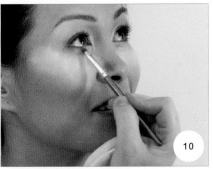

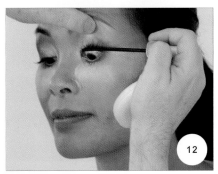

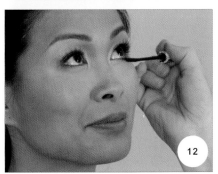

5. It's time to curl your eyelashes and apply the first layer of mascara to your top lashes. (See page 42 to review how to curl properly.)

6. Because you're about to use a bright purple eye shadow, if you are afraid you might drip color, apply a generous amount of powder to the area under your eyes. The powder will catch any spilled eye shadow, and when you are finished, you can brush it all away.

7. Using your #30 contour brush, apply your bright shimmery purple eye shadow to the outside half of your eyelid up into your crease.

8. Grab your #28 blending brush and blend the edges of your purple shadow.

9. Now grab your #13 detail eye shadow brush and apply your midtone eye shadow all along your lower lash line. Once again, start your application from the outside corner, sweeping it across to the inside corner.

10. With that same detail eye shadow brush, apply a generous layer of your bright purple contour color right over your midtone all along your bottom lash line.

11. Using your #14 detail highlighting brush, highlight the inside corner of the lower lash line with your shimmery acid green.

12. Now it's time for another layer of mascara on your top lashes and a layer on your lower lashes. After you finish the rest of your makeup, add yet another layer to the top lashes. Remember, with this look, lush lashes are very important, so you want to really layer your mascara on your top lashes. (See page 44 to review how to layer your mascara properly.)

13. With your #76 detail powder brush, sweep away the powder you laid under your eyes. Any shadow that you dropped during application will go with it.

cheeks

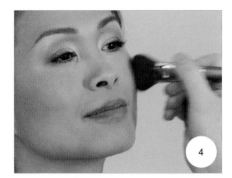

1. Using your #73 bronzer/blush brush, apply your matte bronzer, beginning at the back of your cheekbone. Sweep it forward toward the apple of your cheek and then take the brush back toward your ear. This lays your color in place.

2. Now take your brush and use it in the opposite direction (up and down) to blend. Be sure to blend well, or it won't look natural.

3. Don't forget to add a little at the temples to help shape your face. Sweep the bronzing powder up around the temples and eye sockets. Feel free to blend some bronzer along your jawbone; this also helps create that glow and defines your face.

4. Now for a little extra color, grab your #73 bronzer/blush brush and smile. Then apply your powder blush (the perfect bright sheer peach color) on the apple of your cheek, blending back toward the area that you bronzed. This technique really gives your face that fresh flush that is so perfect.

lips

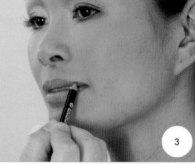

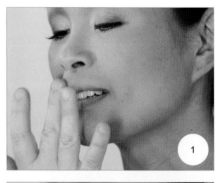

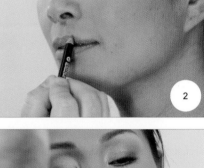

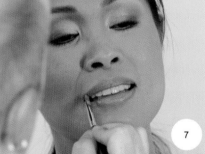

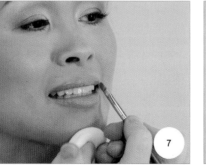

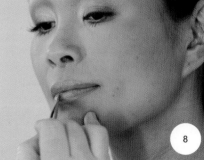

1. You want your lips to be soft, but still well defined. Start by concealing your lip and lip line. This gives you the perfect pale canvas for your subtle lip look.

2. Now, using a barely-there nude lip pencil, line your lips. Begin with a V in the "cupid's bow," or center curve, of the lips. Bring the liner up and around the curves of your bow.

3. Next, starting at the outer corners, move toward the center with your pencil.

4. On the lower lip, first accentuate the lower curve of the lip. Then begin from the outer corners, moving toward the center. Use your entire lip: Take the color to the almost invisible line just at the edge of the colored part of your lips.

5. Make sure you fill in at least halfway toward the center of your lip. This will help your lip liner look more natural and your lip color last longer.

6. Now blend with your #80 lip brush to make it look more natural.

7. Using your lip brush, fill in your entire lip with the perfect peachy nude lipstick. Make sure you blend really well over your lip liner.

8. End with a quick sweep of the perfect sheer peach lip gloss to make your lips shiny, fuller looking, and sexy. Make sure you apply your gloss with your #80 lip brush because if you apply gloss with a brush, it will appear shinier.

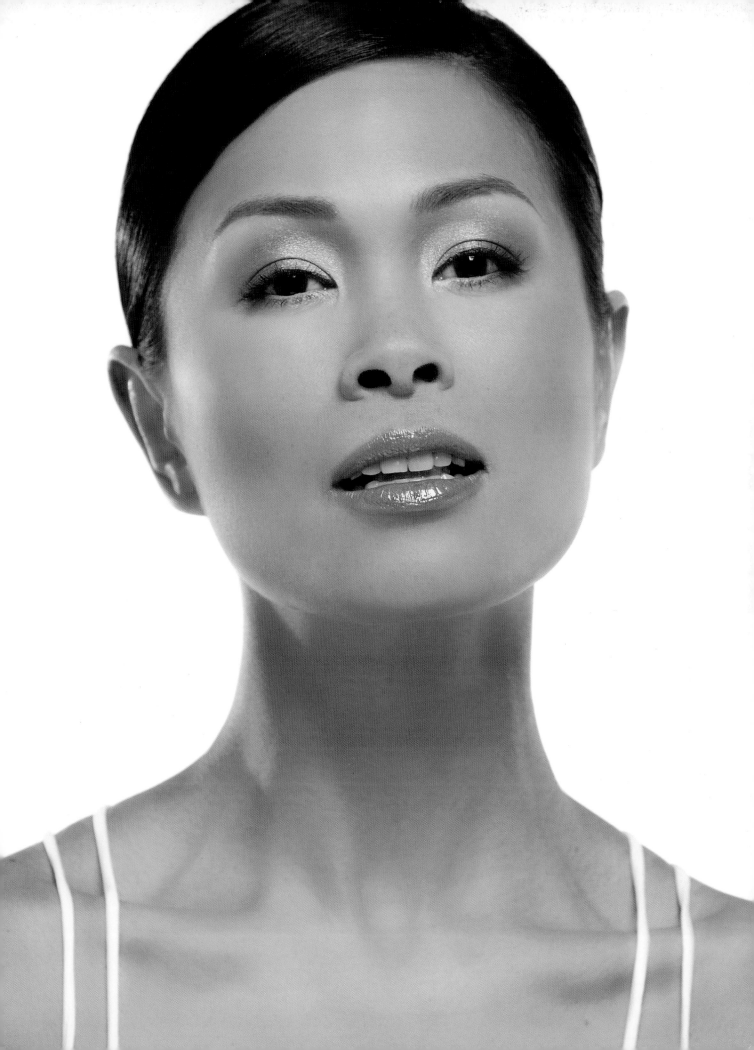

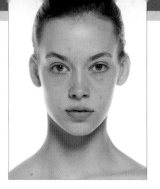

splurge of color

Sometimes a girl just needs a little color in her life or at least just for the day. You'll notice that I wasn't concerned about popping Hannah's eye color because the shadow color I used matched her eye color. (To make them look even bluer, I would need a warm coppery shade.) I just wanted fun, bright color to get your attention. And I did, didn't I?

Keep in mind that anytime you're using bright colors on the eye, you always need to ground them with neutrals first. And because the eyes do grab so much attention, I kept the rest of the face much more subtle.

Here's how to get this look:

eyes

1. To ground your bright eye color, start by creating definition with skin-tone neutral shades. Then you can add the bright shade. Using your #11 midtone brush and starting from the outside corner of your crease, glide your brush across to the inside corner. Use a soft matte taupe shadow (a shade just a bit darker than your skin tone) to get soft definition.

2. Grab your #30 contour brush and some of your midtone eye shadow and define the outer third of your eyelid.

3. Follow with your #28 brush to blend. This starts your lid definition and in this case, grounds all the fun blue you are about to use.

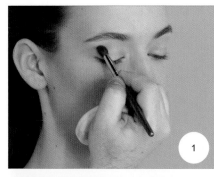

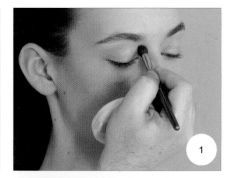

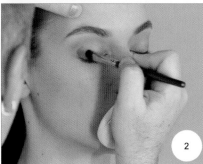

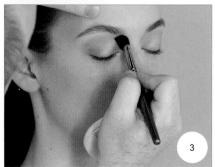

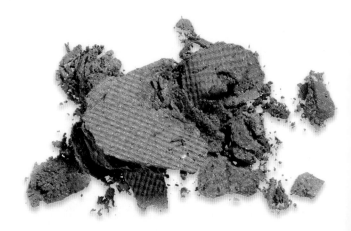

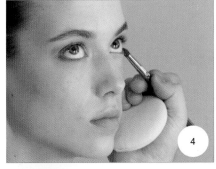

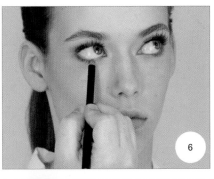

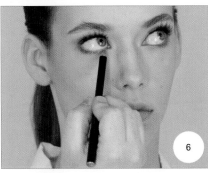

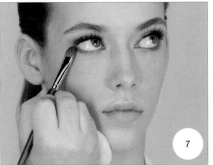

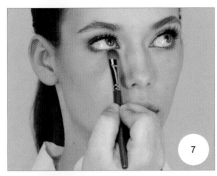

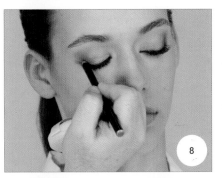

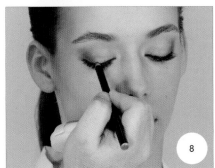

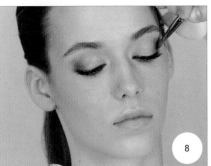

4. Using your #13 detail eye shadow brush, apply your midtone all along your lower lash line. Start from the outside corner and work in toward the inner corner.

5. Next, it's time to curl your eyelashes and apply the first layer of mascara to your top lashes. (See page 42 to review how to curl properly.)

6. Now, it's time for the fun! Using a bright teal blue eyeliner, line along your lower lash line. Because this is not a dark color, you can line from corner to corner without worrying about it closing the eye in and making it look smaller.

7. Using your #22 highlighting brush, blend your eyeliner pencil along the lash line.

8. Do the same lining and blending along the top lash line with your eyeliner. As you're blending, make sure you blend your pencil up toward the crease. Your pencil will make any eye shadow you layer over it later more intense.

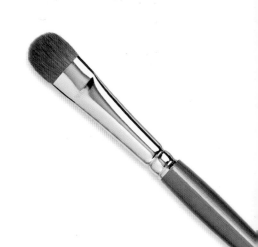

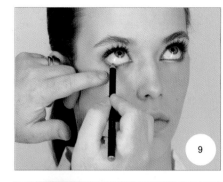

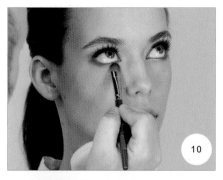

9. Moving back to the lower lid, use your teal eyeliner pencil to line the waterline of your lower lid. (Remember, the waterline is the inner rim above the lower lash line.) This will add just a little bit more drama to the bright eye.

10. Then, using your #22 brush, layer a bright shimmery teal eye shadow over your liner along the bottom lash line.

11. Take your #30 contour brush and layer that same shade of shadow on the top lid and lash line. Start at the base of your lash line and bring the color all the way across the lid and up into the crease.

12. Now you want to create a defined area of color. Use your #30 contour brush to pat that same teal eye shadow on the lid in a half-moon shape, making sure you cover the entire lid. When you pat color on rather than swipe, you'll get more complete coverage and intensity.

13. Next, grab your #28 blending brush and blend just along your crease to slightly blend the line you just created.

14. It's time for another layer of mascara on your top lashes and a layer on your lower lashes. After you finish the rest of your makeup, add yet another layer to the top lashes. Remember, with this look, lush lashes are very important! You want to really layer mascara on your top lashes. (See page 44 to review how to layer your mascara properly.)

We'll further define your eyes at the end of this look.

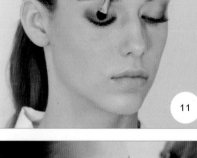

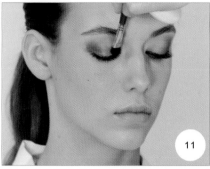

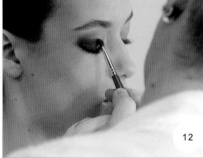

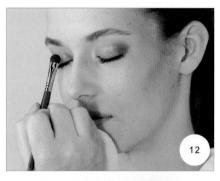

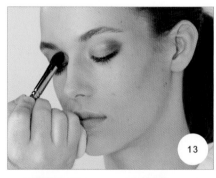

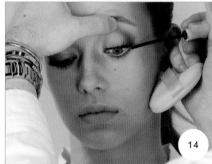

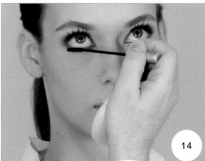

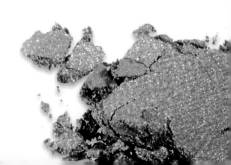

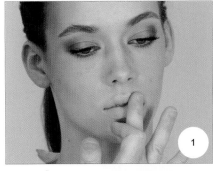

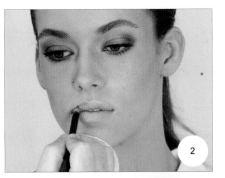

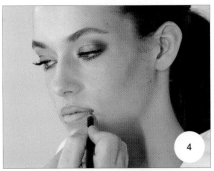

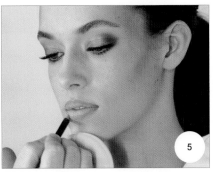

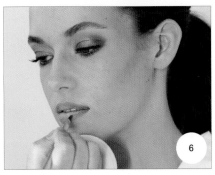

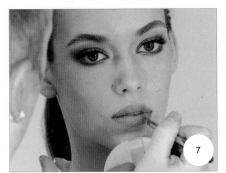

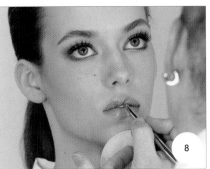

lips

1. You want your lips to be soft, but still well defined. Start by concealing your lip and lip line with concealer or foundation. This gives you the perfect pale canvas for your subtle lip look.

2. Now, using a barely-there nude lip pencil, line your lips. Begin with a V in the "cupid's bow," or center curve, of the lips. Bring the liner up and around the curves of your bow.

3. Next, starting at the outer corners, move toward the center with your pencil.

4. First accentuate the lower curve of the lower lip. Then begin from the outer corners, moving toward the center. Take the color to the almost invisible line at the edge of the colored part of your lips.

5. Make sure you fill in at least halfway toward the center of your lip. This will help your lip liner look more natural and your lip color last longer.

6. Using a #80 lip brush, blend your liner before you apply your lipstick. Again, this step will make your lip liner look more natural.

7. Using your lip brush, which will give you better application and help color last longer, fill in your entire lip with the perfect peachy nude lipstick. Be sure to blend really well over your lip liner.

8. As always, I like to finish with a coat of sheer peach lip gloss to add shine. And I love that sexy shine! Apply your gloss with your #80 lip brush because if you apply gloss with a brush, it will appear shinier. Subtle *and* sexy!

"anytime you're using bright colors on the eye, you need to ground them with neutrals."

cheeks

1. With this look the eye is the focus, so you only want a light dusting of bronzer on your cheeks. Using your #73 bronzer/blush brush, apply your matte bronzer, beginning at the back of your cheekbone. Sweep it forward toward the apple of your cheek and then take the brush back toward your ear. This lays your color in place.

2. Now, take your brush and use it in the opposite direction (up and down) to blend. Be sure to blend well, or it won't look natural.

3. Don't forget to add a little at the temples to help shape your face. Sweep the bronzing powder up around the temples and eye sockets. This always gives the face more color and gives you a glow.

4. Feel free to blend some bronzer along your jawbone. This also helps create that glow and defines your face.

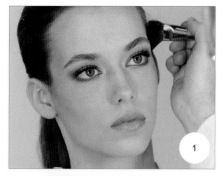
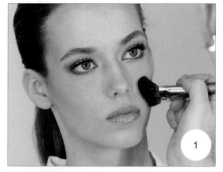
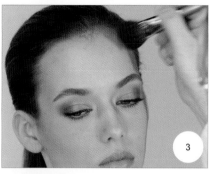
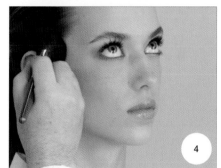
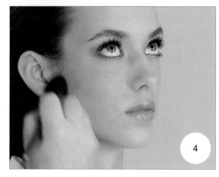

eyes

Here is the final step for your eyes.

15. For the finishing touch, grab your #22 highlighting brush and using a matte beige eye shadow, highlight your brow bone. You do this step last so that it gives the illusion of a bit more defined crease. Keep in mind that for this look, I have used two #22 brushes because I needed one for my highlight and one for my contour.

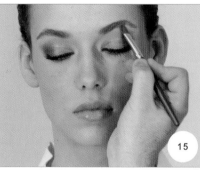
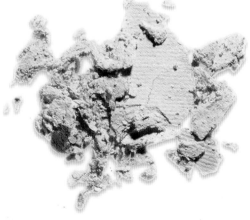

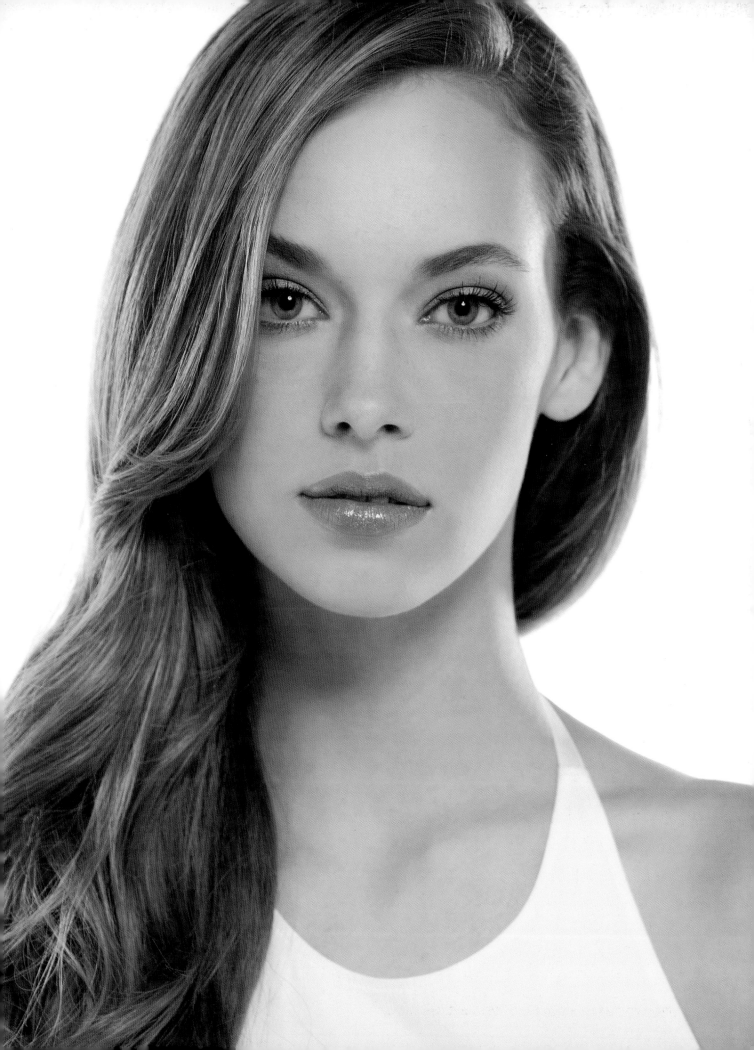

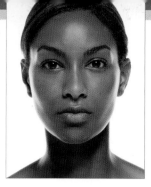

lip service

I always say show off what God gave you, and sometimes you can do it with a little bit of an edge. Let's face it, it's nice to be noticed. Right?

This look pairs simple, very subtle, almost naked eyes with drop-dead lips. Did I say drop-dead? And boy did I deliver! Keep in mind that you must have nice full lips to pull this look off. Medium or thin lips will just look pursed and minimized. And girls, do *not* forget your mascara!

Here's how to get this look:

eyes

1. Because this look is all about the lips, you want your eyes to be understated, but defined. First, using your #22 highlighting brush, apply a matte flesh-colored eye shadow (one a couple of shades lighter than your skin tone to create contrast) to your lid and your brow bone. We don't want your eyes to look made up, but we do want them to have definition, and using highlight and midtone eye shadows will help create contrast that will give your eyelid shape.

2. Using your #11 midtone brush and starting from the outside corner of your crease, glide your brush across to the inside corner. Use a soft matte ginger shadow (a shade just a bit darker than your skin tone) so that you get soft definition. Always follow with your #28 blending brush (the one that is always clean and ready to blend with) and blend your midtone so that there are no hard edges.

3. Now it's time to curl your eyelashes and apply the first layer of mascara to your top lashes. (See page 42 to review how to curl properly.)

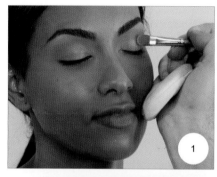

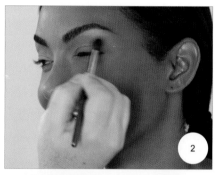

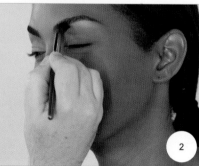

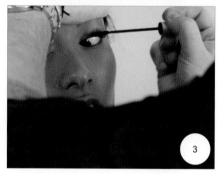

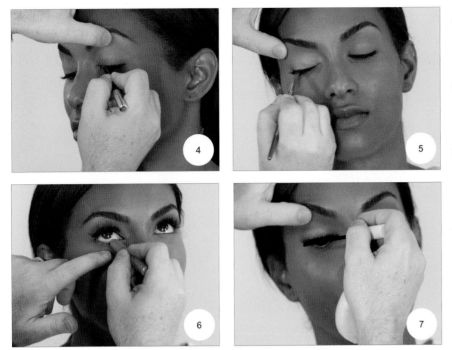

4. Grab a black eyeliner pencil and line your top lash line. Keep it right against your lashes. You do not want your lid to look lined, but you want the definition.

5. To make it look perfect and blend your liner, use your #41 detail eyeliner brush to retrace right along your lash line with a little black eye shadow.

6. To accentuate that bare lower lash line look, grab a concealer pencil and line the waterline of your lower lid. (Remember, the waterline is the inner rim above the lower lash line.)

7. Next, apply another layer of mascara on your top lashes. After you finish the rest of your makeup, add yet another layer to the top lashes. Remember, with this look, lush lashes are very important, so you want to really layer your mascara on your top lashes. (See page 44 to review how to layer your mascara properly.)

cheeks

Because the lips are the focus of this look, I've left Kayann's cheeks totally natural.

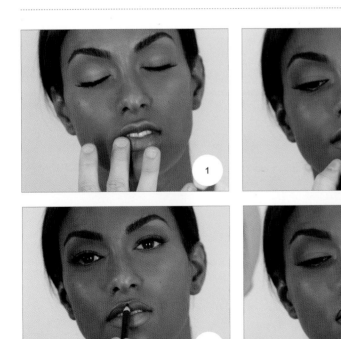

lips

1. This lip look is dramatic, and to help get it perfect, prep your lips first. Using concealer, conceal your lip and along your lip line. Now, powder your lips. This gives you the perfect canvas to apply your dramatic lip look so that the edge of the lip is very crisp.

2. Grab your burgundy lip liner pencil and begin with a V in the "cupid's bow," or center curve, of the lips. Bring the liner up and around the curves of your bow.

3. Next, starting at the outer corners, move toward the center with your pencil.

4. On the lower lip, first accentuate the lower curve of the lip. Then begin from the outer corners, moving toward the center. Take the color to the almost invisible line just at the edge of the colored part of your lips.

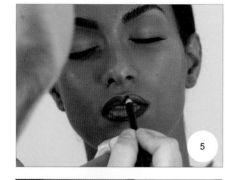

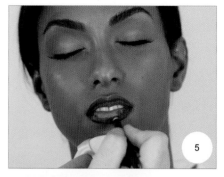

5. Fill in your entire lip with your lip pencil. This will help your lip color last and stay in place because lip liner has a drier texture than lipstick.

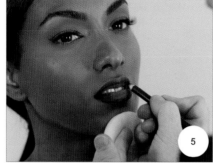

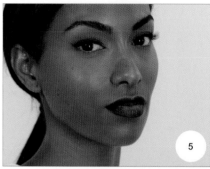

6. With your #80 lip brush, blend your lip liner so that it is even and smooth.

7. Using your lip brush, apply your deep blackberry lipstick to your entire lip. Make sure you blend really well over your lip liner.

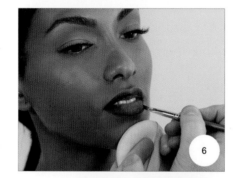

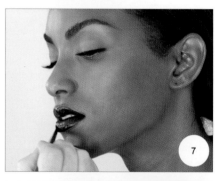

8. Now, take a tissue and blot your lips. This will remove the moisture from the lipstick, but leave a layer of pigment.

9. Then apply another layer of lipstick. Applying these three layers (one of liner and two of lipstick) will help your color be true and intense, as well as last longer.

10. Finish with a thin layer of blackberry lip gloss for shine and dimension. Can you say fabulous?

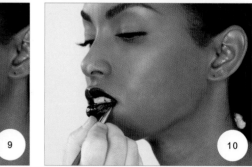

"you'll need full lips to pull off this drop-dead look."

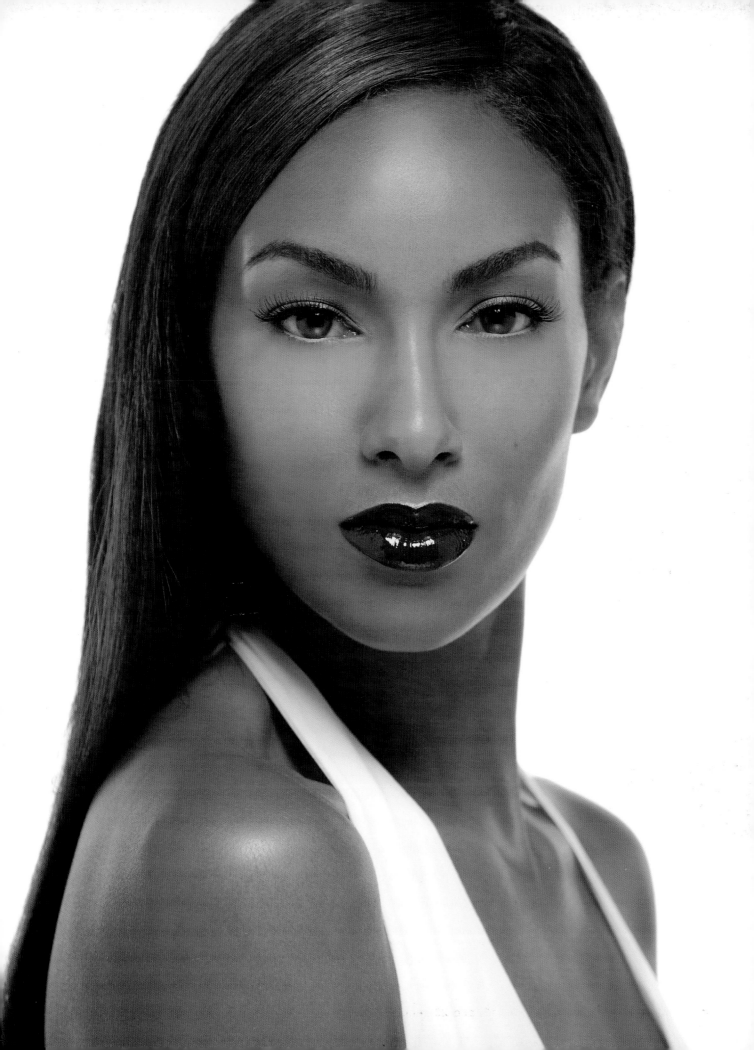

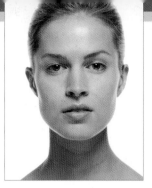

pucker up and blow

Beautiful red lips: I think every girl has wanted them at one time or another. But there's a trick to applying and wearing red lipstick. Barely-there eyes, a defined lash line, and glowing skin are what make the look work. The secret to the perfect red lips is grounding the edge of your lip with a deeper lip liner and choosing a clear, true red lipstick.

Ready to try on Jamie's look? Let's paint!

eyes

1. Using your #22 highlighting brush, apply a crème-to-powder shimmery beige eye shadow, but only to your lid (from the lash line to the crease). You are going to layer crème and powder to make your lid more dramatic.

2. With the same brush, apply a shimmery champagne eye shadow directly on top of the crème you applied to your lid. Apply it to your brow bone, too. When I say brow bone, I mean the area just under the arch of your brow.

3. Using your #41 liner brush, apply black eye shadow as liner all along your top lash line.

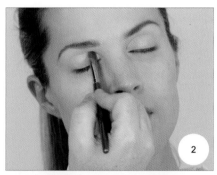
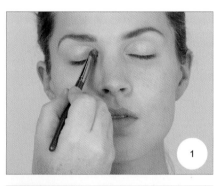
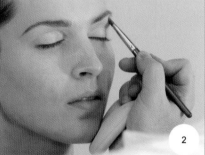
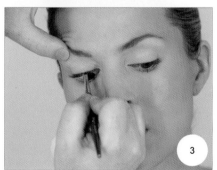

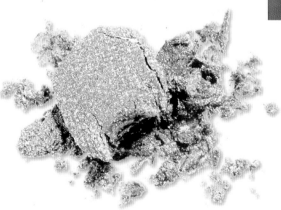

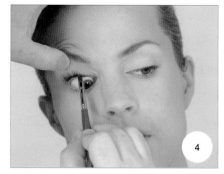

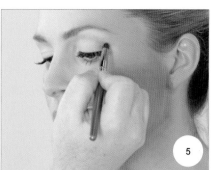

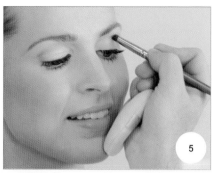

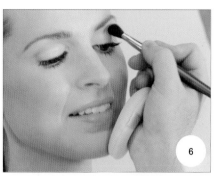

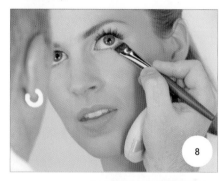

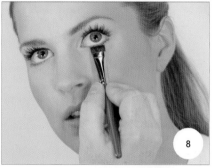

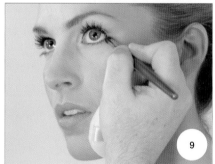

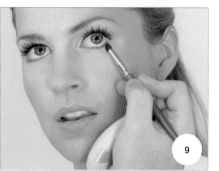

4. Using the same brush, push the same black shadow right at the base of your lashes. (Not on the wet tissue, but right at the base between the lashes.) You don't want your eyes to look lined, but you want definition, and this is the perfect way to get it.

5. With this look, you want your midtone to be very precise, so it doesn't darken your lid but instead defines the shape. Because this look has such an intense lip, you want your lid soft and shimmery. Using your #13 detail shadow brush, apply your matte taupe midtone eye shadow in your crease. Starting from the outside corner of your crease, glide your brush across to the inside corner. Create a distinct line all along your crease.

6. Use your #28 blending brush (the one that is always clean and ready to blend with) and blend your midtone so that there are no hard edges. Be sure to only retrace the same area that you just applied your midtone to, so as to not blend it up and down and darken too much of your lid.

7. It's time to curl your eyelashes and apply the first layer of mascara to your top lashes. (See page 42 to review how to curl properly.)

8. With your #18 brush, apply the faintest bit of dark brown eye shadow, pushing it up into the lashes.

9. To soften and define the lower lash line, using your #13 shadow brush, apply your midtone all along your lower lash line. Starting from the outside corner, work in toward the inner corner.

10. Using your #14 detail highlighting brush, highlight the inside corner of the lower lash line.

11. It's time for another layer of mascara on your top lashes and a layer on your lower lashes. After you finish the rest of your makeup, add yet another layer to the top lashes. Remember that with this look, lush lashes are very important, so you want to really layer your mascara on your top lashes. (See page 44 to review how to layer your mascara properly.)

cheeks

1. With this look, you don't want your cheek color to be noticeable, but you still want subtle definition. You can achieve this with a light application of bronzer. Using your #73 bronzer/blush brush, apply your matte bronzer. Begin at the back of your cheekbone and sweep it forward toward the apple of your cheek. Then take the brush back toward your ear. This lays your color in place.

2. Now take your brush and use it in the opposite direction (up and down) to blend. Be sure to blend well, or it won't look natural.

3. Don't forget to add a little at the temples to help shape your face. Sweep the bronzing powder up around the temples and eye sockets.

4. Feel free to blend some bronzer along your jawbone. This also helps shape and define your face.

lips

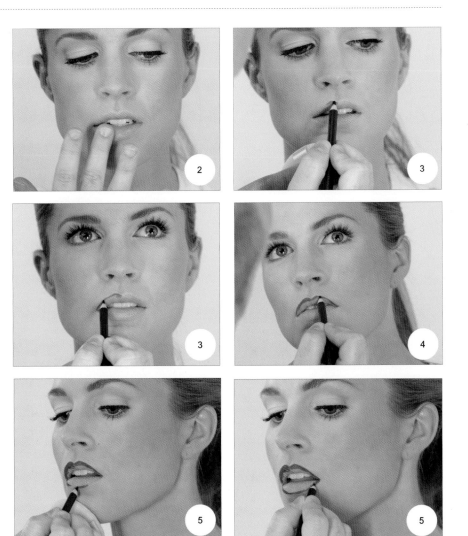

1. This lip is very dramatic, and to help it look its most perfect, you need to prep your lips first. Because this look is all about the lips, you really want them to look sumptuous and smooth, so before you start your color application, moisturize them with lip balm. This will help the color go on smoothly and evenly. After the balm has had a bit of time to soak in, blot off the excess with a tissue so that it won't shorten the staying power of your lipstick.

2. Next, using concealer, conceal your lip and along your lip line. This gives you the ideal canvas to create a perfect lip line.

3. With red lips, the trick is to "ground" them so they don't look like they are floating on your face. To do that, simply use a darker lip liner. Grab your burgundy lip pencil and begin with a V in the "cupid's bow," or center curve, of the lips. Bring the liner up and around the curves of your bow.

4. Now, starting at the outer corners, move toward the center with your pencil.

5. On the lower lip, first accentuate the lower curve of the lip. Then begin from the outer corners, moving toward the center. Remember to use your entire lip: Take the color to the almost invisible line just at the edge of the colored part of your lips.

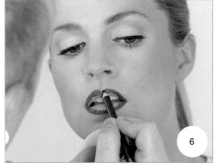

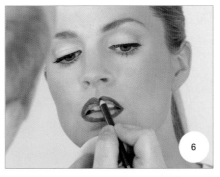

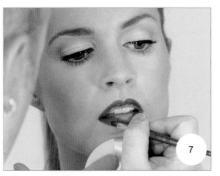

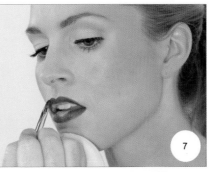

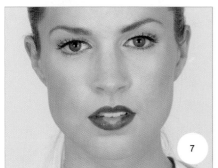

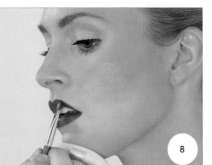

6. Now fill in your entire lip—except for the center of your top and bottom lip—with your lip pencil. By leaving the center without pencil color, you'll get the full impact of the red while grounding it along the edges.

7. Using your #80 lip brush blend, your lip liner while leaving the center of the lip without color. This will make everything look more natural while helping ground your color.

8. Next, using your #80 lip brush, apply the perfect true red lipstick to your entire lip, making sure you blend really well over your lip liner.

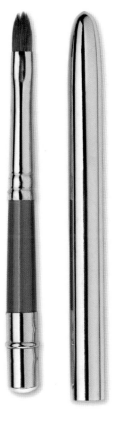

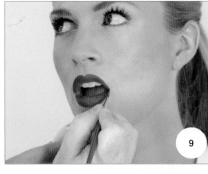

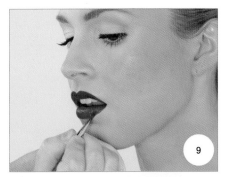

9. Take a tissue and blot your lips. This will remove the moisture from the lipstick, but leave you with a layer of pigment. Then apply another layer of lipstick. Applying these three layers (one of liner and two of lipstick) will help your color be true and intense, as well as last longer.

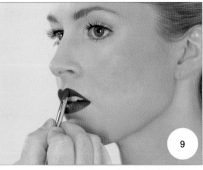

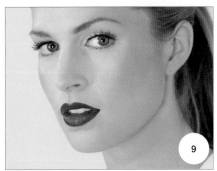

10. Finish with a thin layer of a sheer burgundy lip gloss for shine and shape. I find that a sheer burgundy lip gloss rather that a red one adds more dimension to your red. Be sure to apply your gloss with your #80 lip brush because if you apply gloss with a brush, it will appear shinier.

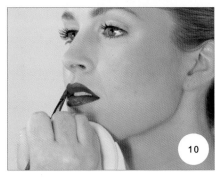

"what girl wouldn't want beautiful red lips?"

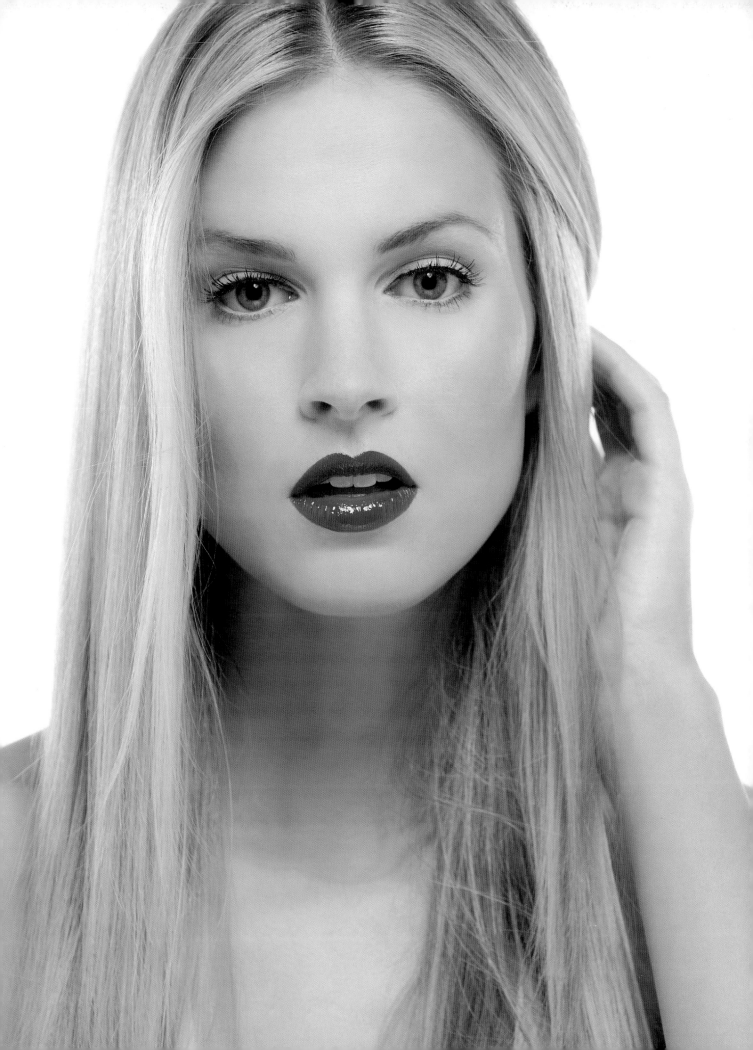

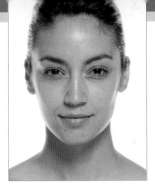

latin lovely

I wanted to take this classic ethnic look and make it modern and fun to wear for everyone. I have taken a look that usually has a stark liquid-lined eye and shown you how to create a softer version, while still staying true to the signature of the look. I've also made it simple for you to create the look's signature lip, deepest around the edges and fading to lighter in the middle. Go ahead, girls—give a modern spin to a look you have preconceived notions about.

Here's how to get this look:

eyes

1. This look is all about eyeliner, but we still want to give your eyelids definition, and using highlight and midtone eye shadows will help create contrast that will give your eyelid shape. First, you need to apply a matte flesh-colored eye shadow to your lid and your brow bone using your #22 highlighting brush.

2. Using your #11 midtone brush and a matte midtone eye shadow and starting from the outside corner of your crease, glide your brush across to the inside corner. Use a soft matte caramel eye shadow (a shade just a bit darker than your skin tone) so that you get soft definition.

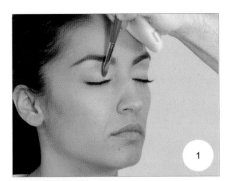

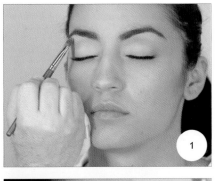

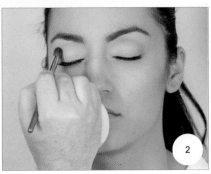

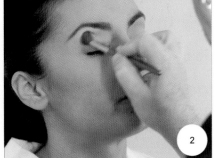

"every girl can use a little Latin fire now and then."

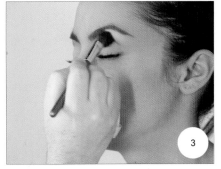 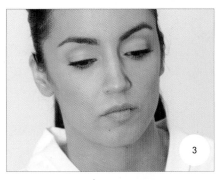

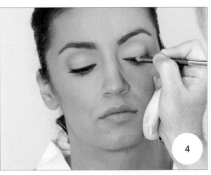 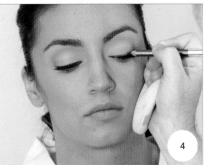

3. Use your #28 blending brush (the one that is always clean and ready to blend with) and blend your midtone so that there are no hard edges. Also, before you move on, curl your eyelashes and apply the first layer of mascara to your top lashes. (See page 42 to review how to curl properly.)

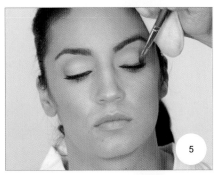 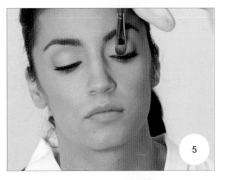

4. Grab your black eyeliner pencil—it's time to start lining! Starting with your upper lash line, line your entire lid all the way from the inside corner to the outside. Keep your liner right against the lash line. You want it to be thinnest at the inside corner, slowly getting thicker as you reach the outer corner.

5. With this look, you want to see a defined line, but you don't want it to look like liquid eyeliner. In other words, you want it to look slightly blurred. To create this effect, simply take another #22 brush (not the same one you highlighted with) and blend your pencil. When blending, blend slightly up—this is what gives you your blur.

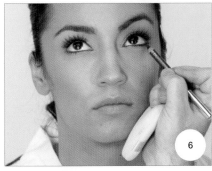 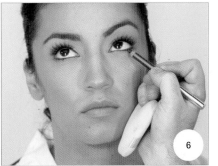

6. Now, line along your bottom lash line. Try to keep the line as close to the lashes as possible.

7. Blend and blur that line with your #22 brush, just like you did along your top lash line.

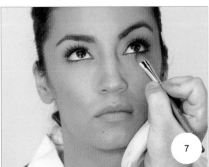 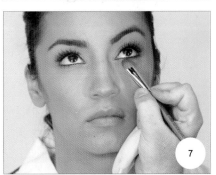

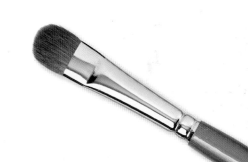

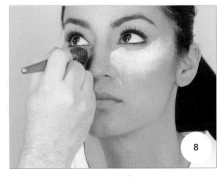

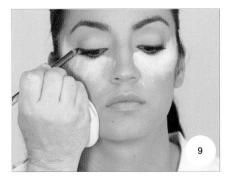

8. Because you're about to use black eye shadow, if you're afraid you might drip color, apply a generous amount of powder to the area under your eyes. The powder will catch any spilled shadow, and when you're finished, you can simply brush it all away.

9. Now for more intensity, line some more with your eyeliner all around your eye.

10. To finish your liner to perfection, using your #18 eyeliner brush, apply black eye shadow all along your lash line, intensifying your liner. Again, as you apply the shadow, once you place your brush down on the lash line, slightly pull up to blend your color.

11. Now do the same all along your bottom lash line, making sure to really push the color into the base of your lower lashes.

12. With your #76 detail powder brush, sweep away the powder you laid under your eye. Any shadow that you dropped during application will go with it.

We'll let your mascara dry and add more at the end of the look.

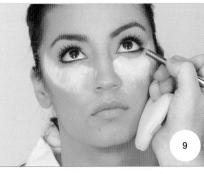

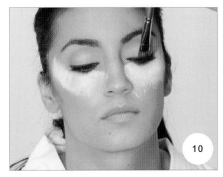

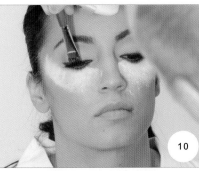

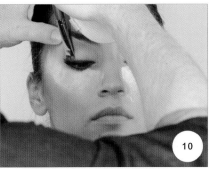

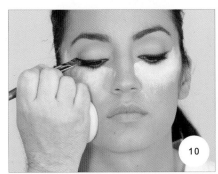

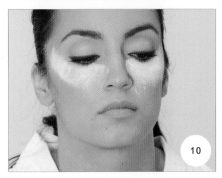

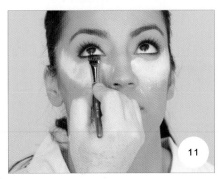

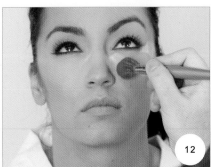

cheeks

1. Using your #73 bronzer/blush brush, apply your matte bronzer. Begin at the back of your cheekbone and sweep it forward toward the apple of your cheek. Then take the brush back toward your ear. This lays your color in place.

2. Now take your brush and use it in the opposite direction (up and down) to blend. Be sure to blend well, or it won't look natural.

3. Sweep the bronzing powder up around the temples and eye sockets to help shape your face.

4. Feel free to blend some bronzer along your jawbone. This also helps create that glow and defines your face.

We'll add more color to your cheeks in a moment.

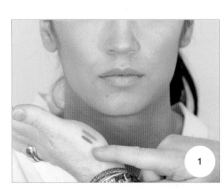

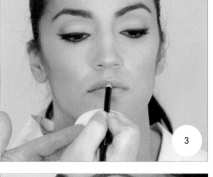

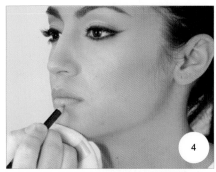

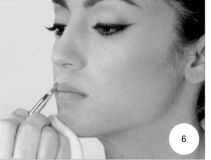

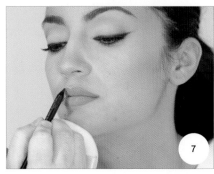

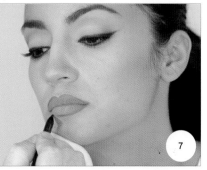

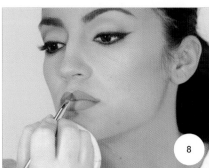

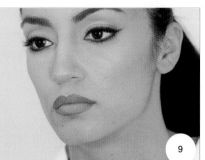

lips

1. With this lip look, your goal is for the outer edge to be the darkest, fading lighter as you get to the center of the lip. To create this look, you are going to line with two different lip liners: first a more neutral shade, followed by a darker shade.

2. First, starting with a dark flesh lip liner, begin with a V in the "cupid's bow," or center curve, of the lips. Bring the liner up and around the curves of your bow.

3. Next, starting at the outer corners, move toward the center with your pencil.

4. On the lower lip, first accentuate the lower curve of the lip. Then begin from the outer corners and move toward the center. Take the color to the almost invisible line just at the edge of the colored part of your lips.

5. Make sure you fill in at least halfway toward the center of your lip. This will help your lip liner look more natural and your lip color last longer.

6. Now blend with your #80 brush to make it look more natural.

7. With a raisin lip liner, reline the outer edge of your lip. Make it a nice wide line so that it will blend well. Blend toward the center, just barely adding color.

8. Now, with your lip brush, blend the two lip liners together at the edge where they meet.

9. You can see after blending how your lips are darkest along the outer edge, fading to nothing in the center. Don't worry, this is the effect you're after!

10. Using your lip brush (because it gives you better application and helps color last longer), fill in your entire lip with the perfect nude lipstick. Make sure you blend really well over your lip liner.

11. End with a quick sweep of the perfect sheer nude lip gloss to make your lips shiny, fuller looking, and sexy. Make sure you apply your gloss with your #80 lip brush because if you apply gloss with a brush, it will appear shinier.

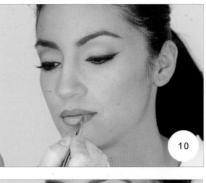
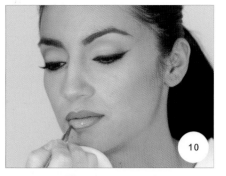
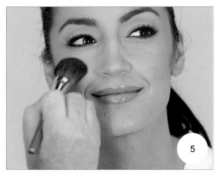
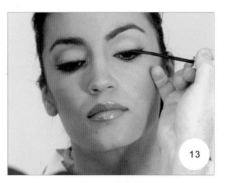

cheeks

Here is the last step for your cheeks.

5. Now for a little extra color, grab your #73 bronzer/blush brush and smile. Then apply your powder blush (the perfect bright sheer apricot color) on the apple of your cheek, blending back toward the area that you bronzed. This technique really gives your face that fresh flush that is so perfect.

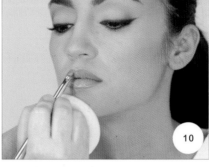
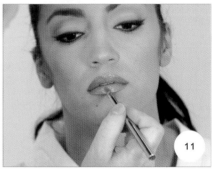

eyes

Here are the final touches for your eyes.

13. Now it's time for another layer of mascara on your top lashes and a layer on your lower lashes. After you finish the rest of your makeup, add yet another layer to the top lashes. Remember, with this look, lush lashes are very important, so you want to really layer your mascara on your top lashes. (See page 44 to review how to layer your mascara properly.)

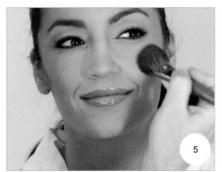

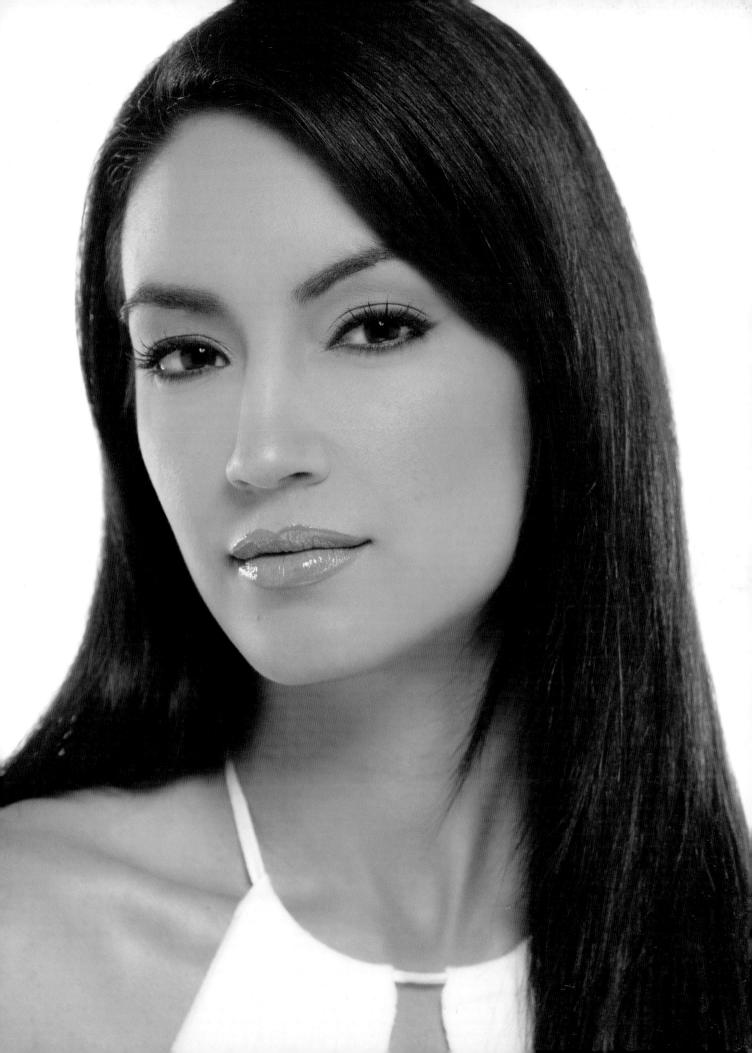

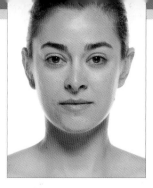

flirty girl

Life is so much more fun when you go through it with a smile on your face and a twinkle in your eye. With eyes like this, you'll be flirting without even trying. This is a simple look to achieve without a lot of work. I think the genius of this look is it simply defines the eyes and gives you that sultry lid, without looking heavy and dark. Anytime you deepen your entire lid, it creates what some might call a bedroom eye. Go ahead, try it and enjoy all the attention!

Here's how to get this look:

eyes

1. Using your #22 highlighting brush, apply a matte beige eye shadow to your brow bone. When I say brow bone, I mean the area just under the arch of your brow.

2. With a #27 eye shadow brush (because you will be applying your color to a large area), apply a dark matte taupe midtone eye shadow. Start at the base of your upper lash line and bring the color up and over your entire lid, all the way up to just under your brow bone. By starting along your lash line and working your way upward, you'll get the highest concentration of color where you laid your brush first. This will make your color deeper at the lash line.

3. Now with the same brush, apply more midtone in a half-moon shape all along your crease.

4. Use your #28 blending brush (the one that is always clean and ready to blend with) and blend your midtone so that there are no hard edges.

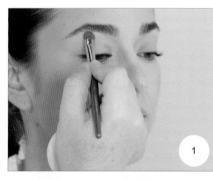
1

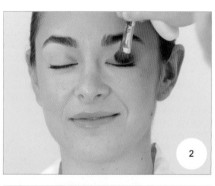
2

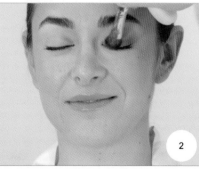
2

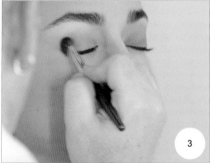
3

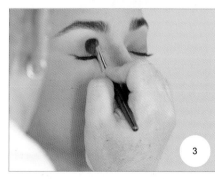
3

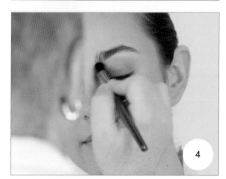
4

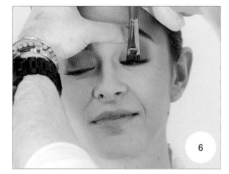

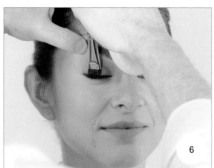

5. It's time to curl your eyelashes and apply the first layer of mascara to your top lashes. (See page 42 to review how to curl properly.)

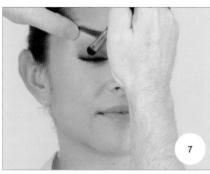

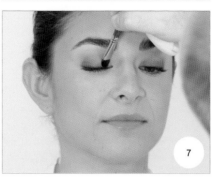

6. With your #18 eyeliner brush, line all along your top lash line with a black eye shadow. As you apply it, pull up slightly with your brush to blend the line. This will create definition without making your eyes looked lined.

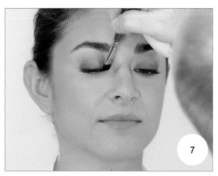

7. Using your #30 contour brush, apply a dark shimmery golden brown eye shadow along your lash line. Start from the outside corner and sweep across to the inside. This will create more definition at the lash line and blend the black shadow you just applied.

We'll let your mascara dry and add more at the end of the look.

cheeks

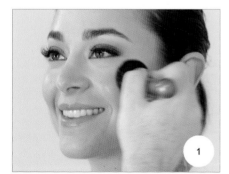

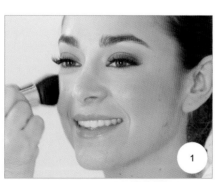

1. Now it's time for a gorgeous glow. You are going to achieve this by layering your blush and using the perfect amount of bronzer. Start with a great crème-to-powder blush. Using your #64 crème blush brush, apply a bright peach blush to the apple of your cheek, starting at the front of the apple and working toward the back.

2. Follow with a light dusting of loose or pressed powder.

3. Using your #73 bronzer/blush brush, apply your matte bronzer. Beginning at the back of your cheekbone, sweep it forward toward the apple of your cheek. Then take the brush back toward your ear. This lays your color in place.

4. Now take your brush and use it in the opposite direction (up and down) to blend. Be sure to blend well, or it won't look natural.

5. Don't forget to add a little at the temples to help shape your face. Sweep the bronzing powder up around the temples and eye sockets. This always gives the face more color and gives you a glow, and that is what this look is all about.

6. Feel free to blend some bronzer along your jawbone. This also helps create that glow and defines your face.

7. To reinforce that lovely flush, smile and apply your powder blush (the perfect bright sheer peach color) with your #73 brush on the apple of your cheek, starting at the front of the apple and working toward the back.

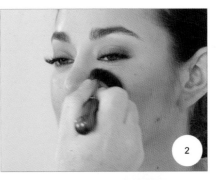

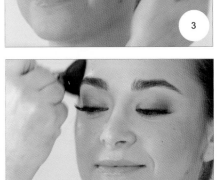

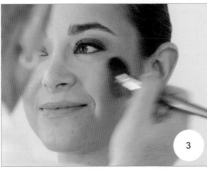

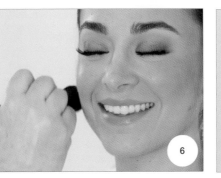

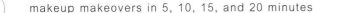

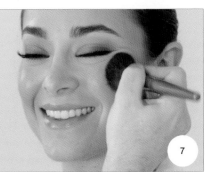

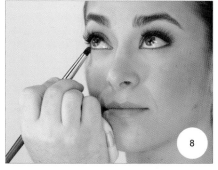

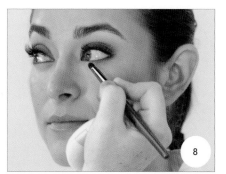

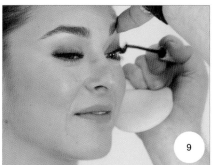

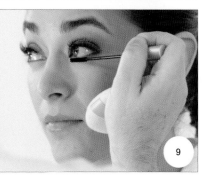

eyes

Here are the final steps for your eyes.

8. Next, using your #13 detail shadow brush, apply your midtone eye shadow all along your lower lash line. Starting from the outside corner, work in toward the inner corner.

9. Now it's time for another layer of mascara on your top lashes and a layer on your lower lashes. (See page 44 to review how to layer your mascara properly.)

"life might get a lot more interesting when you try this 'bedroom eye' look!"

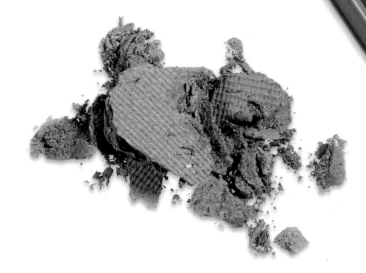

lips

1. I have chosen to use lip liner with this look because I want a very defined lip. Grab your nude pencil and begin with a V in the "cupid's bow," or center curve, of the lips. Bring the liner up and around the curves of your bow.

2. Next, starting at the outer corners, move toward the center with your pencil.

3. On the lower lip, first accentuate the lower curve of the lip. Then begin from the outer corners, moving toward the center. Remember to use your entire lip: Take the color to the almost invisible line just at the edge of the colored part of your lips.

4. Make sure you fill in at least halfway toward the center of your lip. This will help your lip liner look more natural and your lip color last longer.

5. Now blend with your #80 lip brush to make it look more natural.

6. Using your lip brush (because it gives you better application and helps color last longer), fill in your entire lip with the perfect peach lipstick. Make sure you blend really well over your lip liner.

7. End with a quick sweep of the perfect sheer peach lip gloss to make your lips shiny, fuller looking, and sexy. Be sure to apply the gloss with your #80 lip brush because if you apply gloss with a brush, it will appear shinier.

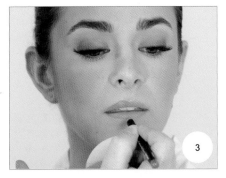

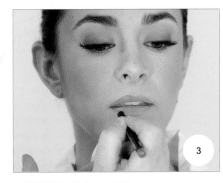

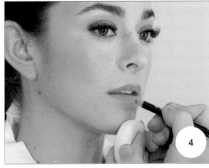

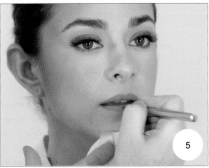

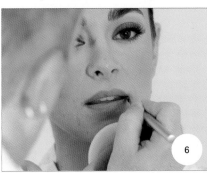

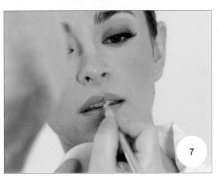

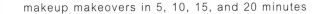

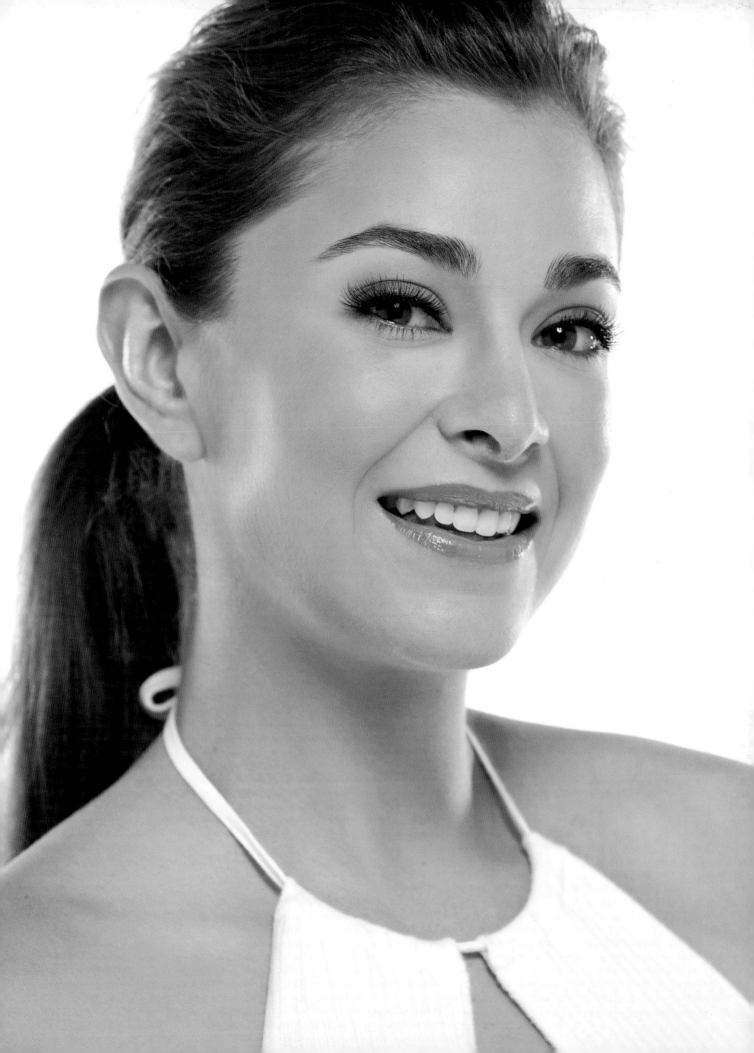

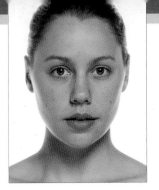

walk the line

Sophisticated, classic, glamorous, timeless: these are all words that describe this look. This is a perfect way to wear a sophisticated, classic look and make it work for the modern-day girl that you are. Just look at that fabulous dramatic liner paired with a shimmery lid and a pale pink pout! Day or evening, dressed up or casual, it works anytime you feel like wearing it.

Here's how to get this look:

eyes

1. Using your #22 highlighting brush and a pale matte beige eye shadow, highlight your lid and brow bone. When I say brow bone, I mean the area just under the arch of your brow.

2. Follow your matte shadow with a shimmer white, layering it on top of your matte shade, but only on your lid, not brow bone. I usually prefer the lid to be a bit more highlighted than the brow bone. This shimmer over the matte will give you a more dramatic highlight.

3. With this look, you want your midtone to be very precise, so as not to darken your lid, but still define the shape. Because this look has such an intense lip, you want your lid to be soft and shimmery. Using your #13 detail shadow brush, apply your matte taupe midtone eye shadow in your crease. Starting from the outside corner of your crease, glide your brush across to the inside corner. Create a distinct line all along your crease.

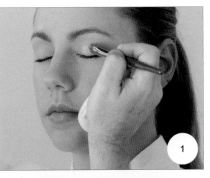

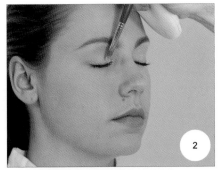

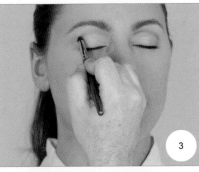

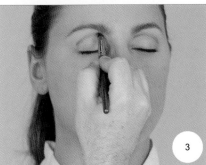

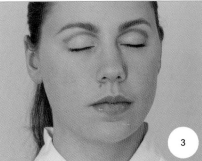

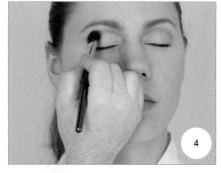

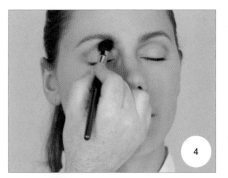

4. Use your #28 blending brush (the one that is always clean and ready to use) and blend your midtone so that there are no hard edges. Then retrace the same area where you just applied your midtone so you don't blend it up and down and darken too much of your lid.

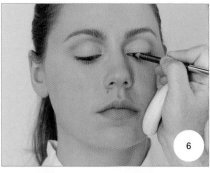

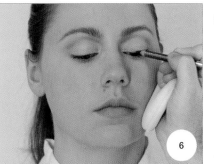

5. It's time to curl your eyelashes and apply the first layer of mascara to your top lashes. (See page 42 to review how to curl properly.)

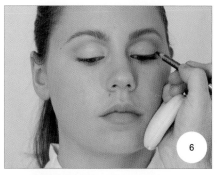

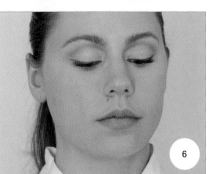

6. Now you want to create that perfect dramatic liner along your top lid. The trick for perfection is layering it in steps. Even pros prefer to layer. First, you begin to create a pattern with a black eyeliner pencil because it is easier to remove and start over if you make a mistake. Starting at the inside corner of your top lash line, slowly move across the lash line. Make sure your line is its narrowest at the inside corner, gradually getting thicker as you reach the outside corner. As you reach the outside corner, you can give it a little "kick" upward.

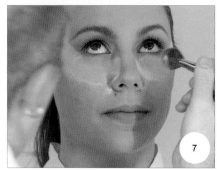

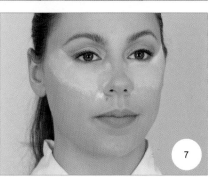

7. Because you are about to use a very dark color, using your #76 powder brush, apply a bit of powder under the eye to catch it. When you are finished, you can just brush the powder and any dripped shadow away and still have flawless skin.

"this timeless look lets you put on the glam anytime, anywhere."

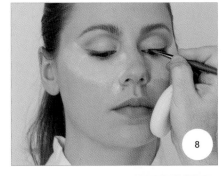
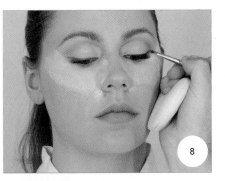

8. Your pencil line probably won't be perfect, but it doesn't have to be because now you're going to trace over it with black eye shadow and your #41 eyeliner brush to perfect your pattern.

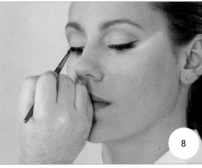
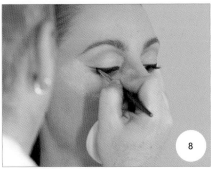

9. I know your line looks perfect now, but it is not dramatic enough. So now it's time to go over your pattern with your liquid or gel eyeliner. Because you've already created the pattern, if your liquid is not perfect, it won't show. Using your #42 eyeliner brush, apply your liquid or gel, starting from the inner corner and working toward the outer corner. Follow your pattern.

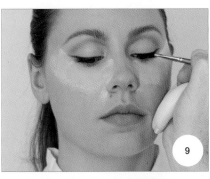
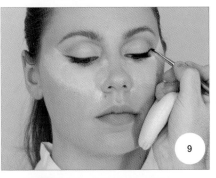

10. With your #76 detail powder brush, sweep away the powder you laid under your eyes. Any shadow that you dropped during application will go with it.

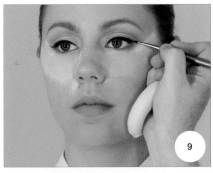
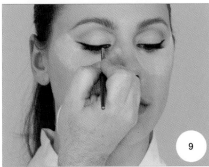

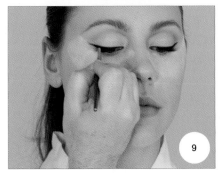
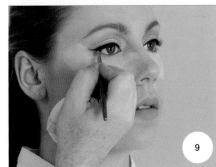

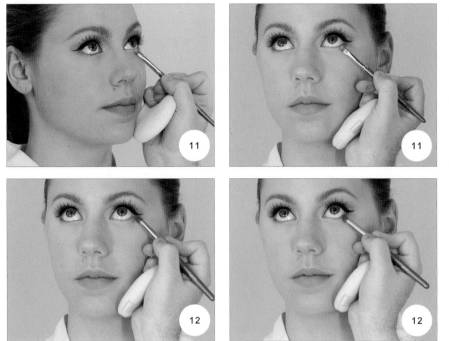

11. Now, with your #14 detail highlighting brush, apply your shimmery white eye shadow all along your lower lash line. Start from the inside corner and work toward the outside corner.

12. Using your #13 detail shadow brush, apply your midtone eye shadow just to the very outside corner along your lower lash line.

13. Finally, it's time for another layer of mascara, but only to your top lashes. You don't want mascara on your bottom lashes with this look. (See page 44 to review how to layer your mascara properly.)

cheeks

1. With this look, you don't want your cheek color to be noticeable, but you still want subtle definition. You can achieve this with a very, very light application of bronzer. Using your #73 bronzer/blush brush, apply your matte bronzer. Beginning at the back of your cheekbone, sweep it forward toward the apple of your cheek. Then take the brush back toward your ear. This lays your color in place.

2. Now take your brush and use it in the opposite direction (up and down) to blend. Be sure to blend well, or it won't look natural.

3. Don't forget to add a little at the temples to help shape your face. Sweep the bronzing powder up around the temples and eye sockets. Feel free to blend some bronzer along your jawbone because this also helps create shape and defines your face.

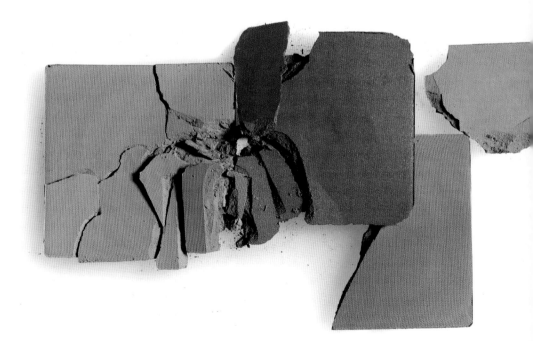

lips

1. With this look, you want your lips to be soft, but still well defined. Start by concealing your lip and lip line. This gives you the perfect pale canvas for your subtle lip look.

2. Using a barely-there pinky nude lip pencil, line your lips. Begin with a V in the "cupid's bow," or center curve, of the lips. Bring the liner up and around the curves of your bow.

3. Next, starting at the outer corners, move toward the center with your pencil.

4. On the lower lip, first accentuate the lower curve of the lip. Then, beginning from the outer corners, move toward the center. Remember to use your entire lip: Take the color to the almost invisible line just at the edge of the colored part of your lips.

5. Make sure you fill in at least halfway toward the center of your lip. This will help your lip liner look more natural and your lip color last longer.

6. Now blend with your #80 lip brush to make it look more natural.

7. Using your lip brush (because it gives you better application and helps color last longer), fill in your entire lip with the perfect pale pink lipstick. Make sure you blend really well over your lip liner.

8. End with a quick sweep of the perfect sheer pink lip gloss to make your lips shiny, fuller looking, and sexy. Be sure to apply your gloss with your #80 lip brush because if you apply gloss with a brush, it will appear shinier.

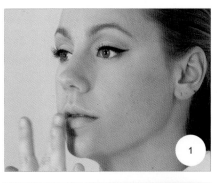

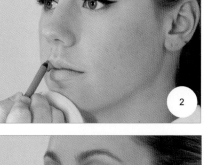

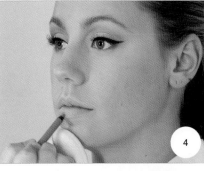

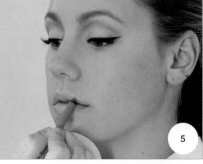

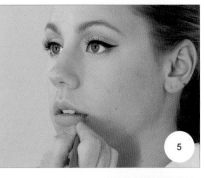

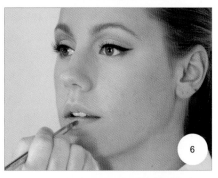

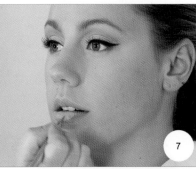

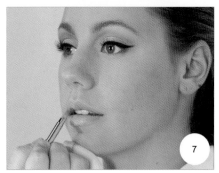

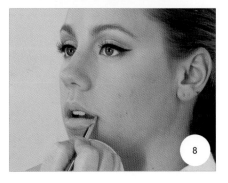

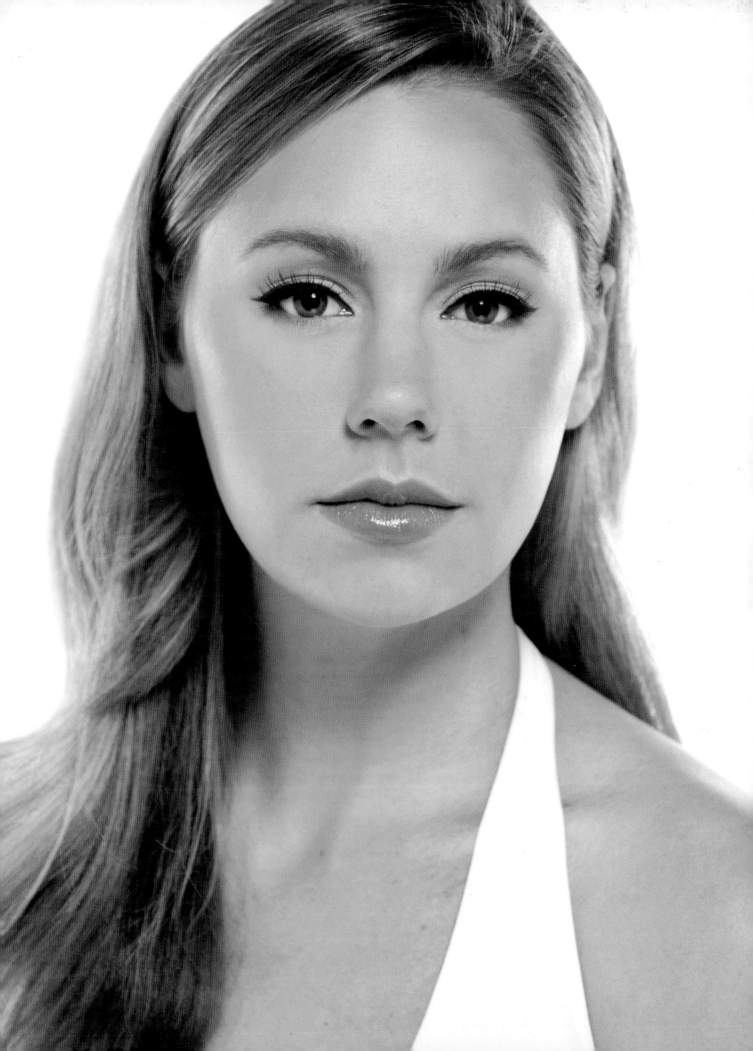

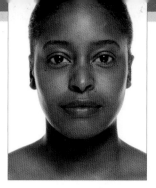

golden girl

Here's another clean, gorgeous, glowing look! Pay attention to the tricks for making your highlight shimmer pop. The whole look is about glow and lashes. I carefully chose shades that give the eyes and face shape without overpowering the look so that when you are finished, it's about flawless glowing skin, bright shimmery eyes, and the perfect, barely-there lip. Keep in mind that some shades of color are universal and some are specific to bronze/ebony skin tone. This is so important when choosing the perfect "there but invisible" shades.

Here's how to get this look:

eyes

1. Using your #22 highlighting brush, apply a crème-to-powder shimmery peachy gold eye shadow, but only to your lid (from your lash line to your crease). You are going to layer crème and powder to make your lid more dramatic.

2. With the same brush, apply a shimmery peachy gold eye shadow directly on top of the crème you applied to your lid and then brush it onto your brow bone.

3. Using your #11 midtone brush and a matte midtone eye shadow, start from the outside corner of your crease and glide your brush across to the inside corner. Use a matte ginger shadow (a shade just a bit darker than your skin tone) so that you get soft definition.

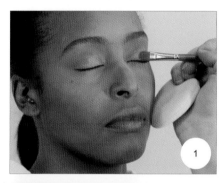

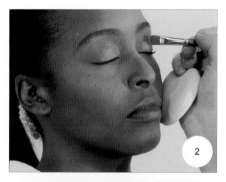

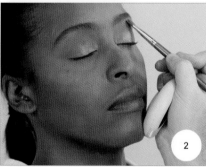

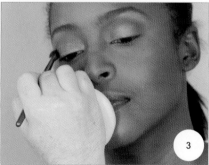

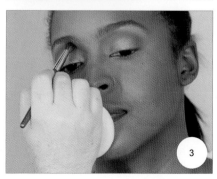

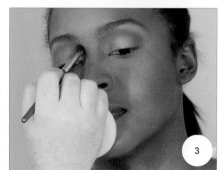

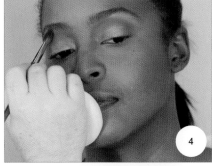

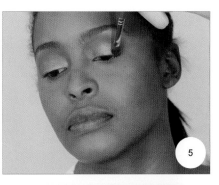

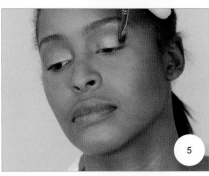

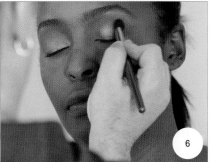

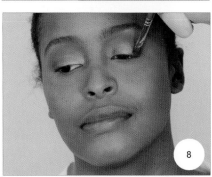

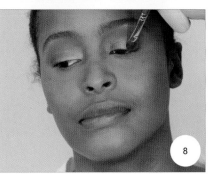

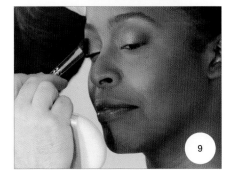

4. Use your #28 blending brush (the one that is always clean and ready to blend with) and blend your midtone so that there are no hard edges.

5. Grab your #30 contour brush and some of your midtone eye shadow and define the outer third of your eyelid.

6. Follow with your #28 brush to blend. This just starts your lid definition.

7. It's time to curl your eyelashes and apply the first layer of mascara to your top lashes. (See page 42 to review how to curl properly.)

8. With your #30 contour brush, apply a dark shimmery brown eye shadow on the outer third of your eyelid and up into the crease. You are layering it over your midtone so it starts to create a blend.

9. Follow again with your clean #28 brush to blend your contour color.

"this whole look is about glow and lashes."

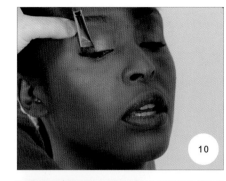
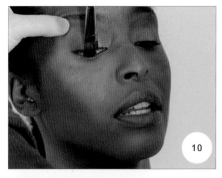

10. With your #18 eyeliner brush, grab some black eye shadow and lay it all along your top lash line for definition. As you apply it, pull up slightly with your brush to blend the line.

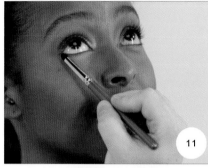
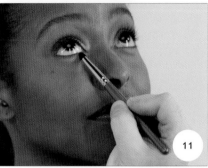

11. Now grab your #13 detail eye shadow brush and apply your midtone eye shadow all along your lower lash line. Once again, start your application from the outside corner, sweeping it across to the inside corner.

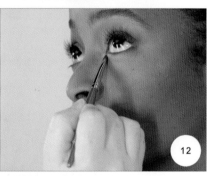
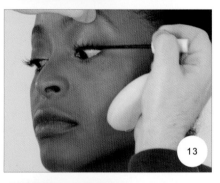

12. Using your #14 detail highlighting brush, highlight the inside corner of the lower lash line. Because there is so little color to this look, this brightens the eye and opens it up to give a wide-eyed effect.

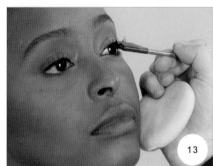
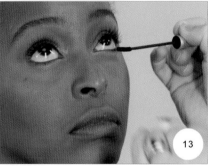

13. Now it's time for another layer of mascara on your top lashes and a layer on your lower lashes. After you finish the rest of your makeup, add yet another layer to your top lashes. Remember, with this look, lush lashes are very important, so you want to really layer your mascara on your top lashes. (See page 44 to review how to layer your mascara properly.)

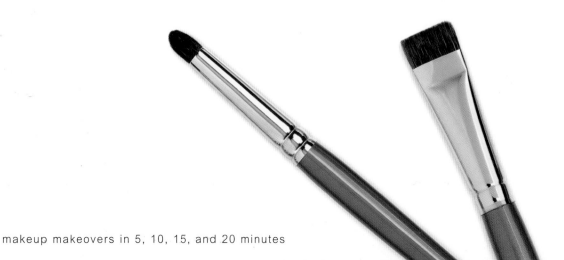

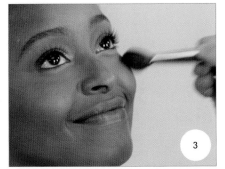

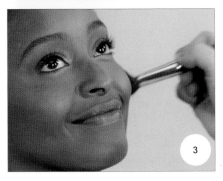

cheeks

1. An important part of this glowing, natural look is a perfectly flushed cheek. You are going to achieve this by layering your blush. Start with a great crème-to-powder blush. Using your #64 crème blush brush, apply a bright apricot blush to the apple of the cheek, starting at the front of the apple and working toward the back.

2. Follow with a light dusting of loose or pressed powder.

3. Now to reinforce that flush, smile and apply your powder blush (the perfect bright sheer apricot color) with your #74 bronzer/blush brush on the apple of your cheek, starting at the front of the apple and working toward the back.

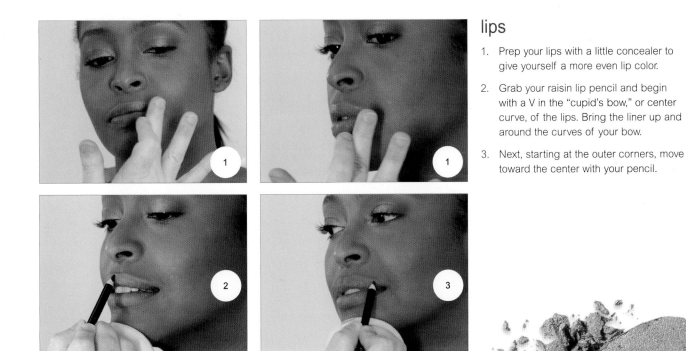

lips

1. Prep your lips with a little concealer to give yourself a more even lip color.

2. Grab your raisin lip pencil and begin with a V in the "cupid's bow," or center curve, of the lips. Bring the liner up and around the curves of your bow.

3. Next, starting at the outer corners, move toward the center with your pencil.

4. On the lower lip, first accentuate the lower curve of the lip. Then begin from the outer corners and move toward the center. Remember to use your entire lip: Take the color to the almost invisible line just at the edge of the colored part of your lips.

5. Make sure you fill in at least halfway toward the center of your lip. This will help your lip liner look more natural and your lip color last longer.

6. Now blend with your #80 lip brush to make it look more natural.

7. Using your lip brush (because it gives you better application and helps the color last longer), fill in your entire lip with the hazelnut lipstick. Make sure you blend really well over your lip liner.

8. Using your lip brush, end with a quick sweep of a sandy beige lip gloss to make your lips shiny and sexy.

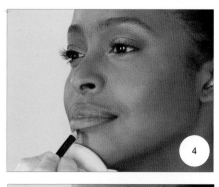

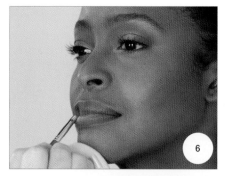

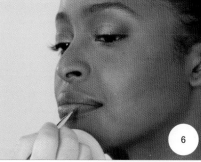

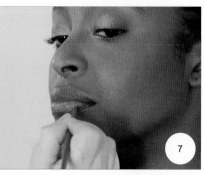

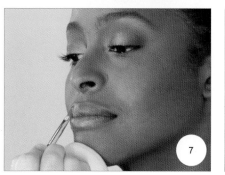

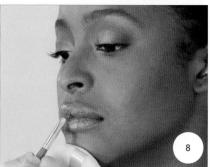

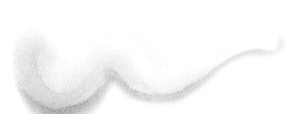

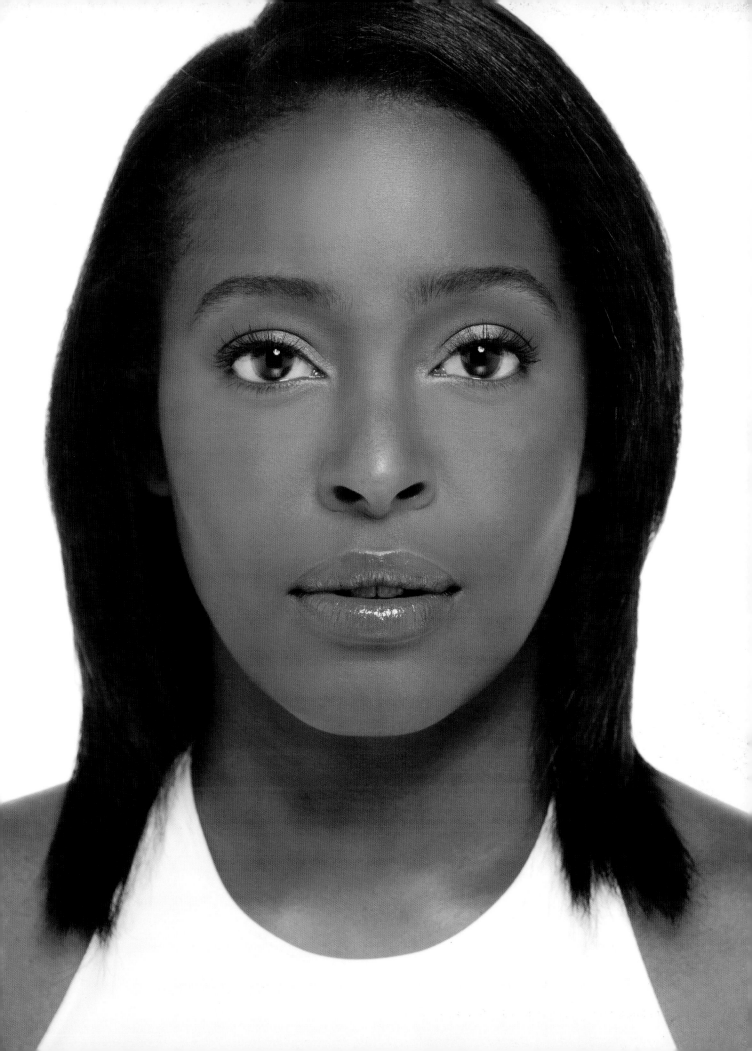

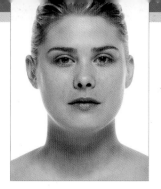

life is a mystery

This look is inspired by Faye Dunaway from the movie *Bonnie and Clyde.* It's timeless, wearable, beautiful, and mysterious. The perfect definition of your eyelid and top lash line creates subtle drama. Mixing the dramatic top lid with the absence and erasing of your bottom lash line creates (I think) a bit of mystery. Even though your eyes are subtle, because your cheeks have a soft flush and your lips are the perfect nude, the eyes are still the focus. We all know that mystery is created in the eyes and nowhere else. Go ahead and be mysterious!

Here's how to get this look:

eyes

1. Using your #22 highlighting brush, apply a matte beige eye shadow to your brow bone. When I say brow bone, I mean the area just under the arch of your brow.

2. With a #27 eye shadow brush (because you'll be applying your color to a large area), apply a dark matte taupe midtone eye shadow. Starting at the base of your upper lash line, bring the color up and over your entire lid, all the way up to just under your brow bone. By starting along your lash line and working your way upward, you will get the highest concentration of color where you laid your brush first, making your color deeper at the lash line.

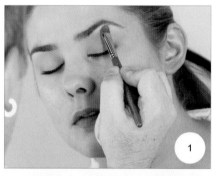

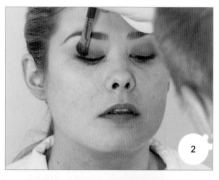

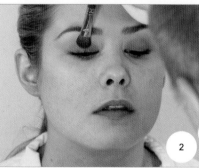

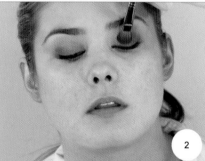

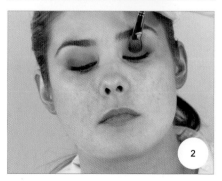

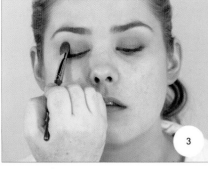

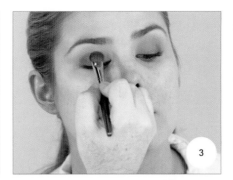

3. Now with the same brush, apply more midtone in a half-moon shape all along your crease.

4. Use your #28 blending brush (the one that is always clean and ready to blend with) and blend your midtone so that there are no hard edges.

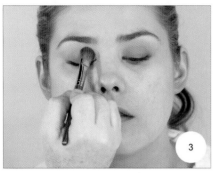

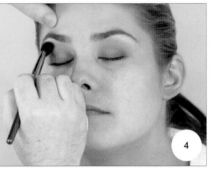

5. It's time to curl your eyelashes and apply the first layer of mascara to your top lashes. (See page 42 to review how to curl properly.)

6. Using a black eyeliner pencil, line all along your top lash line. You can go back over your line with your #41 detail eyeliner brush to smooth the line and make it look perfect.

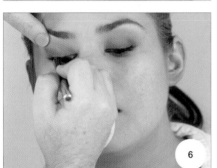

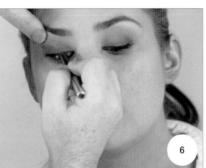

"go ahead and be mysterious!"

7. With a concealer pencil, line your water-line. (Remember, the waterline is the inner rim above the lower lash line.) I don't do this often, but for this look it helps create that "not-there" definition along your lower lash line.

8. With your #14 detail highlighting brush, apply a shimmery white eye shadow all along your lower lash line from the inside corner to the outside corner, right along the lash line.

9. Using your #13 detail shadow brush, apply your midtone just to the very out-side corner along your lower lash line.

10. Now it's time for another layer of mas-cara on your top lashes. After you finish the rest of your makeup, add yet another layer to your top lashes. Remember, with this look, lush lashes are very important, so you want to really layer your mascara on your top lashes. (See page 44 to review how to layer your mascara properly.)

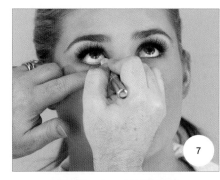

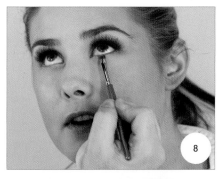

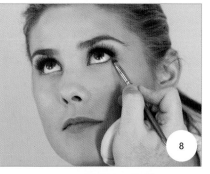

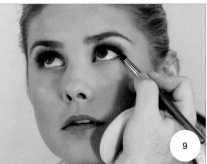

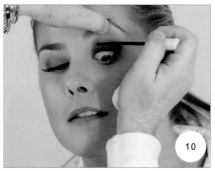

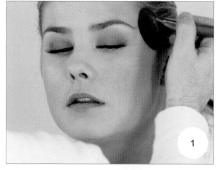

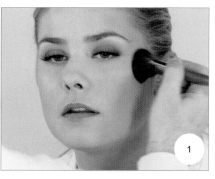

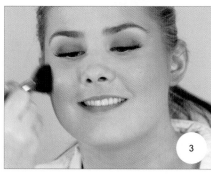

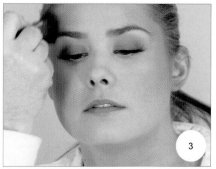

cheeks

1. Using your #73 bronzer/blush brush, apply your matte bronzer, beginning at the back of your cheekbone. Sweep it forward toward the apple of your cheek and then take the brush back toward your ear. This lays your color in place.

2. Now take your brush and use it in the opposite direction (up and down) to blend. Be sure to blend well, or it won't look natural.

3. Don't forget to add a little at the temples to help shape your face. Sweep the bronzing powder up around the temples and eye sockets. This always gives the face more color and gives you a glow.

4. Feel free to blend some bronzer along your jawbone. This also helps create that glow and defines your face.

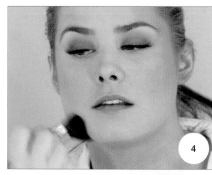

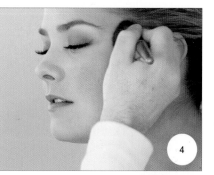

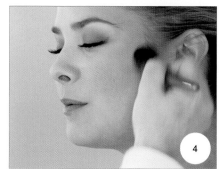

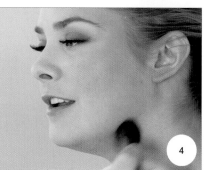

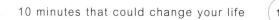

lips

1. For this look, you want your lips to be soft, but still well defined. Start by concealing your lip and lip line. This gives you the perfect pale canvas for your subtle lip look.

2. Using a barely-there nude lip pencil, line your lips. Begin with a V in the "cupid's bow," or center curve, of the lips. Bring the liner up and around the curves of your bow.

3. Next, starting at the outer corners, move toward the center with your pencil.

4. On the lower lip, first accentuate the lower curve of the lip. Then, beginning from the outer corners, move toward the center. Remember to use your entire lip: Take the color to the almost invisible line just at the edge of the colored part of your lips.

5. Make sure you fill in at least halfway toward the center of your lip. This will help your lip liner look more natural and your lip color last longer.

6. Now blend with your #80 lip brush to make it look more natural.

7. Using your lip brush (because it gives you better application and helps color last longer), fill in your entire lip with a soft pink nude lipstick. Make sure you blend really well over your lip liner.

8. End with a quick sweep of the perfect sheer nude lip gloss to make your lips shiny, fuller looking, and sexy. Be sure to apply your gloss with your #80 lip brush because if you apply gloss with a brush, it will look shinier.

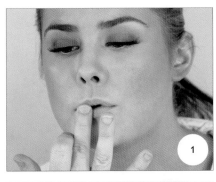

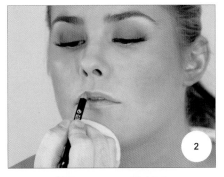

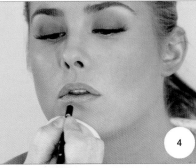

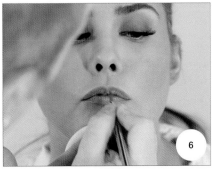

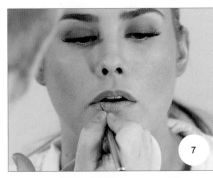

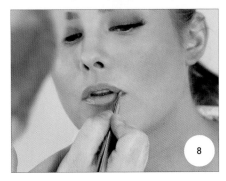

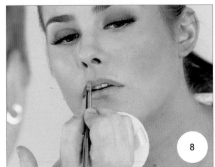

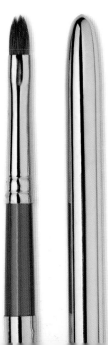

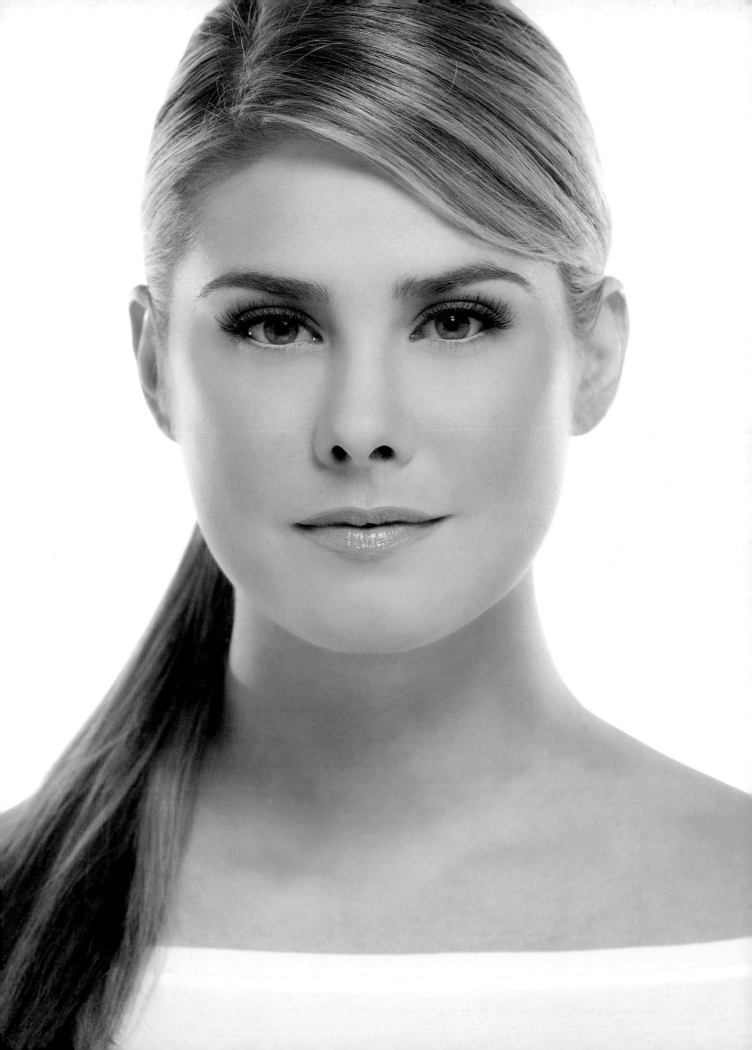

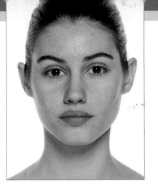

the bold and the beautiful

Did someone say "the perfect pout"?! Shimmery Marilyn Monroe eyes glamorize a modern-day bold lip. I always love mixing retro with a modern twist. With this look, you are taking the classic glamorous 1950s eye shadow application, adding shimmer to it, and mixing it with a dark, edgy lip. The challenge with this look is getting the lips just right. The darker you make your lips, the harder it is to apply the lip treatment properly, so take your time. But don't worry! With my lip-lasting tricks, your dark, fabulous lip color will stay put.

Here's how to get this look:

eyes

1. Using your #22 highlighting brush, apply a crème-to-powder shimmery beige eye shadow, but only to your lid (from the lash line to the crease). You are going to layer crème and powder to make your lid more dramatic.

2. With the same brush, apply a shimmery champagne powder eye shadow directly on top of the crème you applied to your lid. Now apply it to your brow bone.

3. With this look, you want your midtone very precise, so as to not darken your lid, yet define the shape. Because this look has such an intense lip, you want your lid soft and shimmery. Using your #13 detail eye shadow brush, apply your matte taupe midtone eye shadow in your crease: Starting from the outside corner of your crease, glide your brush across to the inside corner. Create a distinct line all along your crease.

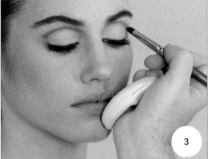

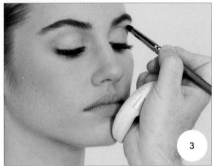

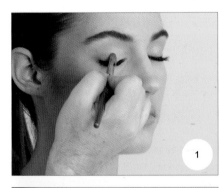

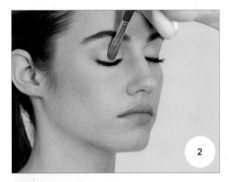

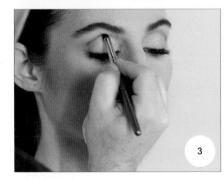

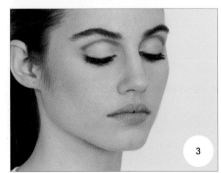

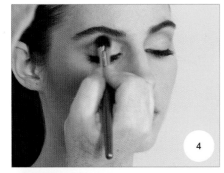

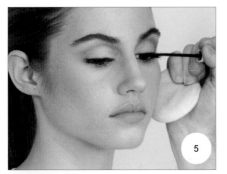

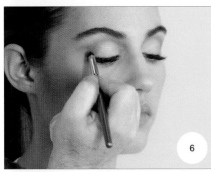

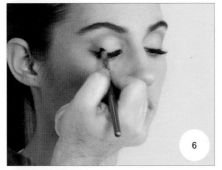

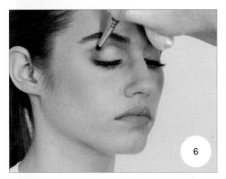

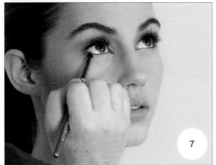

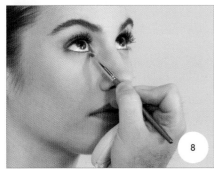

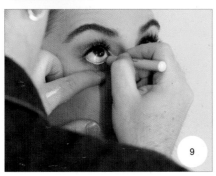

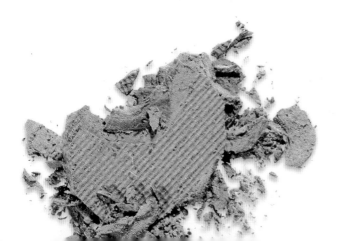

4. Use your #28 blending brush (the one that is always clean and ready to blend with) to blend your midtone so that there are no hard edges. Then retrace the same area that you applied your midtone to in the previous step. Don't blend it up and down or you'll darken too much of your lid.

5. It's time to curl your eyelashes and apply the first layer of mascara to your top lashes. (See page 42 to review how to curl properly.)

6. Now it's time for a little extra definition. Using your #13 detail shadow brush, add some of your midtone eye shadow, but just to the very outermost corner of your eyelid.

7. Using the same brush, apply your midtone all along your lower lash line. Start from the outside corner and work in toward the inside corner.

8. Next, using your #14 detail highlighting brush, highlight the inside corner of the lower lash line.

9. With a concealer pencil, line your waterline. (Remember, the waterline is the inner rim above the lower lash line.) I don't do this often, but for this look it helps create that "wide-eyed" look, which is a big part of this eye effect.

10. Now it's time for another layer of mascara on your top lashes and a layer on your lower lashes. After you finish the rest of your makeup, add yet another layer to the top lashes. Remember, with this look, lush lashes are very important, so you want to really layer your mascara on your top lashes. (See page 44 to review how to layer your mascara properly.)

cheeks

Because the lips are the focus of this look, I've left Alex's cheeks totally natural.

lips

1. This lip look is very dramatic, and to help it look its most perfect, you need to prep your lips first. Because this look is all about the lips, you really want them to look sumptuous and smooth, so before you start your color application, moisturize them with lip balm. This will help the color go on smoothly and evenly. After the balm has had a bit of time to soak in, blot off the excess with a tissue so that it won't shorten the staying power of your lipstick.

2. Next, using concealer, conceal your lip and along your lip line.

3. Now powder your lips. This gives you the perfect canvas to apply your dramatic lip so that the edge of the lip is very crisp.

4. Grab your burgundy lip pencil and begin with a V in the "cupid's bow," or center curve, of the lips. Bring the liner up and around the curves of your bow.

5. Next, starting at the outer corners, move toward the center with your pencil.

6. On the lower lip, first accentuate the lower curve of the lip. Then, beginning from the outer corners, move toward the center. Remember to use your entire lip: Take the color to the almost invisible line just at the edge of the colored part of your lips.

7. Now fill in your entire lip with your lip pencil. This will help your lip color last and stay in place because lip liner is a drier texture than lipstick.

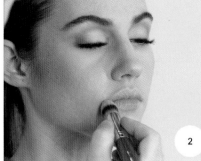

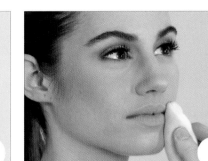

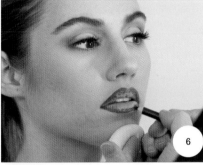

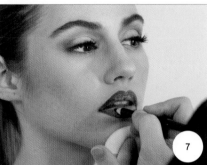

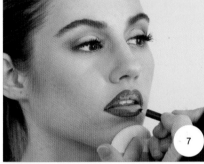

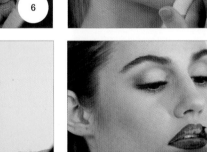

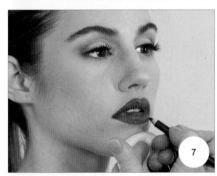

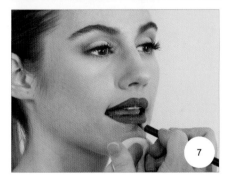

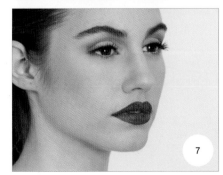

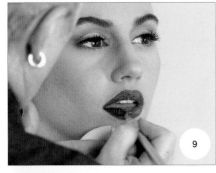 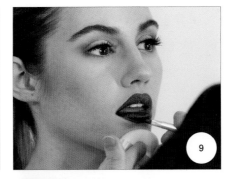

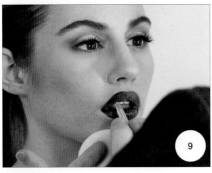 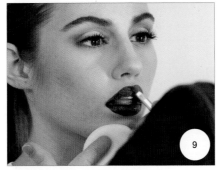

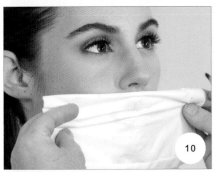 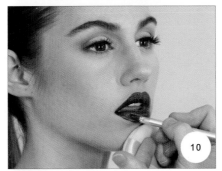

8. With your #80 lip brush, blend your lip liner so that it is even and smooth.

9. Next, using your lip brush, apply your black orchid lipstick to your entire lip, making sure you blend really well over your lip liner.

10. Now take a tissue and blot your lips. This will remove the moisture from the lipstick, but leave you with a layer of pigment. Then apply another layer of lipstick. Applying these three layers (one of liner and two of lipstick) will help your color be true and intense, as well as last much longer.

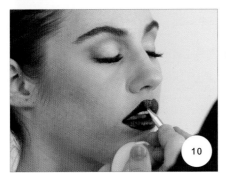 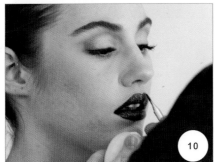

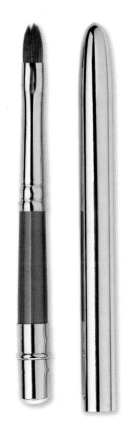

11. Finish with a thin layer of a sheer blackberry lip gloss applied with your lip brush. The gloss will add shine and dimension to your lips.

12. Never worry about not getting a perfect line along your lip when applying a dark or intense color. Grab your #50 concealer brush and go right along your lip line to perfect the edge.

Thrilled with all the looks you can get in just 10 minutes of makeup application? What do you think can happen if you find yourself with a little more time . . . say, 15 minutes? Turn the page and find out. Wow!

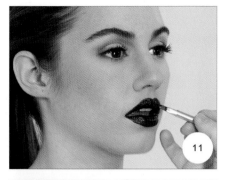

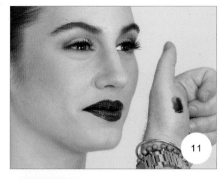

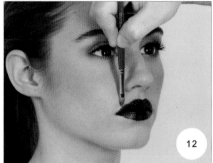

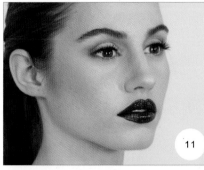

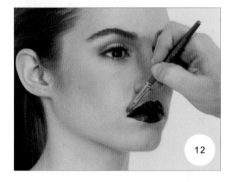

"did someone say 'the perfect pout'?!"

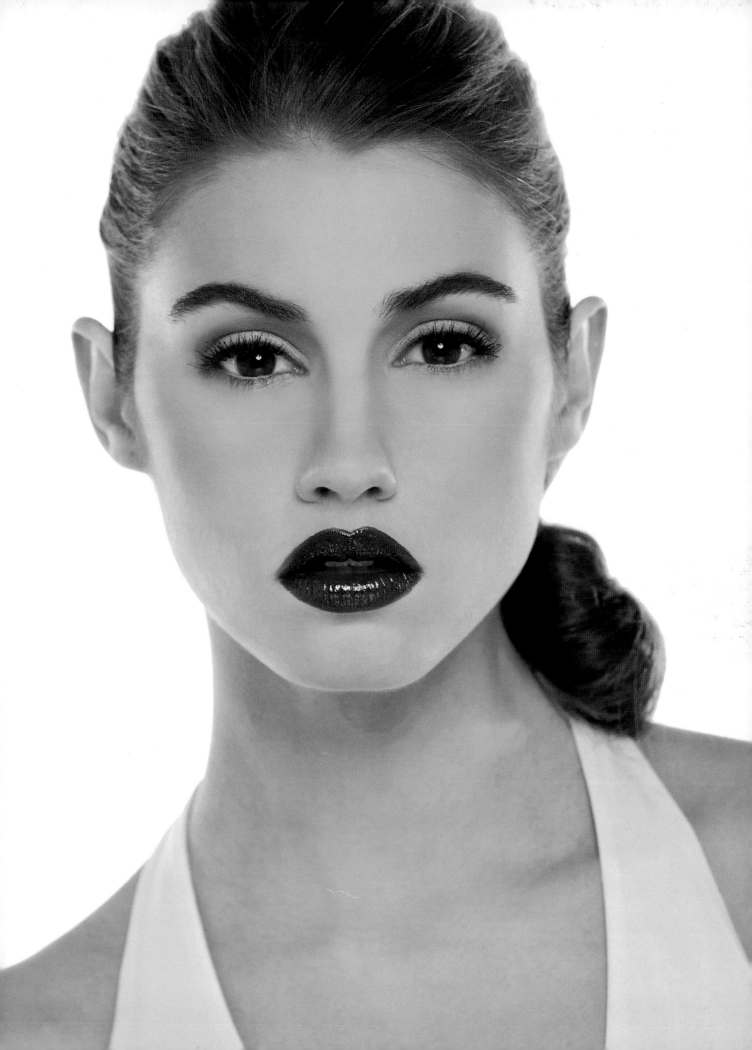

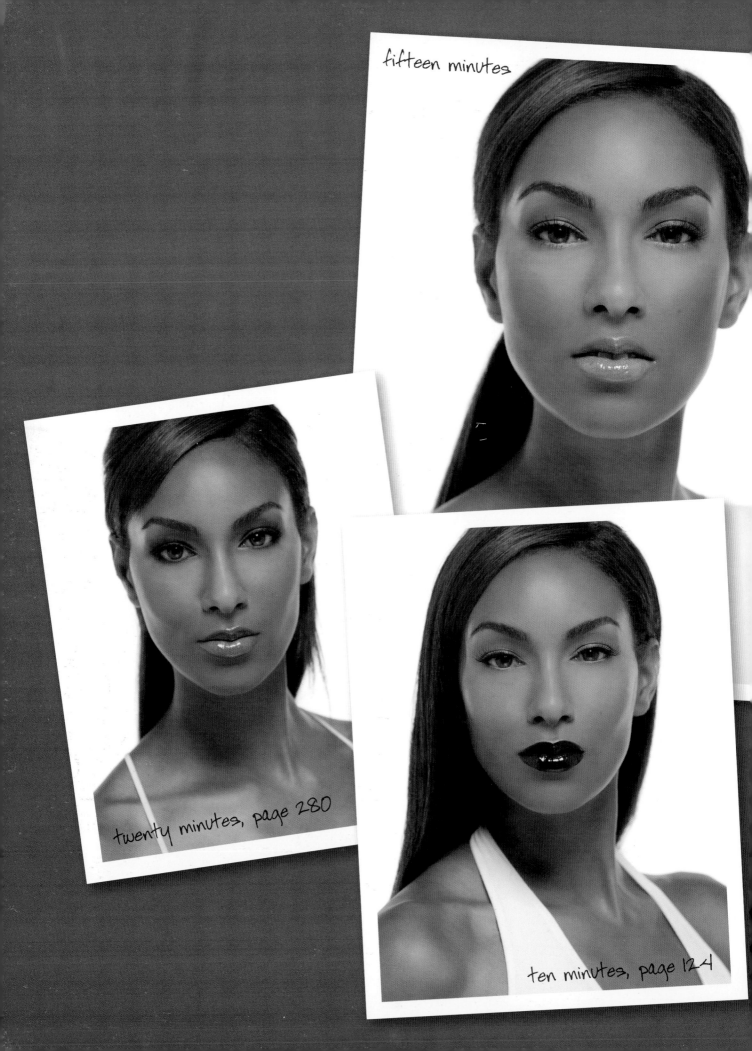

fifteen minutes

twenty minutes, page 280

fifteen minutes

ten minutes, page 124

15 minutes make all the difference

If you've been looking through the 5- and 10-minute chapters, by now you may be wondering what on earth another 5 minutes could possibly add. Why, *everything*, girl! With 15 minutes, you have time for some beautiful basics, plus that essential extra few minutes to add some super-special effects. If you need to look amazing for a meeting or a date, or want to impress your friends on girls' night out, rock that high school or college reunion or just have a little extra time to do something beautiful for yourself, check out the looks in this chapter. You're going to love them!

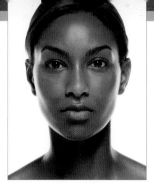

color my world

I love to mix colors. It is super-trendy to use a different color on your top lid from the one you use on your lower lid. Just make sure when doing this that the darker of the two shades is on the top lid. Otherwise, it will drag your eyes down and make you look tired. I have paired complementary opposites so that both shades pop. If I had chosen just an average blue instead of a green-blue, the two shades would have blended together. But because they're opposites, you see the purple *and* the teal, which equals a whole lot of fun!

Here's how to get this look:

eyes

1. With your #22 highlighting brush, high-light your brow bone with a matte flesh-colored eye shadow. Remember, when I say brow bone, I mean the area just under the arch of your brow.

2. Even with bright colors, you still need to ground the color and add shape, so start your eye definition with neutrals. Using your #11 midtone brush and a matte midtone eye shadow and starting from the outside corner of your crease, glide your brush across to the inside corner. Use a matte ginger shadow (a shade just a bit darker than your skin tone) so that you get soft definition.

3. Use your #28 blending brush (the one that is always clean and ready to blend with) and blend your midtone so that there are no hard edges.

4. It's time to curl your eyelashes and apply the first layer of mascara to your top lashes. (See page 42 to review how to curl properly.)

5. Because you are about to use a very bright color, use your #76 powder brush to apply powder under the eye to catch any spills. Once finished, you can just brush the powder and any shadow drips away and still have flawless skin.

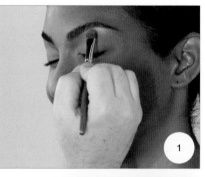

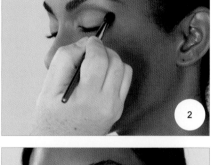

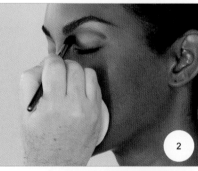

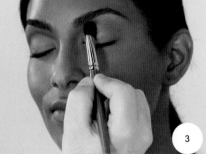

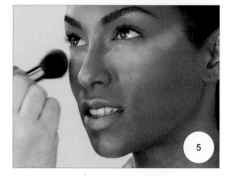

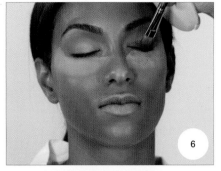

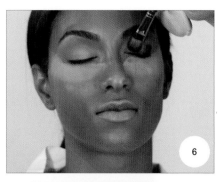

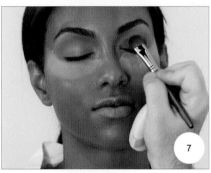

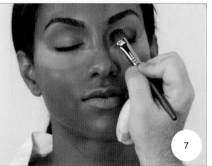

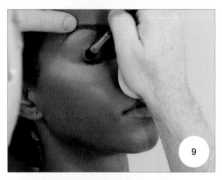

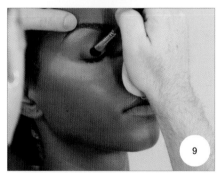

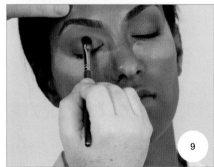

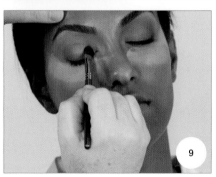

6. With a #27 eye shadow brush (because you will be applying your color to a large area), apply your fabulous shimmer purple eye shadow. Start at the base of your upper lash line and bring the color up and over your entire lid, all the way up to just under your crease.

7. Follow by using the same brush and adding more purple shadow in a half-moon shape right along the crease. When you apply this layer, pat it on so you get more coverage.

8. Now, using your #28 blending brush (the one that is always clean and ready to blend with), blend your color so that there are no hard edges.

9. It's time to add another layer of purple for more fun! Using your #30 contour brush, apply color to the outer third of your lid. Then, with the same brush, pat color in a half-moon shape into the crease.

10. Of course, grab your #28 blending brush and blend.

11. With your teal eyeliner pencil, line along your lower lash line from corner to corner. Keep it as close to the lash line as possible. Because it is a bright (not dark) color, there is no problem with the color going from corner to corner.

12. Next, with the same pencil, line the waterline along your lower lash line. (Remember, the waterline is the inner rim above the lower lash line.)

13. With your #76 detail powder brush, sweep away the powder you laid under your eye. With it will go any purple shadow dropped during application.

14. Grab your #13 detail highlighting brush and layer a bright teal shadow right on top of the eyeliner you just applied. It will intensify the color and blur the line.

15. Now it's time for another layer of mascara on your top lashes and a layer on your lower lashes. After you finish the rest of your makeup, add yet another layer to the top lashes. Remember, with this look, lush lashes are very important, so you want to really layer your mascara on your top lashes. (See page 44 to review how to layer your mascara properly.)

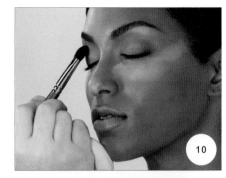

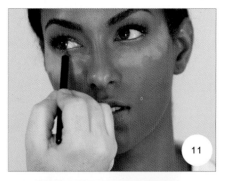

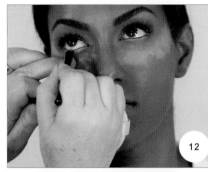

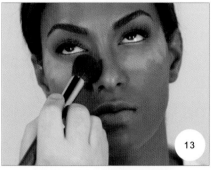

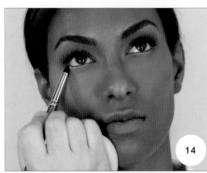

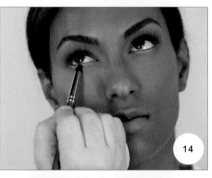

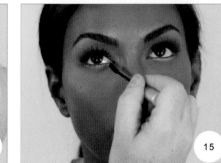

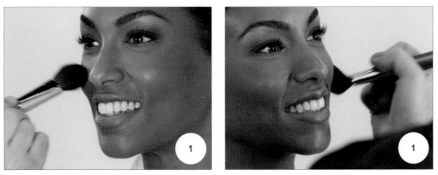

cheeks

1. Now it's time for a little color! Grab your #73 bronzer/blush brush and smile. Then apply your powder blush (the perfect bright apricot color) on the apple of your cheek, blending back toward your ear. This technique really gives your face that fresh flush that is so perfect.

"when you pair complementary opposite colors, both shades pop."

lips

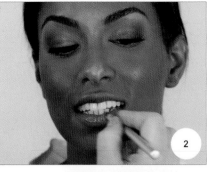

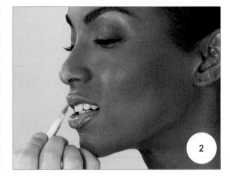

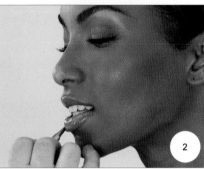

1. For this look, you want your lips to be soft and natural. To help create this effect, start by concealing your lip and lip line. This gives you the perfect pale canvas for your subtle lip look.

2. End with a quick sweep of the perfect sandy beige lip gloss to make your lips shiny, fuller looking, and sexy. Make sure you apply your gloss with your #80 lip brush because if you apply gloss with a brush, it will look shinier. Remember, with this much color on your eye, you want your lips to be barely there.

"with this much color on your eye, you want your lips to be barely there."

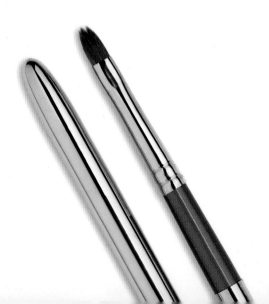

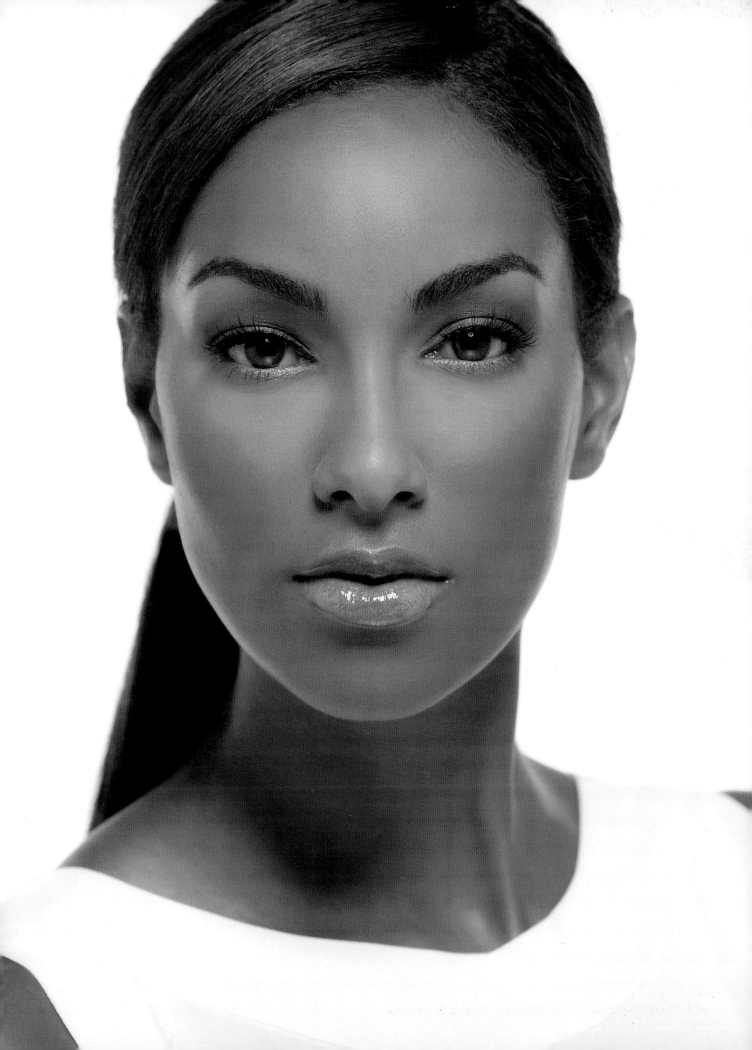

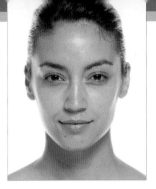

get your glow on

There is nothing more beautiful than a rich, warm glow to the skin and a bright shimmering eye. This look is all about playing matte against shimmer, layering crème and powder, but most of all, creating a natural glow. Anytime you use matte and shimmer opposite each other it intensifies the shine. Anytime you layer powder on crème, it intensifies the color. Playing with textures really creates an amazing result. Okay, girls, go get your glow on!

Here's how to get this look:

eyes

1. Using your #22 highlighting brush, apply a crème-to-powder shimmery beige eye shadow to your lid (just from the lash line to your crease). You are going to layer crème and powder to make your lid more dramatic.

2. With the same brush, apply a shimmery champagne powder eye shadow directly on top of the crème you just applied to your lid.

3. For this look, you want the highlight on your lid to be more dramatic than your brow bone. In order to achieve this, use your #22 brush and apply a matte flesh eye shadow on your brow bone. The fact that it is matte and a bit darker will make it look more subtle. To show you the difference, I have a shimmer on the middle finger and a matte on my index.

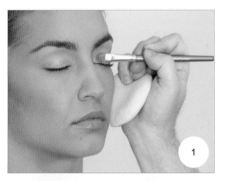

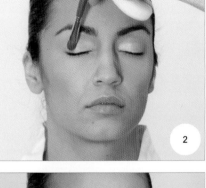

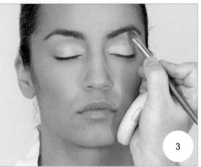

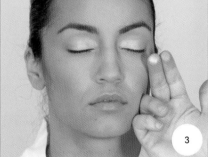

"playing matte against shimmer
creates a natural glow."

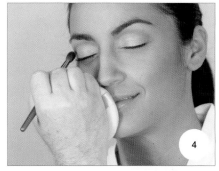

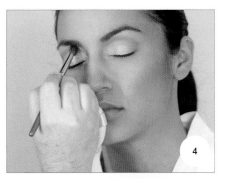

4. Using your #11 midtone brush and a matte midtone eye shadow and starting from the outside corner of your crease, glide your brush across to the inside corner. Use a soft matte caramel shadow (a shade just a bit darker than your skin tone) to get soft definition.

5. Use your #28 blending brush (the one that is always clean and ready to blend with) and blend your midtone so that there are no hard edges.

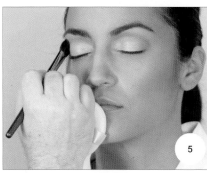

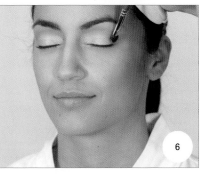

6. Grab your #30 contour brush and some midtone eye shadow and define the outer third of your eyelid. Follow with your #28 brush to blend.

7. To help prevent color from falling under your eye area and darkening the skin you want to look flawless, you can use shadow shields to catch the powder. A shadow shield is another great way to catch the powder fallout. It is a fabric shield that you simply peel and stick on, then remove once you have finished your shadow application.

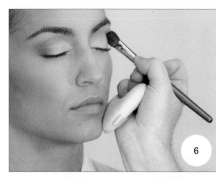

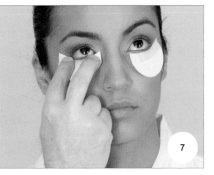

8. For lash line definition, use your #41 detail eyeliner brush and push black eye shadow into the base of your lash line.

9. With your #30 contour brush, apply a dark shimmery brown eye shadow on the outer third of your eyelid and up into the crease. You are layering it over your midtone so it starts to create a blend.

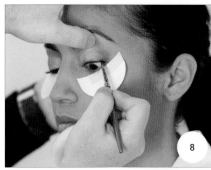

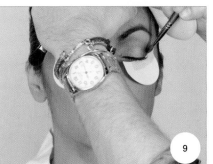

10. Follow again with your #28 brush to blend your contour color.

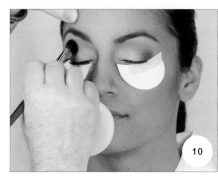

11. Now remove your shadow shield.

12. It's time to curl your eyelashes and apply the first layer of mascara to your top lashes. (See page 42 to review how to curl properly.)

13. Now grab your #13 detail eye shadow brush and apply your midtone eye shadow all along your lower lash line. Once again, start your application from the outside corner, sweeping it across to the inside corner.

14. With that same detail eye shadow brush, apply a layer of your contour color right over your midtone all along your bottom lash line. By layering on your midtone, then your contour on top of it, you are creating a gradation of color, making your lower lash line definition look more natural and blended.

15. Using your #14 detail highlighting brush, highlight the inside corner of the lower lash line. Because there is so little color to this look, this step really brightens the eye and opens it up to give you a wide-eyed effect.

16. Now it's time for another layer of mascara on your top lashes and a layer on your lower lashes. After you finish the rest of your makeup, add yet another layer to the top lashes. Remember, with this look, lush lashes are very important, so you want to really layer your mascara on your top lashes. (See page 44 to review how to layer your mascara properly.)

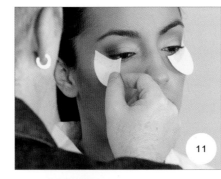

11

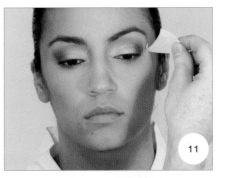

11

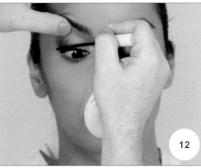

12

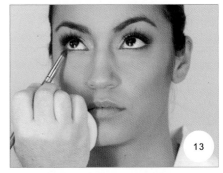

13

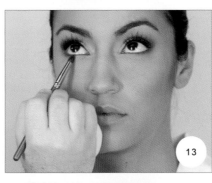

13

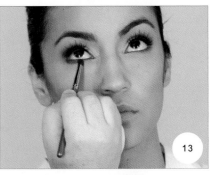

13

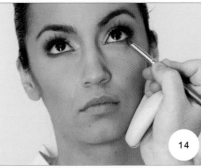

14

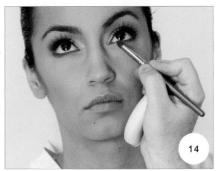

14

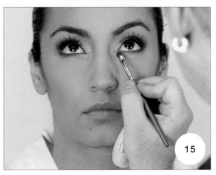

15

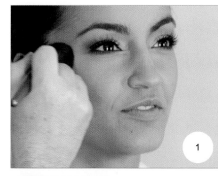

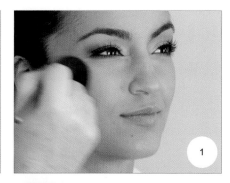

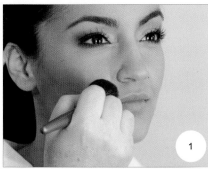

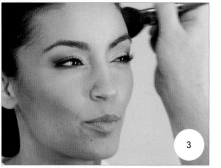

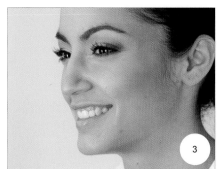

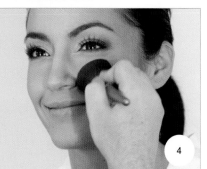

cheeks

1. Using your #73 bronzer/blush brush, apply your matte bronzer. Begin at the back of your cheekbone and sweep it forward toward the apple of your cheek. Then take the brush back toward your ear. This lays your color in place.

2. Now take your brush and use it in the opposite direction (up and down) to blend. Be sure to blend well, or it won't look natural.

3. Don't forget to add a little at the temples to help shape your face. Sweep the bronzing powder up around the temples and eye sockets. This always gives the face more color and gives you a glow.

4. Now for a little extra color, use your #73 bronzer/blush brush and smile. Then apply your powder blush (the perfect bright sheer apricot color) on the apple of your cheek, blending back toward the area that you bronzed. This technique really gives your face that fresh flush that is so perfect.

lips

1. An important part of this look is a pale nude lip. Start by concealing your lip and lip line. This gives you the perfect pale canvas for your subtle lip look.

2. Now, using a barely-there nude lip pencil, line your lips. Begin with a V in the "cupid's bow," or center curve, of the lips. Bring the liner up and around the curves of your bow.

3. Next, starting at the outer corners, move toward the center with your pencil.

4. On the lower lip, first accentuate the lower curve of the lip. Then begin from the outer corners, moving toward the center. Remember to use your entire lip: Take the color to the almost invisible line just at the edge of the colored part of your lips.

5. Make sure you fill in at least halfway toward the center of your lip. This will help your lip liner look more natural and your lip color last longer.

6. Now blend with your #80 lip brush to make it look more natural.

7. Using your lip brush (because it gives you better application and helps the color last longer), fill in your entire lip with the perfect nude lipstick. Make sure you blend really well over your lip liner.

8. End with a quick sweep of a pale nude lip gloss to make your lips shiny, fuller looking, and sexy. Apply your gloss with your #80 lip brush because if you apply gloss with a brush, it will look shinier.

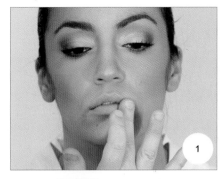

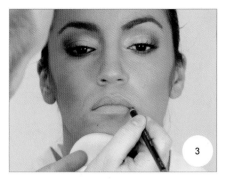

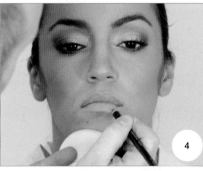

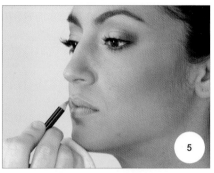

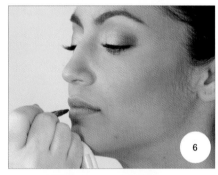

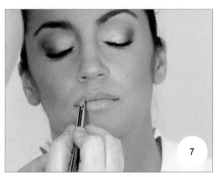

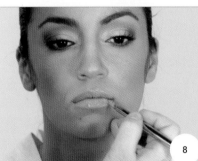

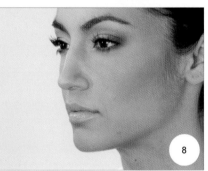

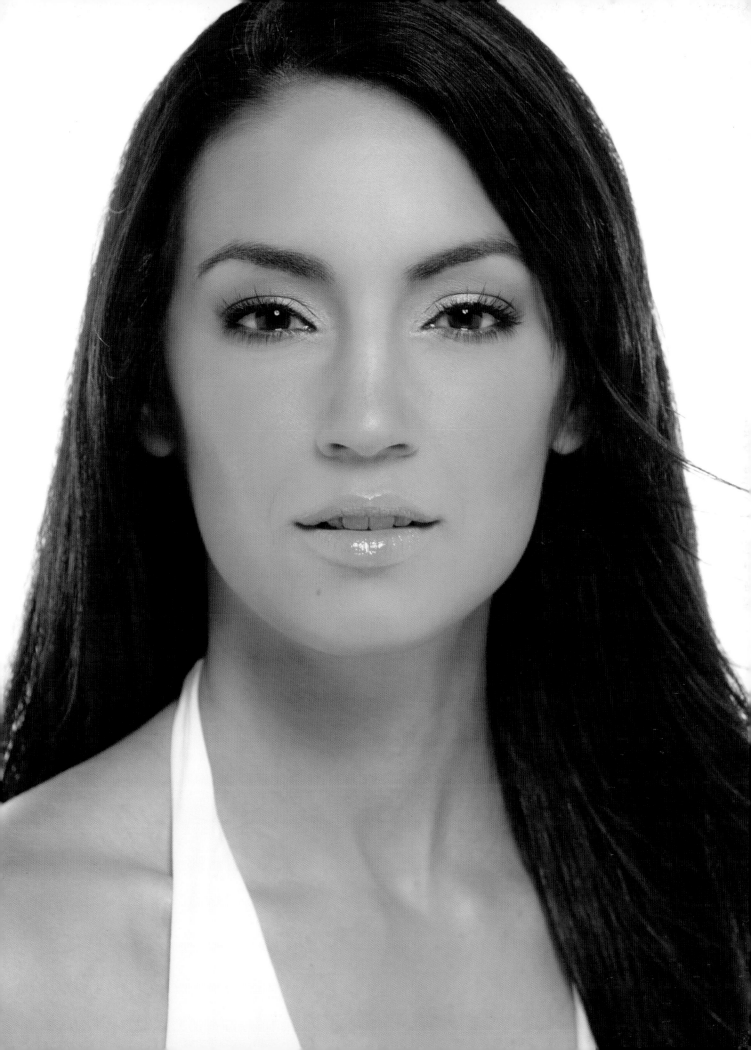

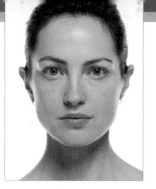

painted lady

For all you glamour girls, there are days you wake up and just want to have fun. A smoky eye is not always for nighttime. Here is a way to wear one during the day without looking like you need a street corner. Smoky is about the application technique, not the color, and by choosing wearable shades, you can smoke wherever and whenever you want.

Here's how to get this look:

eyes

1. Using your #22 highlighting brush and a shimmer beige crème-to-powder eye shadow, highlight just the very inside corner of your lid. You are creating a smoky purple eye, but you want it to be soft, so highlighting the inside corner will soften the look.

2. With the same brush, apply a shimmer champagne powder eye shadow directly over the crème on your lid and onto your brow bone.

3. With a #27 eye shadow brush (because you will be applying your color to a large area), apply a matte taupe midtone eye shadow, starting at the base of your upper lash line and bringing the color up and over your entire lid, all the way up to just under your brow bone.

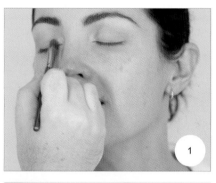

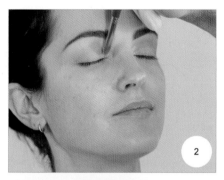

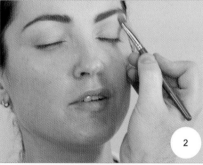

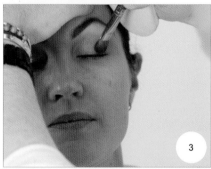

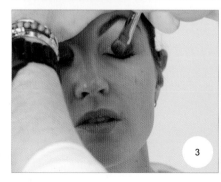

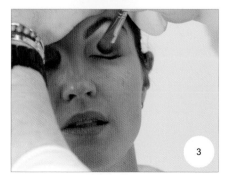

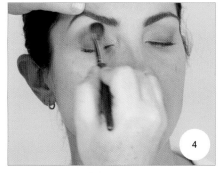

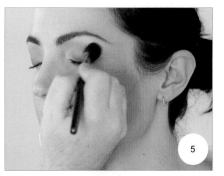

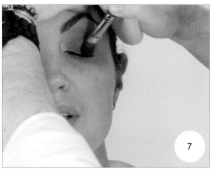

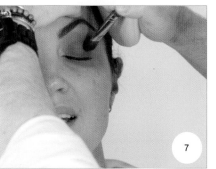

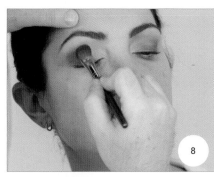

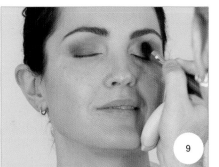

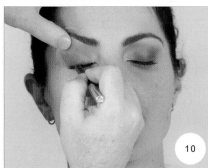

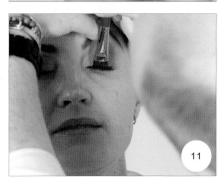

4. Follow by using the same brush and adding more midtone eye shadow in a half-moon shape all along the crease.

5. Now, using your #28 blending brush (the one that is always clean and ready to blend with), blend your midtone so that there are no hard edges.

6. It's time to curl your eyelashes and apply the first layer of mascara to your top lashes. (See page 42 to review how to curl properly.)

7. Okay, it's time for color! With your #27 eye shadow brush and using your purple contour eye shadow, start at the base of your upper lash line and bring the color up and over your entire lid, all the way up to your crease.

8. Using the same brush, add more contour shadow in a half-moon shape right along the crease.

9. Use your #28 blending brush to blend your color.

10. Now it's time for some darker lash line definition. With a black eyeliner, line right along your top lash line from corner to corner.

11. To smudge it out and intensify it at the same time, with your #18 eyeliner brush, apply black eye shadow directly on top of the liner, pulling up as you go along.

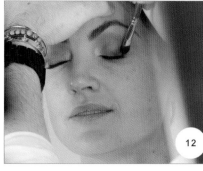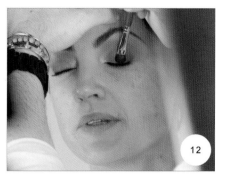

12. For a little more color, apply more purple shadow along your lash line from corner to corner with your #30 contour brush.

13. Follow again with your #28 brush to blend your contour color.

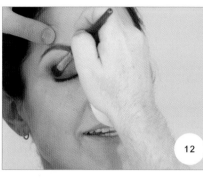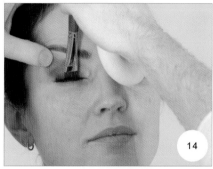

14. To intensify your purple, using your #18 eyeliner brush, apply more contour eye shadow all along your lash line. Once again, pull up with your brush as you move along, creating a blurred definition. By layering the shadow over your liner, you'll create a more intense color at your lash line. And that's our goal!

15. Now grab your #13 detail eye shadow brush and apply your midtone eye shadow all along your lower lash line. Once again, start your application from the outside corner, sweeping it across to the inside corner.

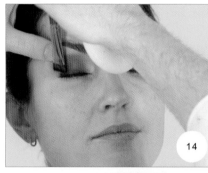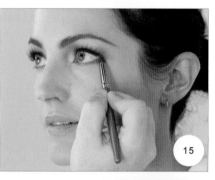

16. Using your #14 detail highlighting brush, highlight the inside corner of the lower lash line. Once again, this step helps soften your smoky eye.

17. With your #18 eyeliner brush, grab a little black eye shadow and push it into your lower lashes and along your lash line. This creates drama without making it look lined.

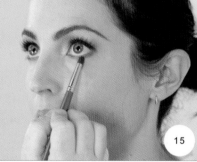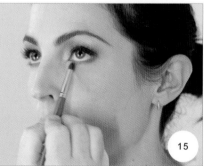

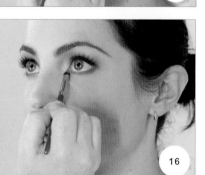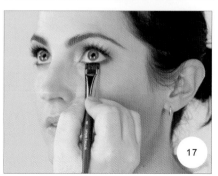

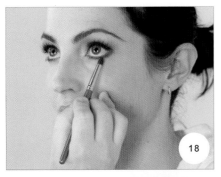

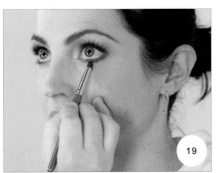

18. Now with your #13 detail eye shadow brush, layer your purple eye shadow along your lower lash line right over where you applied the midtone. This will soften that line even more while creating drama.

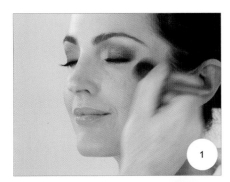

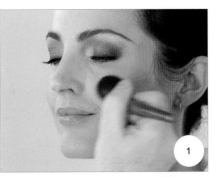

19. It's time for another layer of mascara on your top lashes and a layer on your lower lashes. After you finish the rest of your makeup, add yet another layer to your top lashes. Remember, with this look, lush lashes are very important, so you want to really layer your mascara on your top lashes. (See page 44 to review how to layer your mascara properly.)

cheeks

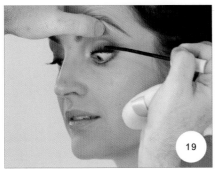

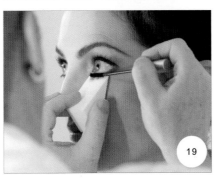

1. Using your #73 bronzer/blush brush, apply your matte bronzer, beginning at the back of your cheekbone. Sweep it forward toward the apple of your cheek and then take the brush back toward your ear. This lays your color in place.

2. Now take your brush and use it in the opposite direction (up and down) to blend. Be sure to blend well, or it won't look natural.

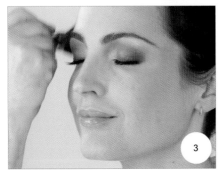

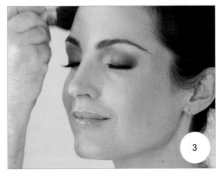

3. Don't forget to add a little at the temples to help shape your face. Sweep the bronzing powder up around the temples and eye sockets. This always gives the face more color and gives you a glow.

4. Feel free to blend some bronzer along your jawbone. This also helps create that glow and defines your face.

We'll add a little extra color to your cheeks at the end of the look.

lips

1. End with nothing more than a quick sweep of the perfect sheer peach lip gloss for just a touch of color (you don't need much with a purple smoky eye!) and to make your lips shiny, fuller looking, and sexy. Make sure you apply your gloss with your #80 lip brush because if you apply gloss with a brush, it will appear shinier.

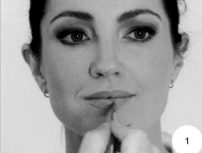

cheeks

Here are the finishing touches for your cheeks.

5. Now for a little extra color, grab your #73 bronzer/blush brush and smile. Then apply your powder blush (the perfect bright sheer peach color) on the apple of your cheek, blending back toward the area that you bronzed. This technique really gives your face that fresh flush that is so perfect.

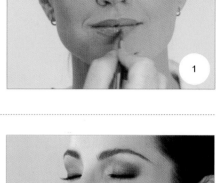

"by choosing wearable shades, you can smoke wherever and whenever you want."

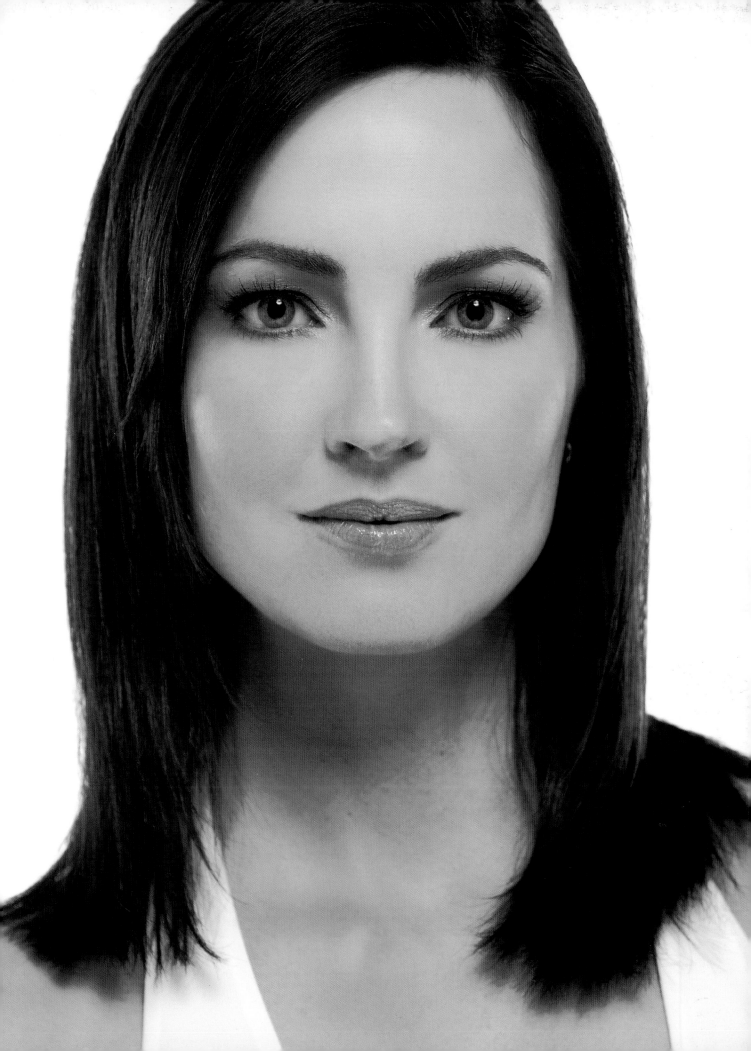

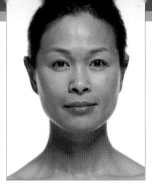

hello, gorgeous

Who needs bright colors when neutral browns, taupes, and coppers can make you look this amazing? At every age, less can always be more. I can't stress enough how your color choices change your life and your look. Do me a favor: I know so many of you think that brown and bronze shades make you look tired. But please try them. Because, as you can see, you are *wrong*! What really pops this look is the beautiful flush that makes it look like Eleanor had a really good night last night (even if she didn't).

　　Here's how to get this look:

eyes

1. Using your #14 detail highlighting brush, apply a crème-to-powder shimmery beige eye shadow to your lid, but only to the area right along your lash line. You are going to layer crème and powder to make your lid more dramatic.

2. With the same brush, apply a shimmery champagne eye shadow powder directly on top of the crème you applied to your lid.

3. For this look, you want the highlight on your lid to be more dramatic than your brow bone. In order to achieve this, you will use your #22 brush and apply a matte beige eye shadow on your brow bone. The fact that it is matte and a bit darker will make it look more subtle.

4. Using your #11 midtone brush and a matte midtone eye shadow and starting from the outside corner of your crease, glide your brush across to the inside corner. Use a dark matte taupe shadow (a shade just a bit darker than your skin tone) so that you get soft definition.

5. Use your #28 blending brush (the one that is always clean and ready to blend with) and blend your midtone so that there are no hard edges.

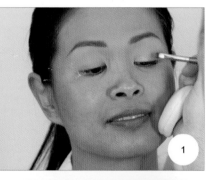

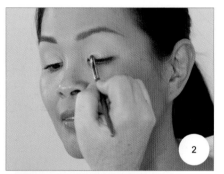

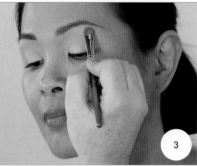

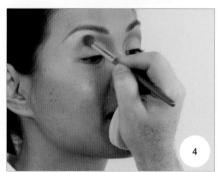

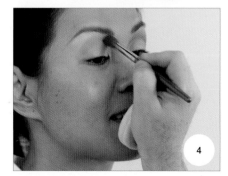

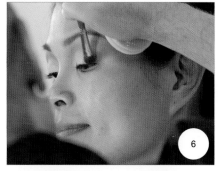

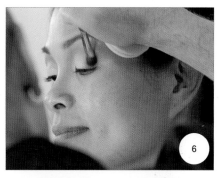

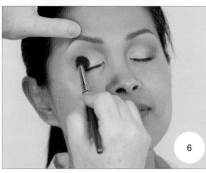

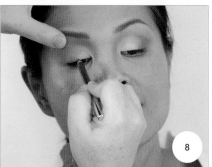

6. Grab your #30 contour brush and some midtone eye shadow and define the outer third of your eyelid. Follow with your #28 brush to blend.

7. It's time to curl your eyelashes and apply the first layer of mascara to your top lashes. (See page 42 to review how to curl properly.)

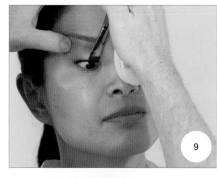

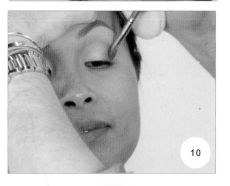

8. To give your lash line a little more punch, start by lining your upper lash line with a black eyeliner. Begin at the inside corner, taking it all the way to the outside corner. Keep it close to your lash line. You want it thinnest on the inside, slowly getting just the slightest bit thicker as you get to the outside corner.

9. With your #18 eyeliner brush, grab some black eye shadow and lay it all along your top lash line to soften the liner you just applied. As you apply it, pull up slightly with your brush to blend the line.

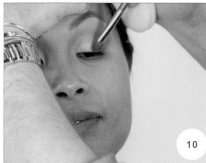

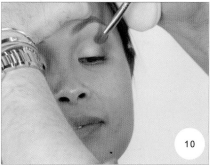

10. With your #30 contour brush, apply a dark shimmery brown eye shadow on the outer third of your eyelid and up into the crease. You are layering it over your midtone so it starts to create a blend.

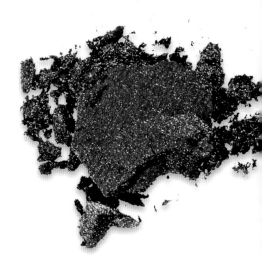

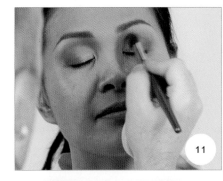

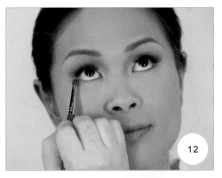

11. Follow again with your #28 brush to blend your contour color.

12. Now grab your #13 detail eye shadow brush and apply your midtone eye shadow all along your lower lash line. Once again, start your application from the outside corner, sweeping it across to the inside corner.

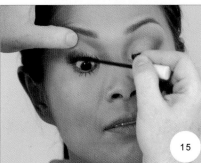

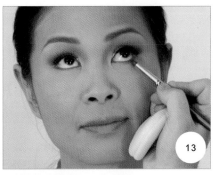

13. With that same detail eye shadow brush, apply a layer of your contour color right over your midtone all along your bottom lash line. By layering on your midtone, then applying your contour on top of it, you are creating a gradation of color, making your lower lash line definition look more natural and blended.

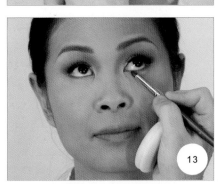

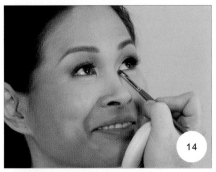

14. Using your #14 detail highlighting brush, highlight the inside corner of the lower lash line. Because there is so little color to this look, this brightens the eye and opens it up to give you a wide-eyed effect.

15. Now it's time for another layer of mascara on your top lashes and a layer on your lower lashes. After you finish the rest of your makeup, add yet another layer to the top lashes. Remember, with this look, lush lashes are very important, so you want to really layer your mascara on your top lashes. (See page 44 to review how to layer your mascara properly.)

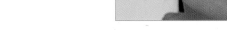

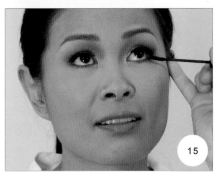

cheeks

This look definitely requires a beautiful flushed cheek. I call it "popping your apples." This is a two-step process with a little secret.

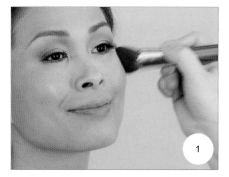

1. First, take a soft peach crème-to-powder blush and using your #64 blush brush, apply it to the apple of your cheek. Remember to start from the front of the apple and brush it toward the back, keeping the color right on your apple. Follow this with a little loose powder to help set the blush.

2. Now grab your #73 bronzer/blush brush and a matte bronzer; begin your application at the back of your cheekbone and sweep it forward toward the apple of your cheek. Then take the brush back toward your ear. This lays your color in place.

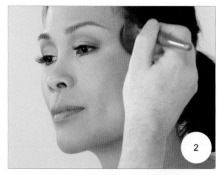

3. Then take your brush and use it in the opposite direction (up and down) to blend. Be sure to blend well, or it won't look natural.

4. Don't forget to add a little at the temples to help shape your face. Sweep the bronzing powder up around the temples and eye sockets. This always gives the face more color and gives you a glow.

5. Feel free to blend some bronzer along your jawbone. This also helps create that glow and softens your face shape.

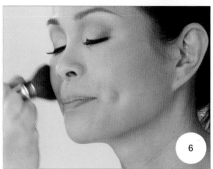

6. Finally, using your #73 brush and a powder blush that matches your crème (a bright sheer peach), apply the blush just to the apple of your cheek. Start at the front of the apple and brush toward the back. By layering powder on top of a crème, your blush will last longer and really give you the perfect flush.

"at every age, less can always be more."

lips

1. You want a pale nude lip for this look. Start by concealing your lip and lip line. This gives you the perfect pale canvas for your subtle lip look.

2. End with a quick sweep of the perfect nude lip gloss to make your lips shiny, fuller looking, and sexy. Make sure you apply your gloss with your #80 lip brush because if you apply gloss with a brush, it will look shinier.

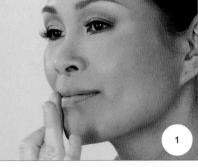

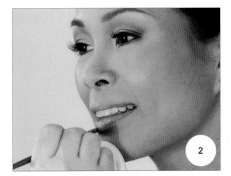

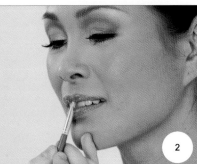

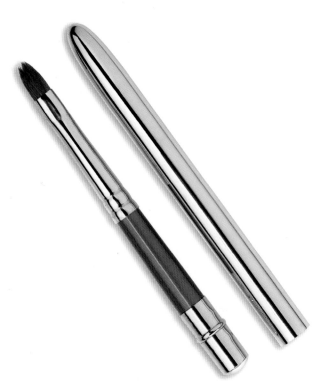

makeup makeovers in 5, 10, 15, and 20 minutes

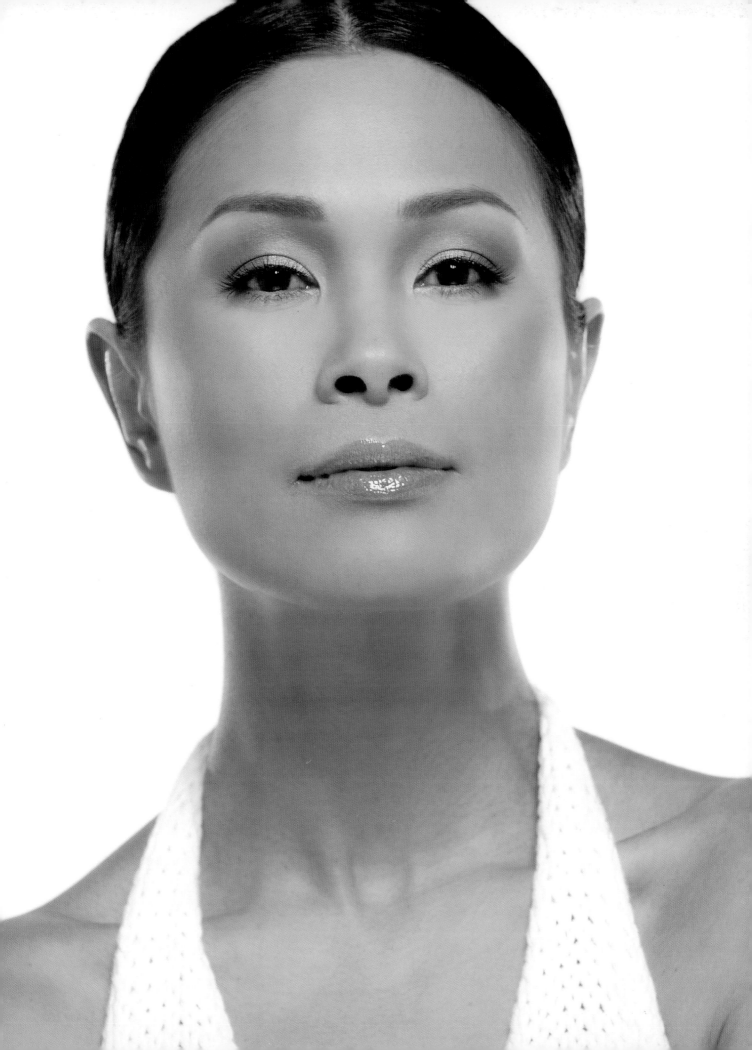

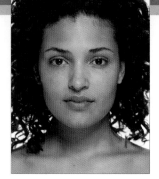

burgundy with envy

This look is a perfect example of how you can take even an intense color like burgundy and use it in a completely natural-looking way. With blending and the perfect pairing of neutrals, you can create that natural look, but with a bit more glamour. This is exactly how you take a natural look and turn up the volume. You know you've seen women who just stand out but don't look made up. It's all about that little extra definition and color. So go ahead and be the woman others envy because they think you wake up looking stunning!

Here's how to get this look:

eyes

1. Using your #22 highlighting brush, apply a crème-to-powder shimmery pale gold eye shadow to your lid (just from the lash line to your crease). You are going to layer crème and powder to make your lid more dramatic.

2. With the same brush, apply a shimmery gold powder eye shadow directly on top of the crème you applied to your lid. Also apply it to your brow bone. When I say brow bone, I mean the area just under the arch of your brow.

3. It's time to curl your eyelashes and apply the first layer of mascara to your top lashes. (See page 42 to review how to curl properly.)

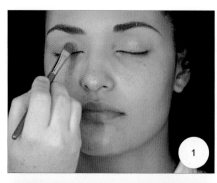

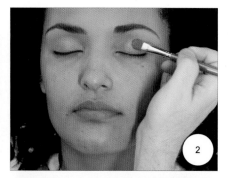

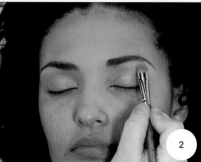

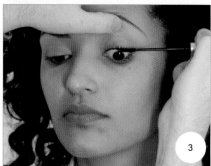

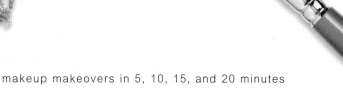

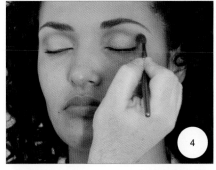

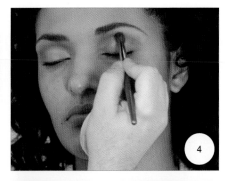

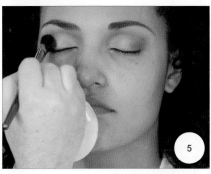

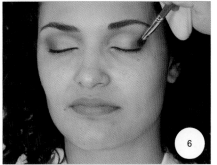

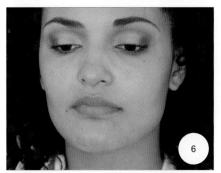

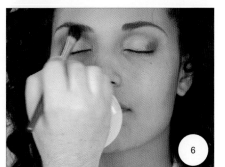

4. Using your #11 midtone brush and a matte midtone eye shadow and starting from the outside corner of your crease, glide your brush across to the inside corner. Use a matte ginger shadow (a shade just a bit darker than your skin tone) so that you get soft definition.

5. Use your #28 blending brush (the one that is always clean and ready to blend with) and blend your midtone so that there are no hard edges.

6. Grab your #30 contour brush and some midtone eye shadow and define the outer third of your eyelid. Follow with your #28 brush to blend.

7. To start your lash line definition, use your #41 eyeliner brush and push black eye shadow into the base of your lash line.

8. To give your lash line a little more punch, start by lining your upper lash line with a black eyeliner. Begin at the inside corner, taking it all the way to the outside corner. Keep it really close to your lash line. You want it to be thinnest on the inside, then to slowly get just the slightest bit thicker as you get to the outside corner.

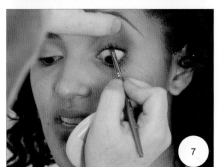

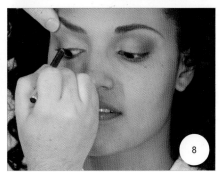

"this is how you take a natural look and turn up the volume."

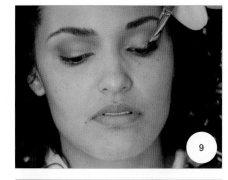

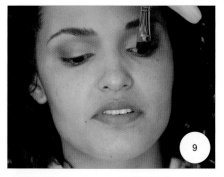

9. With your #18 eyeliner brush, grab some black eye shadow and lay it all along your top lash line to soften the liner you just applied. As you apply it, pull up slightly with your brush to blend the line.

10. With your #30 contour brush, apply a dark shimmery burgundy eye shadow on the outer third of your eyelid and up into the crease. You are layering it over your midtone eye shadow so it starts to create a blend.

11. Follow again with your #28 brush to blend your contour color.

12. Now grab your #13 detail eye shadow brush and apply your midtone eye shadow all along your lower lash line. Once again, start your application from the outside corner, sweeping it across to the inside corner.

13. With that same detail eye shadow brush, apply a layer of your contour color right over your midtone all along your bottom lash line. By layering on your midtone and then applying your contour on top of it, you are creating a gradation of color, making your lower lash line definition look more natural and blended.

14. Using your #14 detail highlighting brush, highlight the inside corner of the lower lash line. This brightens the eye and opens it up to give you a wide-eyed effect.

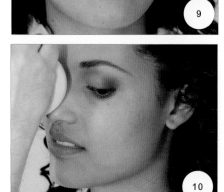

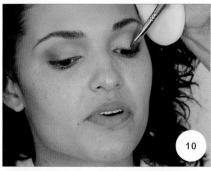

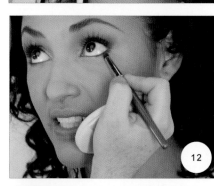

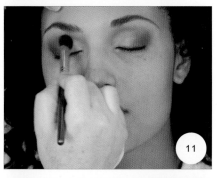

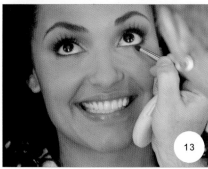

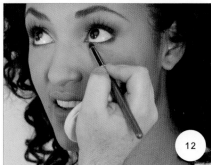

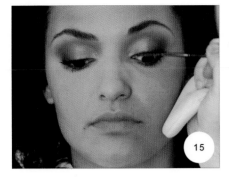

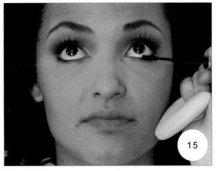

15. Now it's time for another layer of mascara on your top lashes and a layer on your lower lashes. After you finish the rest of your makeup, add yet another layer to the top lashes. Remember, with this look, lush lashes are very important, so you want to really layer your mascara on your top lashes. (See page 44 to review how to layer your mascara properly.)

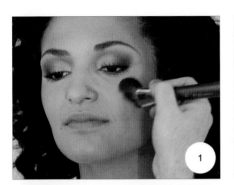

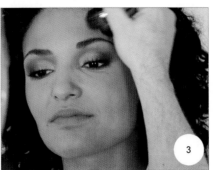

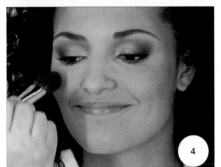

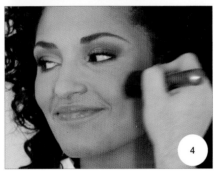

cheeks

1. Using your #73 bronzer/blush brush, apply your matte bronzer. Beginning at the back of your cheekbone, sweep it forward toward the apple of your cheek. Then take the brush back toward your ear. This lays your color in place.

2. Now take your brush and use it in the opposite direction (up and down) to blend. Be sure to blend well, or it won't look natural.

3. Don't forget to add a little at the temples to help shape your face. Sweep the bronzing powder up around the temples and eye sockets. This always gives the face more color and gives you a glow.

4. Now, for a little extra color, grab your #73 bronzer/blush brush and smile. Then apply your powder blush (the perfect bright sheer apricot color) on the apple of your cheek, blending back toward the area that you bronzed. This technique really gives your face that fresh flush that is so perfect.

lips

1. An important part of this look is a pale nude lip. Start by concealing your lip and lip line. This gives you the perfect pale canvas for your subtle lip look.

2. End with a quick sweep of the perfect sandy beige lip gloss to make your lips shiny, fuller looking, and sexy. Make sure you apply your gloss with your #80 lip brush because if you apply gloss with a brush, it will appear shinier.

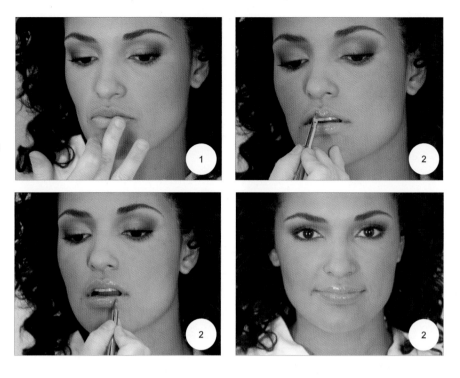

"go ahead and be the woman others envy because they think you wake up looking stunning!"

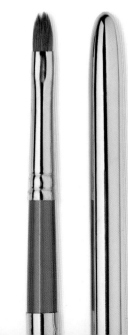

makeup makeovers in 5, 10, 15, and 20 minutes

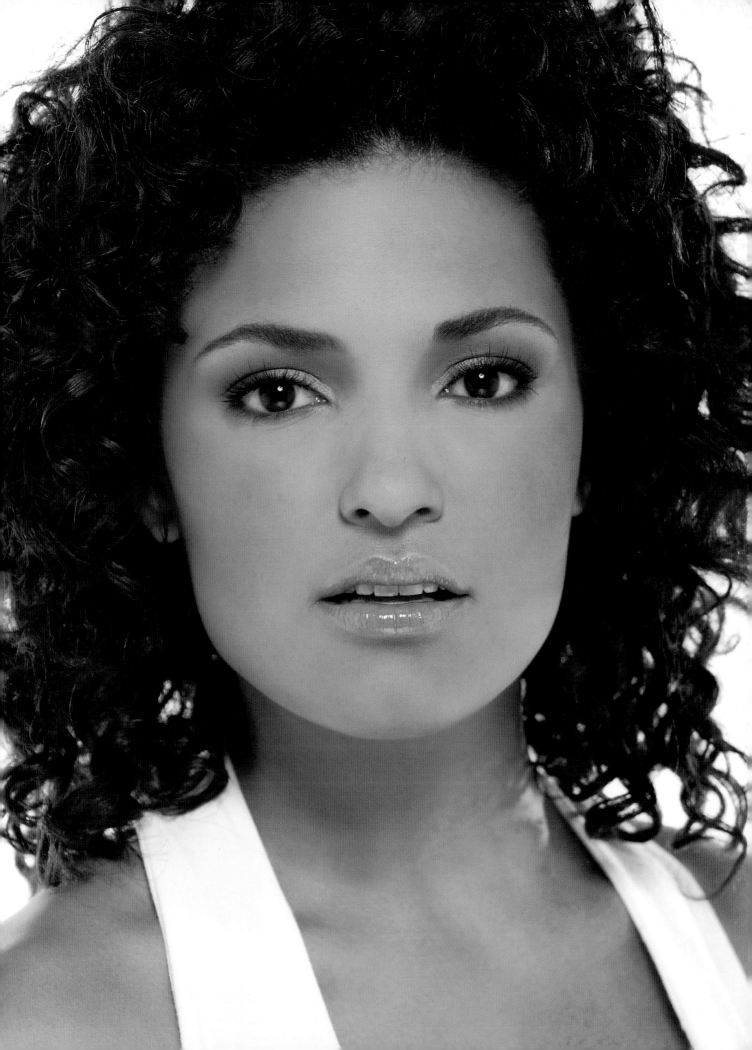

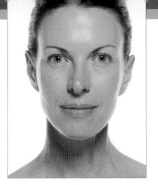

blushing beauty

So many women think it's all about how much makeup you put on, but it is not! This look is the perfect example of a completely fresh, youthful glow that is all about picking the perfect shades. The right shades are what truly make the difference. This look is completely polished without appearing overly made up: subtly defined eyes, the perfect peach glow, and that gorgeous peach pucker.

Here's how to get this look:

eyes

1. Using your #22 highlighting brush, apply a crème-to-powder shimmery beige eye shadow to your lid (only from the lash line to your crease). You are going to layer crème and powder to make your lid more dramatic.

2. With the same brush, apply a shimmery champagne eye shadow powder directly on top of the crème you applied to your lid. Also apply it to your brow bone. When I say brow bone, I mean the area just under the arch of your brow.

3. Using your #11 midtone brush and a matte midtone eye shadow and starting from the outside corner of your crease, glide your brush across to the inside corner. Use a matte taupe shadow (a shade just a bit darker than your skin tone) so that you get soft definition.

4. Use your #28 blending brush (the one that is always clean and ready to blend with) and blend your midtone so that there are no hard edges.

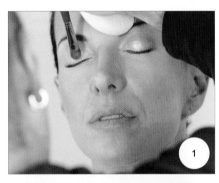

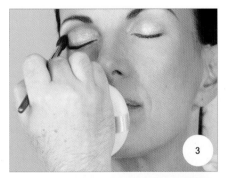

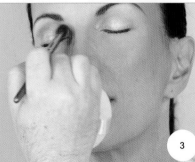

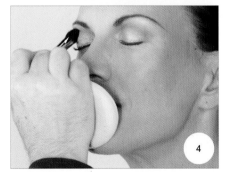

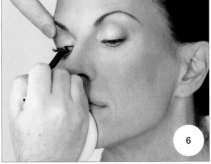

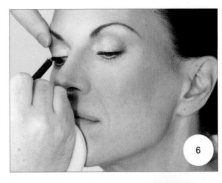

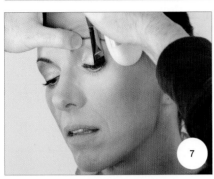

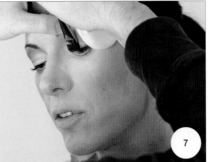

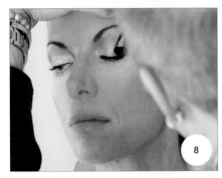

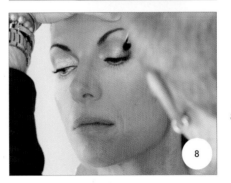

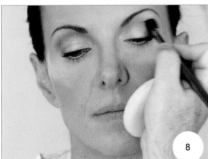

5. It's time to curl your eyelashes and apply the first layer of mascara to your top lashes. (See page 42 to review how to curl properly.)

6. For lash line definition, you want a little more punch. Start by lining your upper lash line with a black eyeliner. Keep it really close to your lash line.

7. With your #18 eyeliner brush, grab some dark brown eye shadow and lay it all along your top lash line to soften the liner you just applied. As you apply it, pull up slightly with your brush to blend the line. Layering brown shadow over black eyeliner creates a softer look than black does, yet a more intense look than brown.

8. Grab your #30 contour brush and some midtone eye shadow and define the outer third of your eyelid. Follow with your #28 brush to blend.

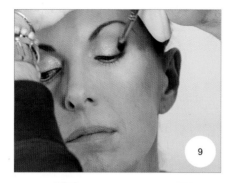

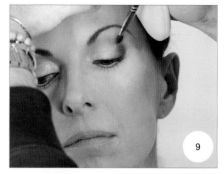

9. With your #30 contour brush, apply a dark brown eye shadow on the outer third of your eyelid and up into the crease. You are layering it over your midtone so it starts to create a blend.

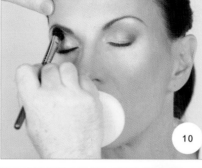

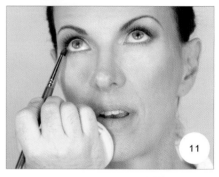

10. Follow again with your #28 brush to blend your contour color.

11. Now grab your #13 detail eye shadow brush and apply your midtone eye shadow all along your lower lash line. Once again, start your application from the outside corner, sweeping it across to the inside corner.

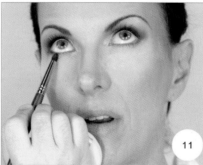

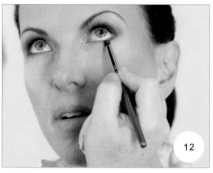

12. With that same detail eye shadow brush, apply a layer of your contour color right over your midtone all along your bottom lash line. By layering on your midtone, and then putting your contour on top of it, you're creating a gradation of color, making your lower lash line definition look more natural and blended.

13. Next, using your #14 detail highlighting brush, highlight the inside corner of the lower lash line. Because there is so little color to this look, this step really brightens the eye and opens it up to give you a wide-eyed effect.

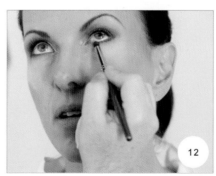

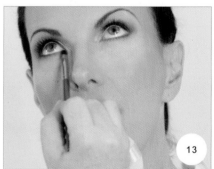

We'll add the final layers of mascara at the end of the look.

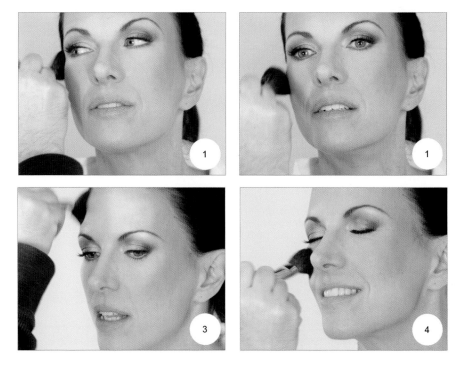

cheeks

1. Using your #73 bronzer/blush brush, apply your matte bronzer. Begin at the back of your cheekbone and sweep it forward toward the apple of your cheek. Then take the brush back toward your ear. This lays your color in place.

2. Now, take your brush and use it in the opposite direction (up and down) to blend. Be sure to blend well, or it won't look natural.

3. Don't forget to add a little at the temples to help shape your face. Sweep the bronzing powder up around the temples and eye sockets. This always gives the face more color and gives you a glow.

4. Now for a little extra color, using your #73 brush again, smile and apply your powder blush (the perfect bright sheer peach color) on the apple of your cheek, blending back toward the area that you bronzed. This technique really gives your face that fresh flush that is so perfect.

"the right shades are what truly make the difference."

lips

1. I have chosen to use lip liner with this look because I want a very defined lip. Grab your nude pencil and begin with a V in the "cupid's bow," or center curve, of the lips. Bring the liner up and around the curves of your bow.

2. Next, start at the outer corners, moving toward the center with your pencil.

3. On the lower lip, first accentuate the lower curve of the lip. Then begin from the outer corners, moving toward the center. Remember to use your entire lip: Take the color to the almost invisible line just at the edge of the colored part of your lips.

4. Make sure you fill in at least halfway toward the center of your lip. This will help your lip liner look more natural and your lip color last longer.

5. Now blend with your #80 lip brush to make it look more natural.

6. Using your #80 lip brush (because it gives you better application and helps color last longer), fill in your entire lip with the perfect peach lipstick. Make sure you blend really well over your lip liner.

7. End with a quick sweep of the perfect sheer peach lip gloss to make your lips shiny, fuller looking, and sexy. Make sure you apply your gloss with your #80 lip brush because if you apply gloss with a brush, it will appear shinier.

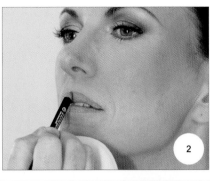
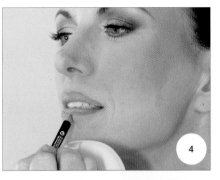
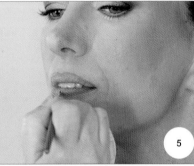
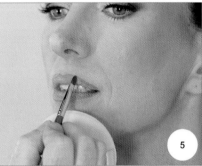
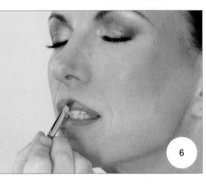
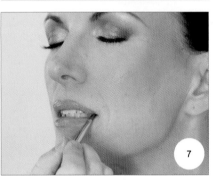
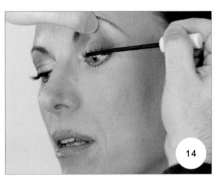

eyes

Here are the final steps for your eyes.

14. Now it's time for another layer of mascara on your top lashes and a layer on your lower lashes. After you finish the rest of your makeup, add yet another layer to the top lashes. Remember, with this look, lush lashes are very important, so you want to really layer your mascara on your top lashes. (See page 44 to review how to layer your mascara properly.)

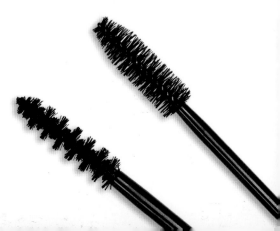

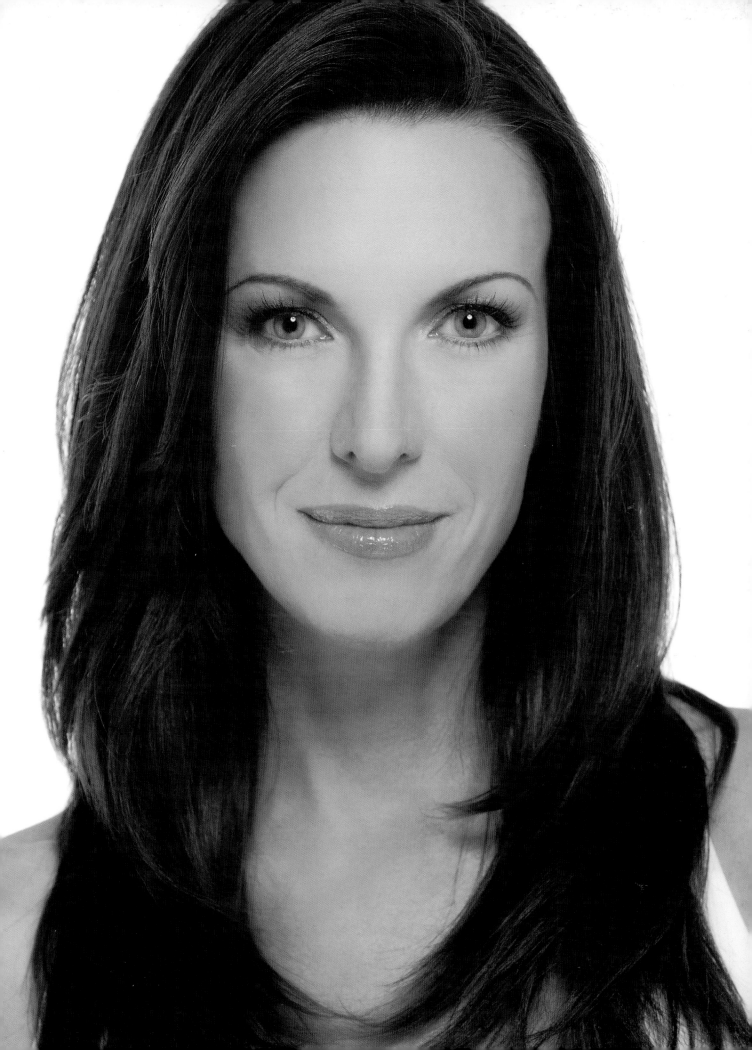

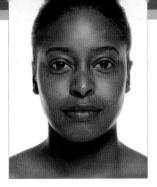

smoke signal

I would normally never do an intense eye with an intense lip, but in this case, it works. One of the reasons why is that Amanda's skin tone is deep enough to pull it off. Second is the fact that I toned down her smoky eye by highlighting the inside corners of her eyes. It is definitely an evening look, but can you imagine the attention you will get when you enter the room? Go ahead, try it—it's nice being the most glamorous girl in the room!

Here's how to get this look:

eyes

1. With your #22 highlighting brush, apply a shimmery peachy gold eye shadow to your eyelid and brow bone.

2. Using your #11 midtone brush and a matte midtone eye shadow and starting from the outside corner of your crease, glide your brush across to the inside corner. Use a matte ginger shadow (a shade just a bit darker than your skin tone) so that you get soft definition.

3. Use your #28 blending brush (the one that is always clean and ready to blend with) and blend your midtone so that there are no hard edges.

4. It's time to curl your eyelashes and apply the first layer of mascara to your top lashes. (See page 42 to review how to curl properly.)

5. Because you are about to use a very dark color, use your #76 powder brush and apply a bit of powder under the eye to catch any eye shadow. Now, when you are finished, you can just brush the powder and any dripped shadow away and still have flawless skin.

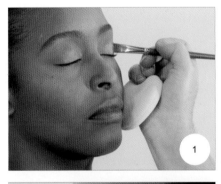

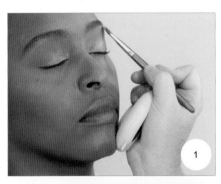

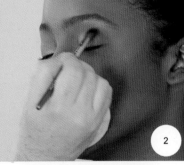

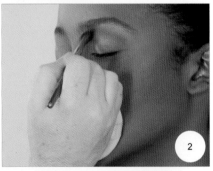

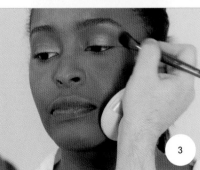

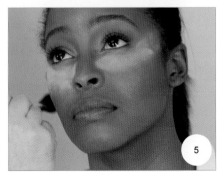

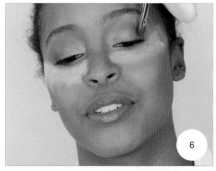

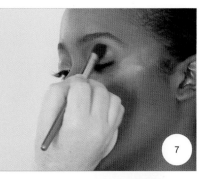

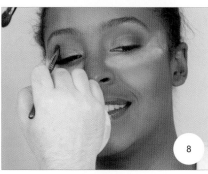

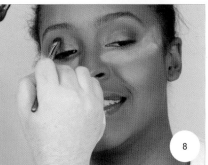

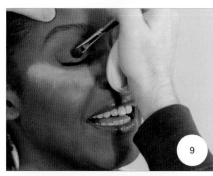

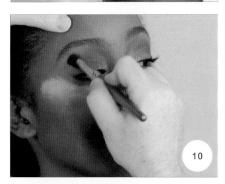

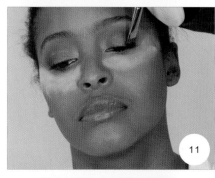

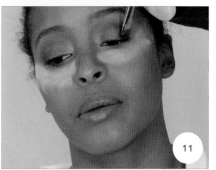

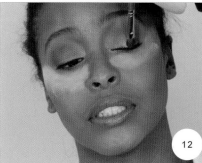

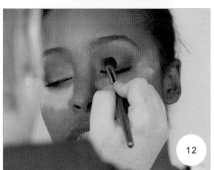

6. With your #30 contour brush, apply a dark gray shimmery eye shadow on the outer third of your eyelid and up into the crease. Pat the shadow on so you get more intense color application. You are layering it over your midtone so it starts to create a blend.

7. Follow again with your #28 brush to blend your contour color.

8. Follow with the same brush and apply eye shadow in your crease in a half-moon shape.

9. Now it's time for another layer of your contour for more drama. Using your #30 contour brush, pat more eye shadow on the outer half of your lid. Remember, if you pat shadow on, it gives you a more intense application of color.

10. Using your #28 blending brush, blend your contour shadow, making sure you blend toward the inside corner. This will give you the perfect gradation of color that actually covers the outer two-thirds of your eyelid.

11. With your #18 eyeliner brush, grab some black eye shadow and lay it all along your top lash line to create a subtle hint of a line. As you apply it, pull up slightly with your brush to blend the line.

12. Add a little more of your contour shadow to the outer third of your eyelid with your #30 eye shadow brush. This creates a bit more depth. Follow with your #28 brush to blend.

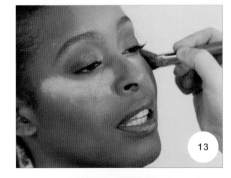

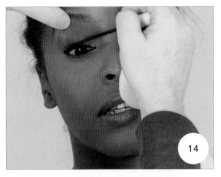

13. With your #76 detail powder brush, sweep away the powder you laid under your eye. Any eye shadow that you dropped during application will go with it.

14. Apply another layer of mascara to your top lash line.

15. Now grab your #13 detail eye shadow brush and apply your midtone eye shadow all along your lower lash line. Once again, start your application from the outside corner, sweeping it across to the inside corner.

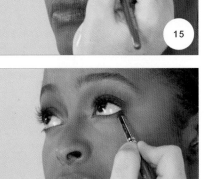

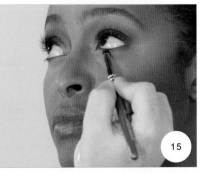

16. With that same detail eye shadow brush, apply a layer of your contour color right over your midtone all along your bottom lash line. By layering on your midtone and then applying your contour on top of it, you are creating a gradation of color, making your lower lash line definition look more natural and blended.

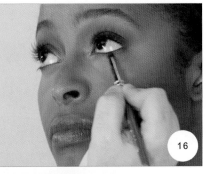

17. With your #18 eyeliner brush, grab a little black eye shadow and lay it into your lower lashes and along your lash line. This creates drama without it looking lined.

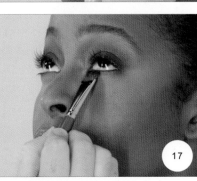

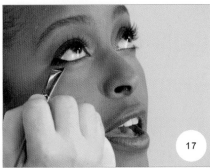

18. Using your #14 detail highlighting brush, highlight the inside corner of the lower lash line. Once again, this step helps soften your smoky eye.

19. Now it's time for another layer of mascara on your top lashes and a layer on your lower lashes. After you finish the rest of your makeup, add yet another layer to the top lashes. Remember, with this look, lush lashes are very important, so you want to really layer your mascara on your top lashes. (See page 44 to review how to layer your mascara properly.)

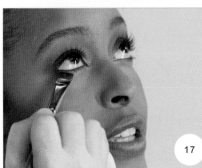

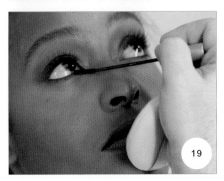

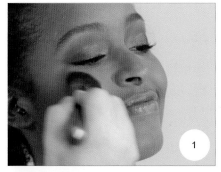

cheeks

1. Now it's time for a soft, glowy cheek! You are going to achieve this by layering your blush. Start with a great crème-to-powder blush. Using your #64 crème blush brush, apply a bright apricot blush to the apple of the cheek, starting at the front of the apple and working toward the back.

2. Follow with a light dusting of loose or pressed powder.

3. Now to reinforce that flush, smile and apply your powder blush (the perfect bright sheer apricot color) with your #74 bronzer/blush brush on the apple of your cheek, starting at the front of your apple and working toward the back.

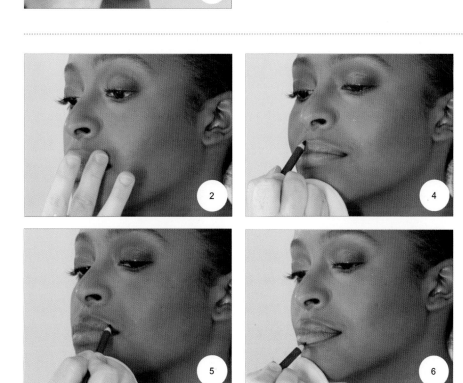

lips

1. This lip is very dramatic, and to help it look its most perfect, you need to prep your lips first. You want them to be sumptuous and smooth, so before you start your color application, moisturize them with lip balm. This will help the color go on smoothly and evenly. After the balm has had time to soak in, blot off the excess with a tissue so that it won't shorten the staying power of your lipstick.

2. Now, using concealer, conceal your lip and along your lip line.

3. Next, powder your lips. This gives you the perfect canvas to now apply your dramatic lip, so that the edge of the lip is very crisp.

4. Grab your burgundy lip pencil and begin with a V in the "cupid's bow," or center curve, of the lips. Bring the liner up and around the curves of your bow.

5. Next, starting at the outer corners, move toward the center with your pencil.

6. On the lower lip, first accentuate the lower curve of the lip. Then begin from the outer corners, moving toward the center. Use your entire lip: Take the color to the almost invisible line just at the edge of the colored part of your lips.

7. Now fill in your entire lip with your lip pencil. This will help your lip color last and stay in place because lip liner is a drier texture than lipstick.

8. With your #80 lip brush, blend your lip liner so that it is even and smooth.

9. Next, using your lip brush, apply your deep berry lipstick to your entire lip, making sure you blend really well over your lip liner.

10. Now take a tissue and blot your lips. This will remove the moisture from the lipstick, but leave a layer of pigment. Then apply another layer of lipstick. Applying these three layers (one of liner and two of lipstick) will help your color be true and intense, as well as last longer.

11. End with a quick sweep of the perfect rich burgundy lip gloss to make your lips shiny, fuller looking, and sexy. Make sure you apply your gloss with your #80 lip brush because if you apply gloss with a brush, it will appear shinier.

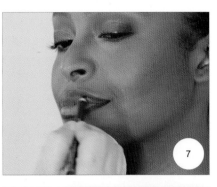

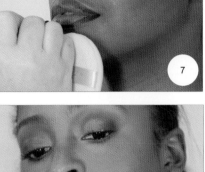

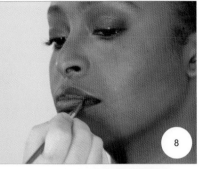

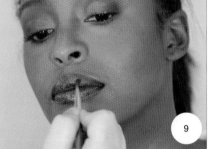

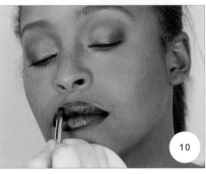

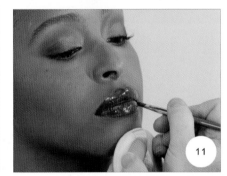

"it's nice being the most glamorous girl in the room!"

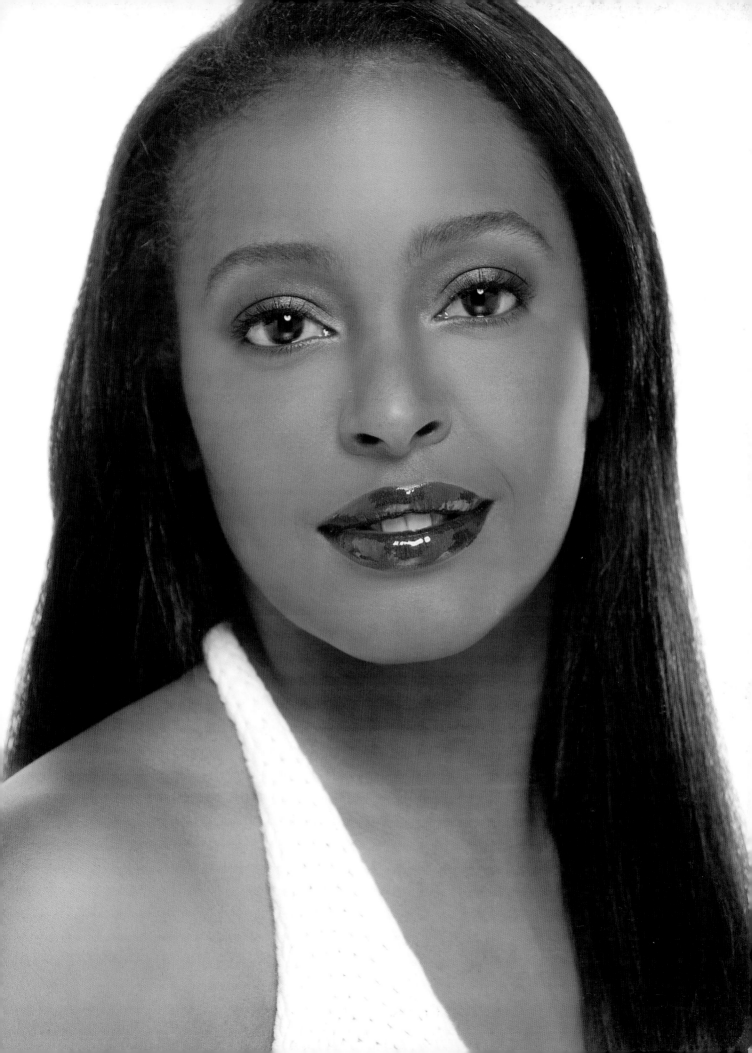

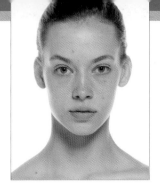

ray of light

Pretty is pretty, and this look is understated yet glamorous! I always love when you can create a look that naturally defines everything without appearing heavily made up. I think the flushed cheeks, the subtle lip, and the well-defined lash line are always perfect. This look is glowy natural on steroids. It is also perfect for girls of every age. It's never wrong to look beautiful!

Here's how to get this look:

eyes

1. Using your #22 highlighting brush, apply a crème-to-powder shimmery beige eye shadow to your lid (just from the lash line to your crease). Layering crème and powder will make your lid more dramatic.

2. With the same brush, apply a shimmery champagne eye shadow powder directly on top on the crème you applied to your lid and also apply it to your brow bone. When I say brow bone, I mean the area just under the arch of your brow.

3. It's time to curl your eyelashes and apply the first layer of mascara to your top lashes. (See page 42 to review how to curl properly.)

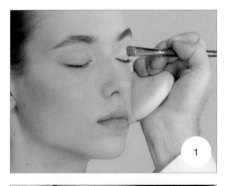

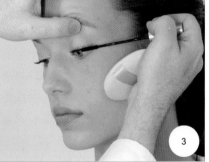

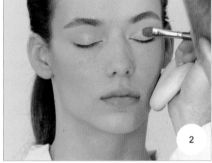

"it's never wrong to look beautiful!"

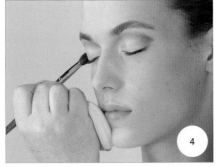

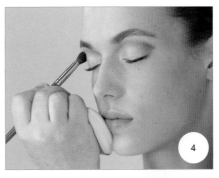

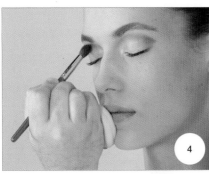

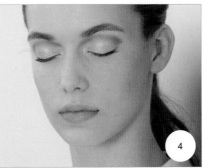

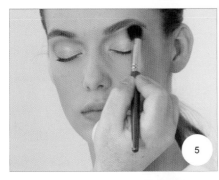

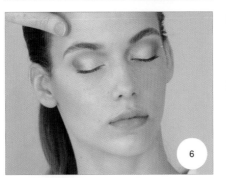

4. Using your #11 midtone brush and a matte midtone eye shadow and starting from the outside corner of your crease, glide your brush across to the inside corner. Use a matte taupe shadow (a shade just a bit darker than your skin tone) so that you get soft definition.

5. Use your #28 blending brush (the one that is always clean and ready to blend with) to blend your midtone so that there are no hard edges.

6. Grab your #30 contour brush and some midtone eye shadow and define the outer third of your eyelid. Follow with your #28 brush to blend.

7. With your #30 contour brush, apply a dark brown eye shadow on the outer third of your eyelid and up into the crease. You are layering it over your midtone so it starts to create a blend.

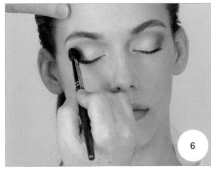

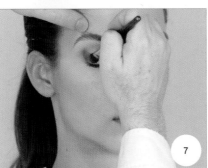

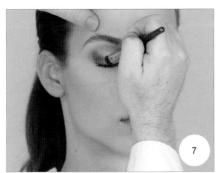

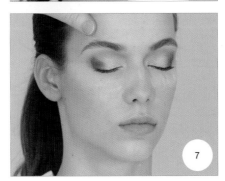

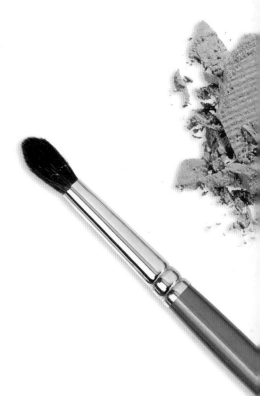

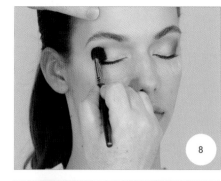

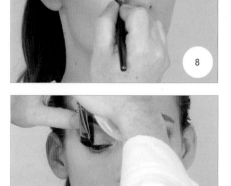

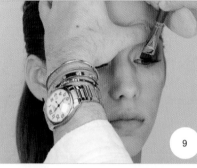

8. Follow again with your #28 brush to blend your contour color.

9. With your #18 eyeliner brush, grab some black eye shadow and lay it all along your top lash line for definition. As you apply it, pull up slightly with your brush to create a very blended smudged line.

10. Now it is time for another layer of mascara on your top lashes.

11. Now grab your #13 detail eye shadow brush and apply your midtone eye shadow all along your lower lash line. Once again, start your application from the outside corner, sweeping it across to the inside corner.

12. With that same detail eye shadow brush, apply a layer of your contour color right over your midtone all along your bottom lash line. By layering on your midtone and then your contour on top of it, you are creating a gradation of color, making your lower lash line definition look more natural and blended.

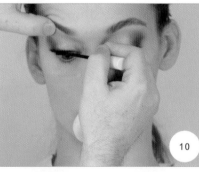

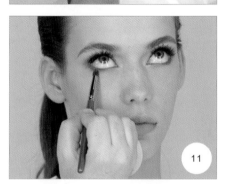

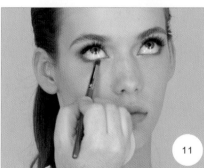

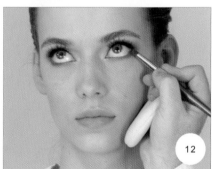

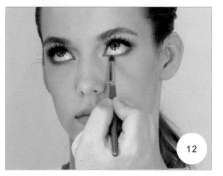

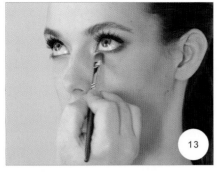

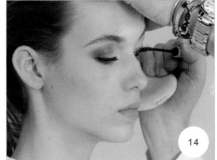

13. Using your #22 detail highlighting brush, highlight the inside corner of the lower lash line. Because there is so little color to this look, this step really brightens the eye and opens it up to give you a wide-eye effect.

14. Now it's time for another layer of mascara on your top lashes and a layer on your lower lashes. After you finish the rest of your makeup, add yet another layer to your top lashes. Remember, with this look, lush lashes are very important, so you want to really layer your mascara on your top lashes. (See page 44 to review how to layer your mascara properly.)

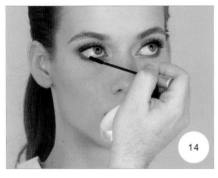

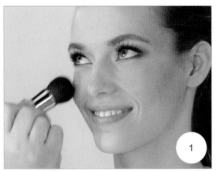

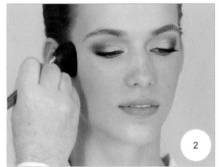

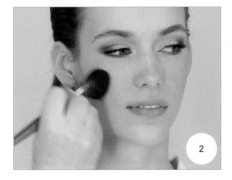

cheeks

This look requires a beautiful flushed cheek. I call it "popping your apples." This is a two-step process with a secret.

1. The first thing you want to do is take a soft peach crème-to-powder blush, and with your #64 blush brush, apply it to the apple of your cheek. Remember to start from the front of the apple and brush it toward the back. Keep the color right on your apple. Follow this with a little loose powder to help set the blush.

2. Grab your #73 cheek brush and bronzer (the same shade you used on your eyes) and apply the bronzer, beginning at the back of your cheekbone. Sweep it forward toward the apple of your cheek and then take the brush back toward your ear. This lays your color in place.

3. Now take your brush and use it in the opposite direction (up and down) to blend. Be sure to blend well, or it won't look natural.

4. Don't forget to add a little at the temples to help shape your face. Sweep the bronzing powder up around the temples and eye sockets. This always gives the face more color and gives you a glow.

5. Feel free to blend some bronzer along your jawbone because this also helps create that glow and softens the shape of your face.

6. Finish by using your #73 brush and a powder blush that matches your crème (a bright sheer peach), applying it just to the apple of your cheek. Start at the front of the apple and brush toward the back. By layering powder on top of a crème, your color will last longer and really give you the perfect flush.

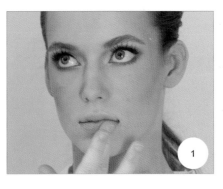

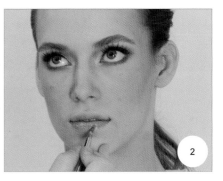

lips

1. For this look, you want your lips to be soft and natural. To help create this effect, start by concealing your lip and lip line. This gives you the perfect pale canvas for your subtle lip look.

2. End with a quick sweep of the perfect sheer peach lip gloss to make your lips shiny, fuller looking, and sexy. Make sure you apply your gloss with your #80 lip brush because if you apply gloss with a brush, it will appear shinier.

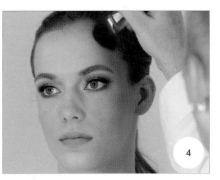

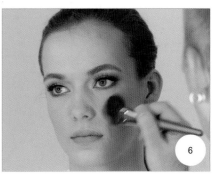

"This look is glowy natural on steroids."

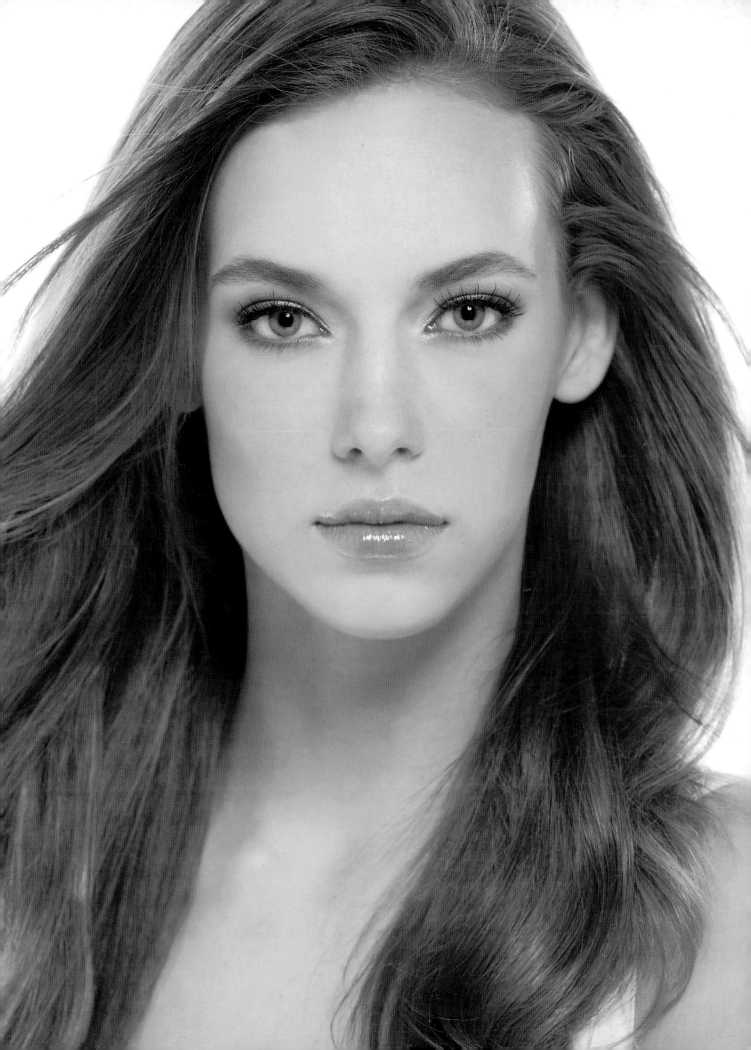

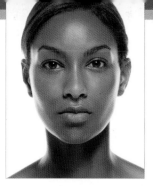

bronze goddess

Bronze is beautiful! No matter what your skin tone, a gorgeous, natural bronzy look is breathtaking. Here, warm coppery shades mix with flawless skin and a quiet flush to the cheek. This look has become a classic and works on all skin tones by simply making great color choices. Nothing is more completely appropriate and beautiful for any occasion than the perfect "no-makeup makeup" look.

Here's how to get this look:

eyes

1. Using your #22 highlighting brush, apply a crème-to-powder shimmery peachy gold eye shadow to your lid (just from the lash line to your crease). You are going to layer crème and powder to make your lid more dramatic.

2. With the same brush, apply a shimmery peachy gold eye shadow powder directly on top of the crème you applied to your lid and to your brow bone. When I say brow bone, I mean the area just under the arch of your brow.

3. Using your #11 midtone brush and a matte midtone eye shadow and starting from the outside corner of your crease, glide your brush across to the inside corner. Use a matte ginger shadow (a shade just a bit darker than your skin tone) so that you get soft definition.

4. Use your #28 blending brush (the one that is always clean and ready to blend with) and blend your midtone so that there are no hard edges.

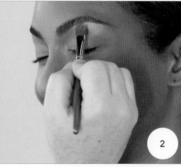

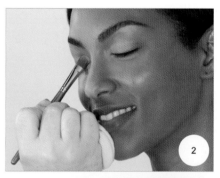

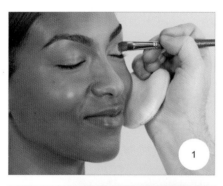

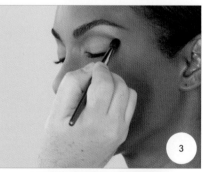

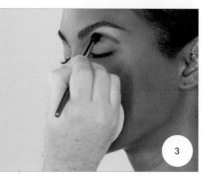

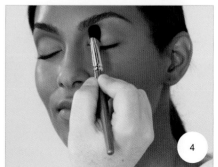

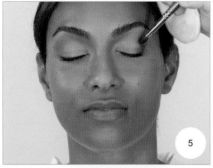

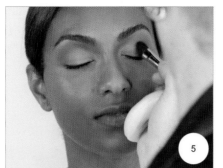

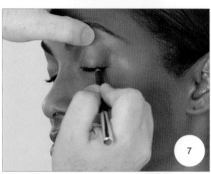

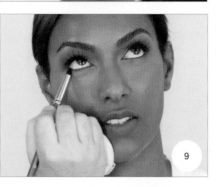

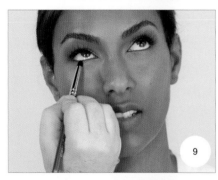

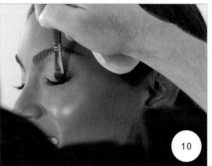

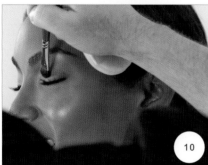

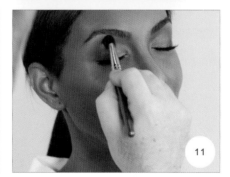

5. Grab your #30 contour brush and some midtone eye shadow and define the outer third of your eyelid. Follow with your #28 brush to blend.

6. It's time to curl your eyelashes and apply the first layer of mascara to your top lashes. (See page 42 to review how to curl properly.)

7. To give your lash line a little more punch, line your upper lash line with a black eyeliner. Begin at the inside corner, taking it all the way to the outside corner. Keep it really close to your lash line. You want it to be thinnest on the inside and slowly get just the slightest bit thicker as you get to the outside corner.

8. With your #18 eyeliner brush, grab some black eye shadow and lay it all along your top lash line to soften the liner you just applied. As you apply it, pull up slightly with your brush to blend the line.

9. Now grab your #13 detail eye shadow brush and apply your midtone eye shadow all along your lower lash line. Start your application from the outside corner, sweeping it across to the inside corner.

10. With your #30 contour brush, apply a dark shimmery burgundy eye shadow on the outer third of your eyelid and up into the crease. You are layering it over your midtone so it starts to create a blend.

11. Follow again with your #28 brush to blend your contour color.

15 minutes make all the difference

12. Again, with your #13 detail eye shadow brush, apply a layer of your contour color right over your midtone all along your bottom lash line. By layering on your midtone, then applying your contour on top of it, you are creating a gradation of color, making your lower lash line definition look more natural and blended.

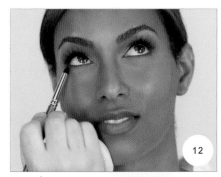

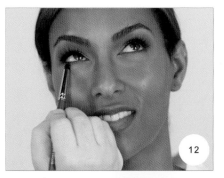

13. Using your #14 detail highlighting brush, highlight the inside corner of the lower lash line. Because there is so little color to this look, this brightens the eye and opens it up for a wide-eyed effect.

14. Now it's time for another layer of mascara on your top lashes and a layer on your lower lashes. After you finish the rest of your makeup, add yet another layer to the top lashes. Remember, with this look, lush lashes are very important, so you want to really layer your mascara on your top lashes. (See page 44 to review how to layer your mascara properly.)

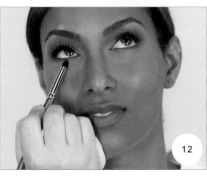

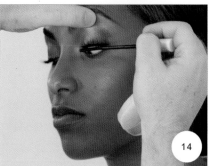

cheeks

1. Now it's time for a little extra color! Grab your #73 bronzer/blush brush and smile. Then apply your powder blush (the perfect bright apricot color) on the apple of your cheek, blending back toward the area that you bronzed. This technique really gives your face that fresh flush that is so perfect.

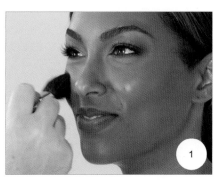

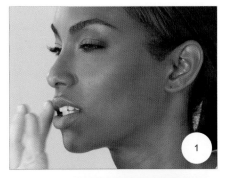

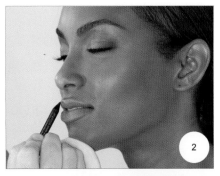

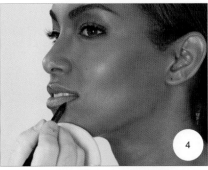

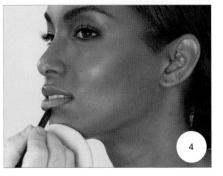

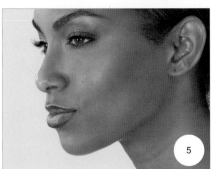

lips

1. You want your lips to be soft, but still well defined. Start by concealing your lip and lip line. This gives you the perfect pale canvas for your subtle lip look.

2. Using a raisin lip pencil, line your lips. Begin with a V in the "cupid's bow," or center curve, of the lips. Bring the liner up and around the curves of your bow.

3. Next, starting at the outer corners, move toward the center with your pencil.

4. On the lower lip, first accentuate the lower curve of the lip. Then, beginning from the outer corners, move toward the center. Remember to use your entire lip: Take the color to the almost invisible line just at the edge of the colored part of your lips.

5. Now, fill in your entire lip except the center of the top and bottom lip. This will create a slightly puckered look and help your lip color last longer.

"No matter what your skin tone, a gorgeous, natural bronzy look is breathtaking."

6. Blend with your #80 lip brush to make it look more natural.

7. Using your lip brush (because it gives you better application and helps color last longer), fill in your entire lip with the perfect shimmery pale ginger lipstick. Make sure you blend really well over your lip liner.

8. End with a quick sweep of the perfect sheer raisin lip gloss to make your lips shiny, fuller looking, and sexy. Be sure to apply your gloss with your #80 lip brush because if you apply gloss with a brush, it will appear shinier.

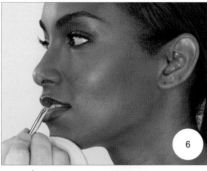

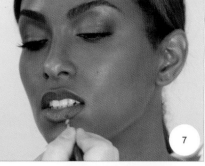

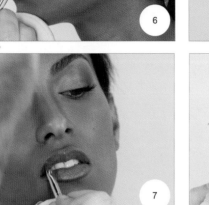

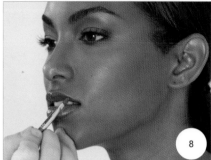

"bronze is beautiful!"

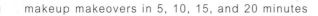

makeup makeovers in 5, 10, 15, and 20 minutes

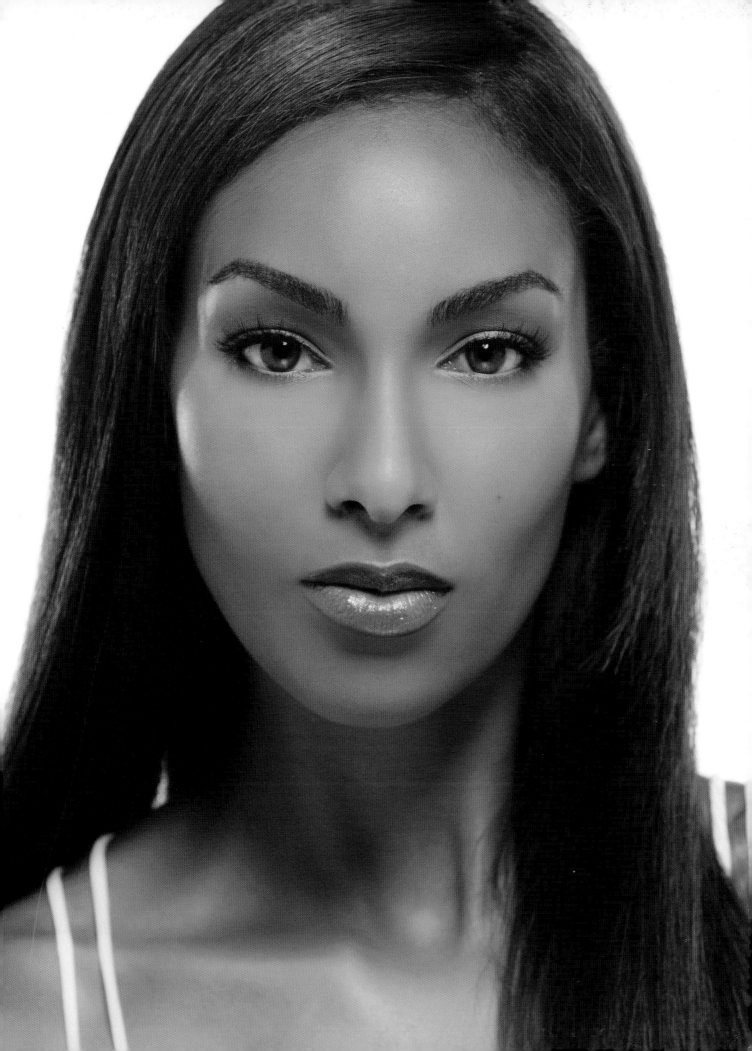

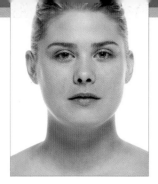

that girl's a looker

This is a modern-day nod to the 1980s, without the frost and without the blue. Okay, maybe it's not so '80s. (See, I told you it's modern!) This look is about glamour, and if you are a makeup maven you could wear it day or night. But for most, this will probably be an evening staple. This application would work with a ton of color options: Just replace the purple with the color of your dreams. Go ahead, girls, get your glamour on!

Here's how to get this look:

eyes

1. Using your #22 highlighting brush, apply a crème-to-powder shimmery beige eye shadow to your lid (only from your lash line to your crease). Layering crème and powder makes your lid more dramatic.

2. With the same brush, apply a shimmery champagne eye shadow powder directly on top of the crème you applied to your lid and also apply it to your brow bone. When I say brow bone, I mean the area just under the arch of your brow.

3. You want your midtone eye shadow very precise, so it won't darken your lid but will define the shape. We want to ground your bright color yet keep purple as the focus, so by keeping your midtone so precise, the purple will shine through. Using your #13 detail shadow brush, apply your matte taupe eye shadow in your crease, starting from the outside corner of your crease and gliding your brush across to the inside corner.

4. Use your #28 blending brush (the one that is always clean and ready to blend with) to blend your midtone so that there are no hard edges. Just retrace the same area that you just applied your midtone to, so as not to blend it up and down and darken too much of your lid.

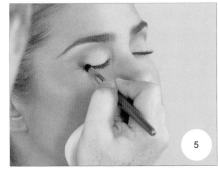

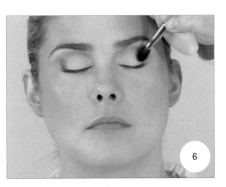

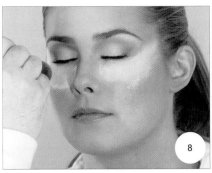

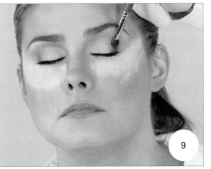

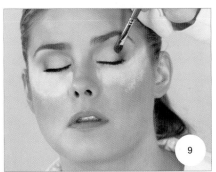

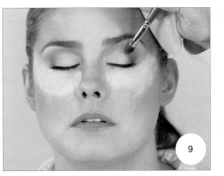

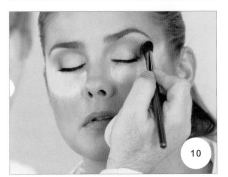

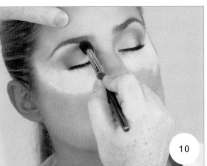

5. With your #13 detail shadow brush, apply midtone eye shadow just to the very outer edge of your lid.

6. Of course, follow with your #28 blending brush and blend toward the inside. This gives you just a hint of definition and color.

7. It's time to curl your eyelashes and apply the first layer of mascara to your top lashes. (See page 42 to review how to curl properly.)

8. Because you are about to use a very bright color, use your #76 powder brush to apply a bit of powder under the eye to catch it. Then, when you are finished, you can just brush the powder and any eye shadow dripping away and still have flawless skin.

9. Using your #30 contour brush, apply your bright purple shadow to the outer third of your eyelid. Pat it on rather than swipe! Remember, if you pat color on, it will be more intense.

10. With your #28 blending brush, blend over the purple to soften the edges and create a gradation. Blend from the outer corner in.

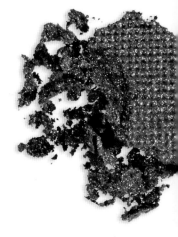

"go ahead, girls, get your glamour on!"

11. Go ahead and apply another layer of the purple for intensity and drama.

12. Blend once more with your #28 brush.

13. To increase contrast, add another layer of your shimmery champagne eye shadow to the inner two-thirds of your eyelid with your #22 highlighting brush.

14. For even more drama, line the waterline of your lower lid with a fun purple eyeliner. (Remember, the waterline is the inner rim above the lower lash line.)

15. Now grab your #13 detail eye shadow brush and apply your midtone eye shadow all along your lower lash line. Once again, start your application from the outside corner, sweeping it across to the inside corner. Immediately follow it with your bright fun purple. When applying the purple, use your #30 contour brush because you want your application to smudge out further for a more dramatic look. Apply the color to the outer two-thirds of your lower lash line.

16. With your #14 detail highlighting brush, apply your shimmery champagne eye shadow to the inner third of your eyelid.

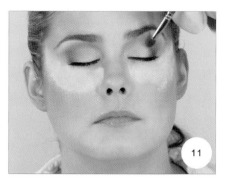
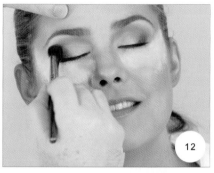
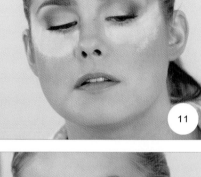
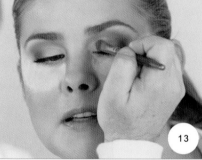
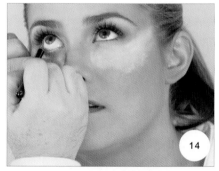
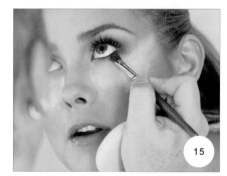
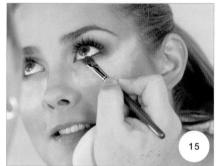
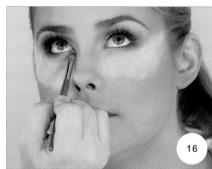
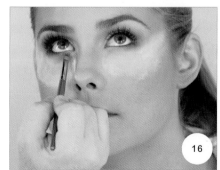

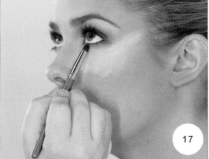

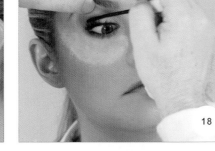

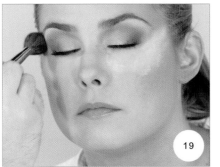

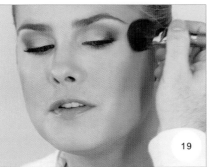

17. Next, grab your #13 detail eye shadow brush and blend where your highlight and contour meet.

18. Now it's time for another layer of mascara on your top lashes and a layer on your lower lashes. After you finish the rest of your makeup, add yet another layer to the top lashes. Remember, with this look, lush lashes are very important, so you want to really layer your mascara on your top lashes. (See page 44 to review how to layer your mascara properly.)

19. Finally, with your #76 detail powder brush, sweep away the powder under your eyes. Any eye shadow that dripped will disappear with it as well.

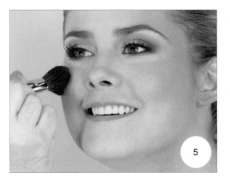

cheeks

1. Using your #73 bronzer/blush brush, apply your matte bronzer, beginning at the back of your cheekbone. Sweep it forward toward the apple of your cheek and then take the brush back toward your ear. This lays your color in place.

2. Now take your brush and use it in the opposite direction (up and down) to blend. Be sure to blend well, or it won't look natural.

3. Don't forget to add a little at the temples to help shape your face. Sweep the bronzing powder up around the temples and eye sockets. This always gives the face more color and gives you a glow.

4. Feel free to blend some bronzer along your jawbone, which also helps create that glow and defines your face.

5. Now, for a little extra color, grab your #73 bronzer/blush brush and smile. Apply your powder blush (the perfect bright sheer peach color) on the apple of your cheek, blending back toward the area that you bronzed. This technique really gives your face that fresh flush that is so perfect.

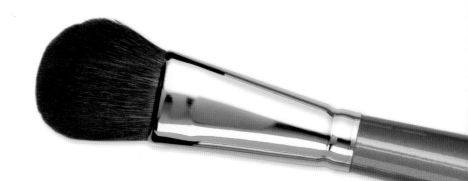

lips

1. Color, color everywhere? Because your eyes are colorful and the focus of this look, you want a barely-there lip with just a hint of color. To help create this effect, start by concealing your lip and lip line. This gives you the perfect pale canvas for your subtle lip look.

2. Using a pale nude lip liner, line your lips. Begin with a V in the "cupid's bow," or center curve, of the lips. Bring the liner up and around the curves of your bow.

3. Next, starting at the outer corners, move toward the center of the bow.

4. On the lower lip, first accentuate the lower curve of the lip. Then begin from the outer corners, moving toward the center. Remember to use your entire lip: Take the color to the almost invisible line just at the edge of the colored part of your lips.

5. Now, using the same pencil, fill in your entire lip. This will help your lip color last longer.

6. Using a #80 lip brush, blend your liner.

7. End with a quick sweep of the perfect sheer peach lip gloss to make your lips shiny, fuller looking, and sexy. Make sure you apply your gloss with your #80 lip brush because if you apply gloss with a brush, it will appear shinier. This gives you just the perfect hint of color while still looking almost naked.

Think you couldn't look any more stunning than this? Wait until you see what just 5 more minutes can do for you! In the next chapter, you'll find the ultimate in glamour and beauty for those times when you *really* want—or need—to make an unforgettable impression.

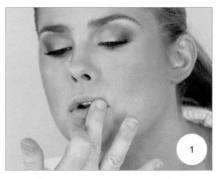

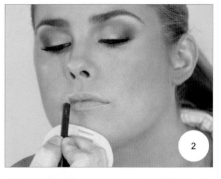

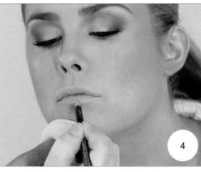

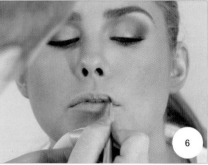

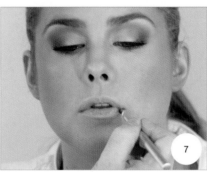

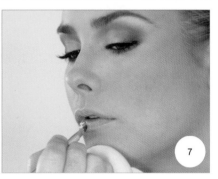

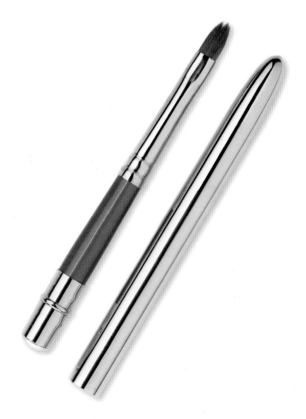

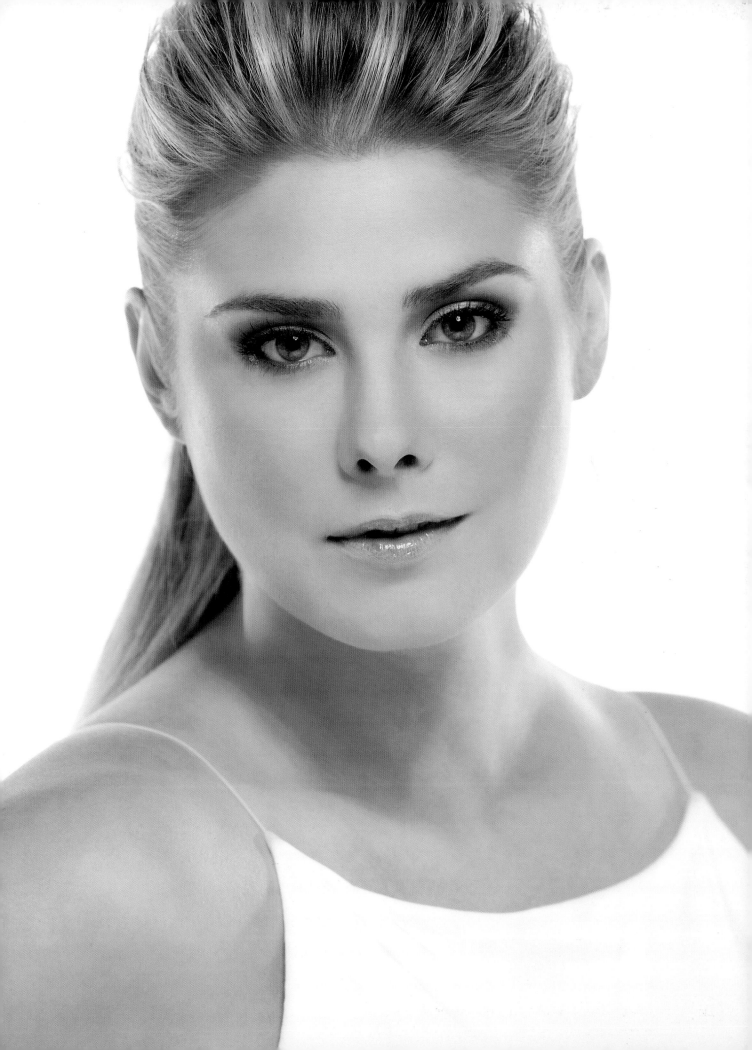

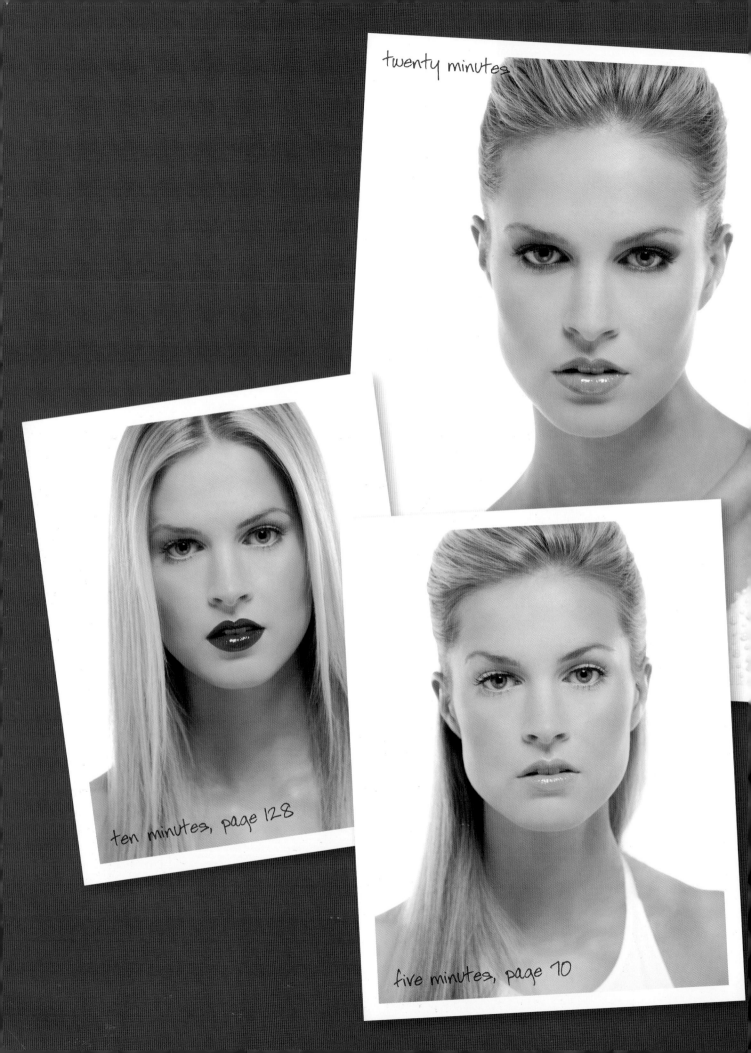

twenty minutes

ten minutes, page 128

five minutes, page 70

7

20 minutes: could I really look that fabulous?

Girls, are you ready for perfection? If your answer is yes, it's time for the ultimate, the makeovers to end all makeovers. And yes, you can create any look in this chapter in just 20 minutes! Without more ado, let me present ten luscious looks that can change your life.

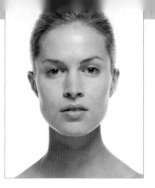

quiet elegance

You don't have to go dark to go dramatic. This look is the perfect example of how you can create a fabulous nighttime look without the whole eye looking dark. More often, it's about knowing what to darken than darkening everything. Add a beautiful lip and flawless skin, and you have perfect glamour.

　　Here's how to get this look:

eyes

1. Using your #22 highlighting brush, apply a crème-to-powder shimmery beige eye shadow to your lid (just from your lash line to your crease). You are going to layer crème and powder to make your lid more dramatic.

2. With the same brush, apply a shimmery champagne eye shadow powder directly on top of the crème you applied to your lid and to your brow bone. (Remember, when I say brow bone, I mean the area just under the arch of your brow.)

3. Using your #11 midtone brush and a matte midtone eye shadow and starting from the outside corner of your crease, glide your brush across to the inside corner. Use a matte taupe shadow (a shade just a bit darker than your skin tone) so that you get soft definition.

4. Use your #28 blending brush (the one that is always clean and ready to blend with) and blend your midtone so that there are no hard edges.

5. Grab your #30 contour brush and some midtone eye shadow and define the outer third of your eyelid. Follow with your #28 brush to blend.

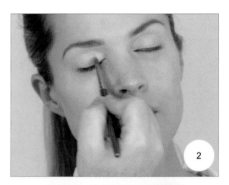

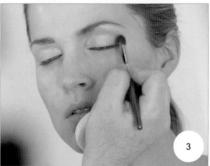

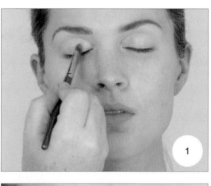

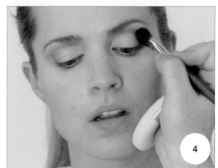

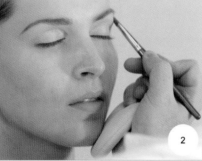

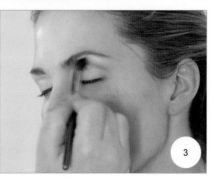

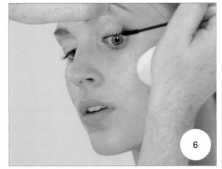

6

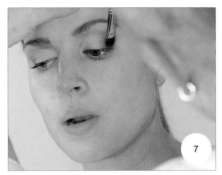

7

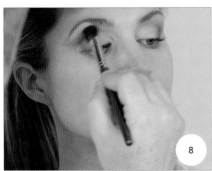

7

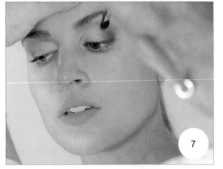

7

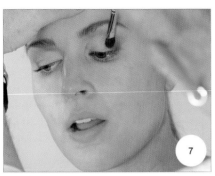

8

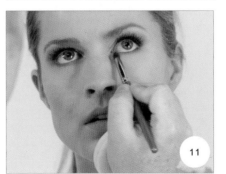

9

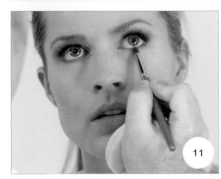

11

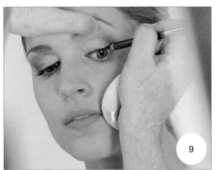

11

6. It's time to curl your eyelashes and apply the first layer of mascara to your top lashes. (See page 42 to review how to curl properly.)

7. With your #30 contour brush, apply a shimmery bronze eye shadow on the outer third of your eyelid and up into the crease. You are layering it over your mid-tone so it starts to create a blend.

8. Follow again with your #28 brush to blend your contour color.

9. Apply black eyeliner all along your top lash line, starting at the inside corner of your top lash line and slowly moving across the lash line. Make sure your line is its most narrow at the inside corner, gradually getting thicker as you reach the outside corner.

10. You can go back over your line with your #41 detail eyeliner brush to smooth your line and make it look perfect.

11. Now, grab your #13 detail eye shadow brush and apply your midtone eye shadow all along your lower lash line. Once again, start your application from the outside corner, sweeping it across to the inside corner.

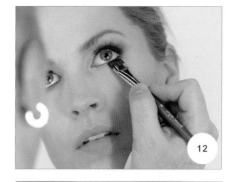

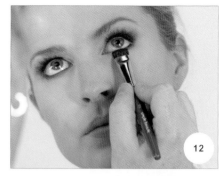

12. With your #18 brush, lay black eye shadow right into the base of your lower lashes.

13. Follow with your #13 brush and retrace with your shimmery bronze all along your lower lash line, again from the outside corner to the inside corner, to blend it all together.

14. Now it's time for another layer of mascara on your top lashes and a layer on your lower lashes. After you finish the rest of your makeup, add yet another layer to your top lashes. Remember, with this look, lush lashes are very important, so you want to really layer your mascara on your top lashes. (See page 44 to review how to layer your mascara properly.)

15. Now with a black eyeliner, line the water-line of your lower lid. (Remember, the waterline is the inner rim above the lower lash line.) This will add just a little bit more drama.

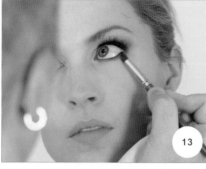

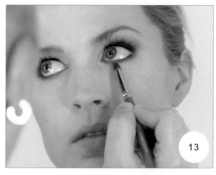

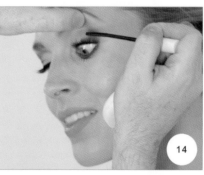

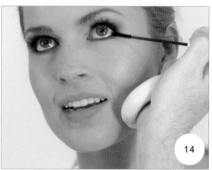

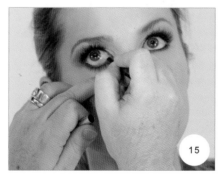

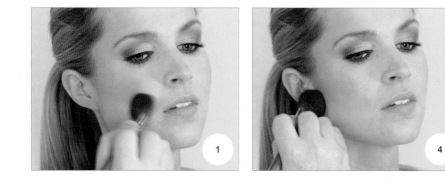

cheeks

1. Using your #73 bronzer/blush brush, apply your matte bronzer. Begin at the back of your cheekbone and sweep it forward toward the apple of your cheek. Then take the brush back toward your ear. This lays your color in place.

2. Now take your brush and use it in the opposite direction (up and down) to blend. Be sure to blend well, or it won't look natural.

3. Don't forget to add a little at the temples to help shape your face. Sweep the bronzing powder up around the temples and eye sockets. This always gives the face more color and gives you a glow.

4. Also, feel free to blend some bronzer along your jawbone. This also helps create that glow and defines your face.

"you don't have to go dark to go dramatic."

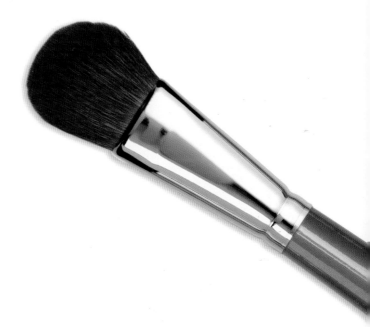

lips

1. Here, you want your lips to be soft, but well defined. Start by concealing your lip and lip line. This gives you the perfect pale canvas for your subtle lip look.

2. Now, using a barely-there nude lip pencil, line your lips. Begin with a V in the "cupid's bow," or center curve, of the lips. Bring the liner up and around the curves of your bow.

3. Next, starting at the outer corners, move toward the center with your pencil.

4. On the lower lip, first accentuate the lower curve of the lip. Then begin from the outer corners, moving toward the center. Remember to use your entire lip: Take the color to the almost invisible line just at the edge of the colored part of your lips.

5. Make sure you fill in at least halfway toward the center of your lip. This will help your lip liner look more natural and your lip color last longer.

6. Using a #80 lip brush, blend your liner before you apply your lip gloss. This will also make it look more natural.

7. End with a quick sweep of the perfect sheer peach lip gloss to make your lips shiny, fuller looking, and sexy. Make sure you apply your gloss with your #80 lip brush because if you apply gloss with a brush, it will look shinier.

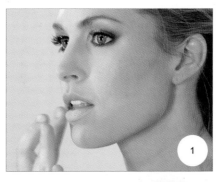
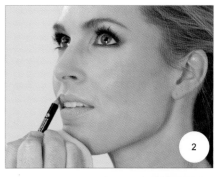
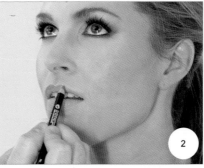
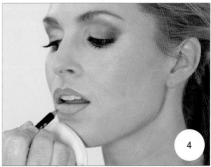
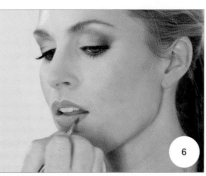
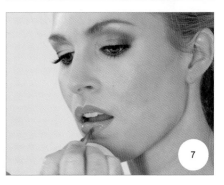

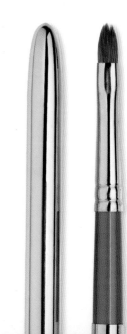

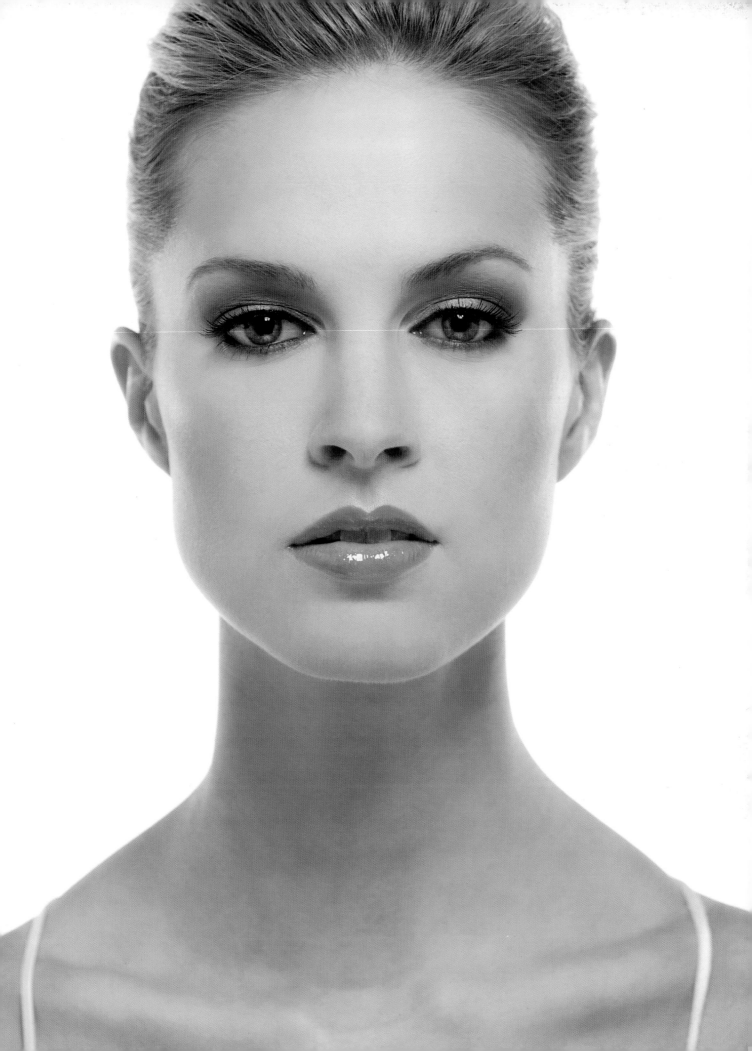

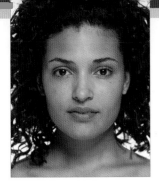

delicate glamour

An evening look does not have to push the limits to be dramatic. As I always say, sometimes you just need to know what to draw attention to. This look is all about the power of retro glamorous eyes and lips. The eyelid has the subtlest definition and a strong, defined lash line. Let's not forget a mouth that grabs attention, but in all the right ways. Yes, you too can create that perfect "modern retro" look for evening!

Here's how to get this look:

eyes

1. Using your #22 highlighting brush, apply a shimmery gold eye shadow to your lid to create a soft sheen.

2. Next, with the same brush, apply a matte flesh eye shadow to your brow bone. (Remember, when I say brow bone, I mean the area just under the arch of your brow.)

3. With this look, you want your midtone eye shadow to be very precise so as not to darken your lid, yet define the shape. Because this look has such an intense lip and dramatic liner, you want your lid soft and shimmery. Using your #13 detail eye shadow brush, apply your matte ginger midtone eye shadow in your crease. Starting from the outside corner of your crease, glide your brush across to the inside corner, creating a distinct line all along your crease.

4. Use your #28 blending brush (the one that is always clean and ready to blend with) and blend your midtone so that there are no hard edges. Just retrace the same area that you just applied your midtone to, rather than blending it up and down and darkening too much of your lid.

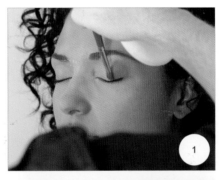

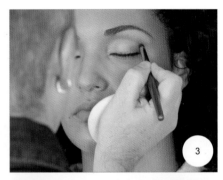

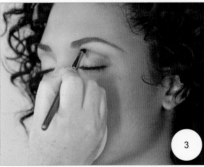

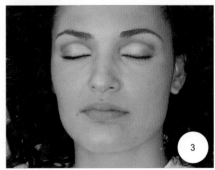

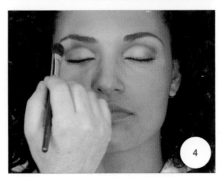

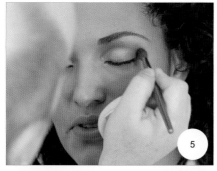

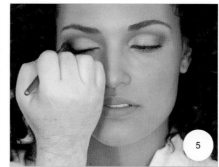

5. With your #11 shadow brush, apply midtone just to the very outer edge of your lid. Now blend with your #28 brush, making sure to be careful and keeping the color to the very outer edge of your lid.

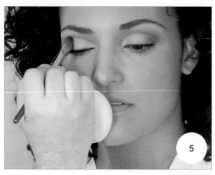

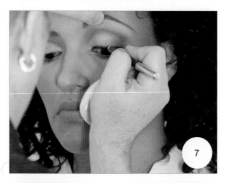

6. It's time to curl your eyelashes and apply the first layer of mascara to your top lashes. (See page 42 to review how to curl properly.)

7. Now you want to create that perfect dramatic liner along your top lid. The trick to perfection is layering it in steps. Even pros prefer to layer. First step, you begin to create a pattern with a black eyeliner pencil because it is easier to remove and start over if you make a mistake. Starting at the inside corner of your top lash line, slowly move across the lash line. Make sure your line is its most narrow at the inside corner, gradually getting thicker as you reach the outside corner. As you reach the outside corner, you can give it a little "kick" upward.

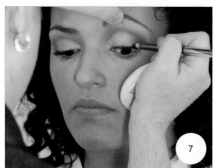

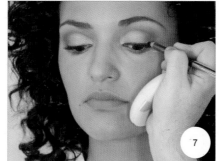

8. Because you are about to use a very dark eye shadow to fine-tune your liner, using your #76 powder brush, apply a bit of powder under the eye to catch any shadow spills. When you are finished, you can just brush the powder and any shadow drips away and you still have flawless skin.

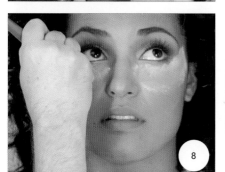

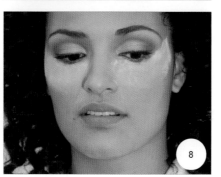

"sometimes you just need to know what to draw attention to."

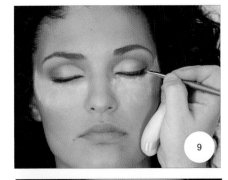

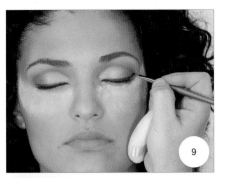

9. Your penciling probably won't be perfect, and it doesn't have to be because you are now going to trace over it with a matte black eye shadow and your #41 eyeliner brush to perfect your pattern.

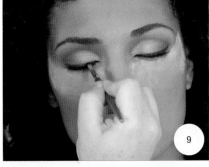

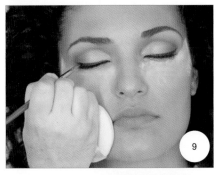

10. I know your line looks perfect now, but it's still not dramatic enough! So you need to go over your pattern with your liquid or gel eyeliner. Because you created the pattern, even if your liquid isn't perfect, it won't show. Using your #42 eyeliner brush, apply your liquid or gel, starting from the inside corner and working toward the outside corner. Follow your pattern. That wasn't so hard, was it?

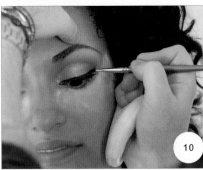

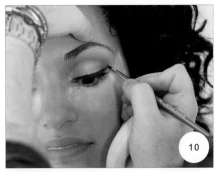

11. Next, with your #76 brush, remove the powder from under your eye, and with it will go all the shadow fallout.

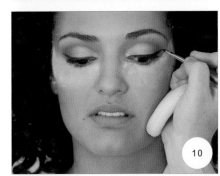

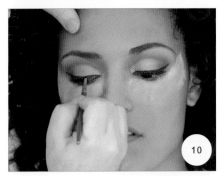

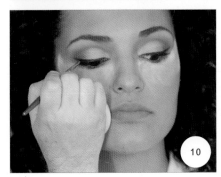

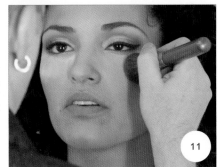

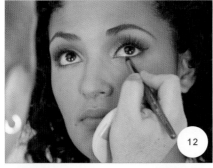

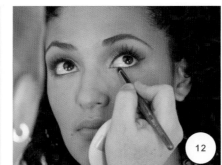

12. Now grab your #13 detail eye shadow brush and apply your midtone eye shadow all along your lower lash line. Start your application from the outside corner, sweeping it across to the inside corner. This will give you subtle definition and give a modern twist to this classic eye application.

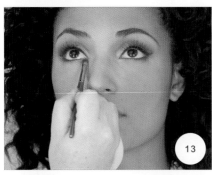

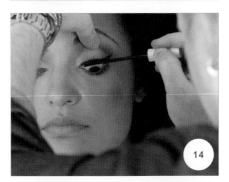

13. Using your #14 detail highlighting brush, highlight the inside corner of the lower lash line. Because there is so little color to this look, this step really brightens the eye and opens it up to give you a wide-eyed effect.

14. Now it's time for another layer of mascara on your top and your lower lashes. (See page 44 to review how to layer your mascara properly.)

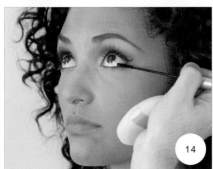

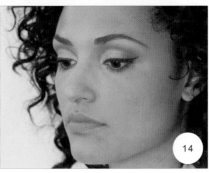

cheeks

Because this look is all about the eyes and lips, I prefer to leave the cheeks completely natural.

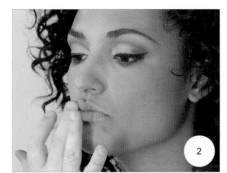

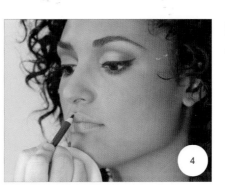

lips

1. This lip is very dramatic, and to help it look its most perfect, you need to prep your lips first. You want them to appear sumptuous and smooth, so before you start your color application, moisturize them with lip balm. This will help the color go on smoothly and evenly. After the balm has had a bit of time to soak in, blot off the excess with a tissue so that it won't reduce the staying power of your lipstick.

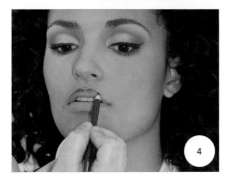

2. Now, using concealer, conceal your lip and along your lip line.

3. Next, powder your lips. This gives you the perfect canvas to now apply your dramatic lip, so that the edge of the lip is very crisp.

4. Grab your burgundy lip pencil and begin with a V in the "cupid's bow," or center curve, of the lips. Bring the liner up and around the curves of your bow.

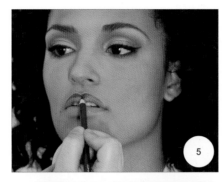

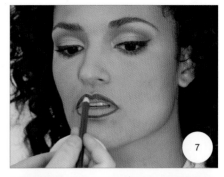

5. Next, starting at the outer corners, move toward the center with your pencil.

6. On the lower lip, first accentuate the lower curve of the lip. Then begin from the outer corners, moving toward the center. Remember to use your entire lip: Take the color to the almost invisible line just at the edge of the colored part of your lips.

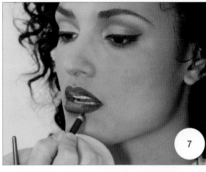

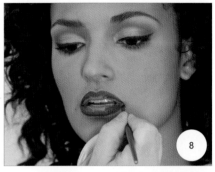

7. Now fill in your entire lip with your lip pencil, except the very center. This will help create dimension in a really dark lip. The lip liner will help your lip color last and stay in place because lip liner is a drier texture than lipstick.

8. With your #80 lip brush, blend your lip liner so that it is even and smooth.

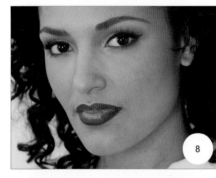

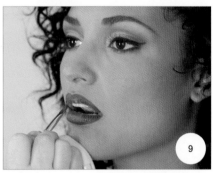

9. Next, using your lip brush, apply your deep russet lipstick to your entire lip, making sure you blend really well over your lip liner.

10. Now take a tissue and blot your lips. This will remove the moisture from the lipstick, but leave you with a layer of pigment. Then apply another layer of lipstick. Applying these three layers (one of liner and two of lipstick) will help your color be true and intense, as well as last longer.

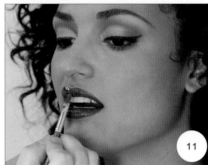

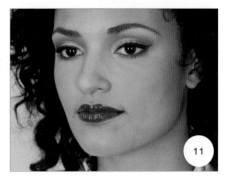

11. End with a quick sweep of the perfect burgundy lip gloss to make your lips shiny, fuller looking, and sexy. Make sure you apply your gloss with your #80 lip brush because if you apply gloss with a brush, it will look shinier.

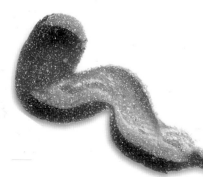

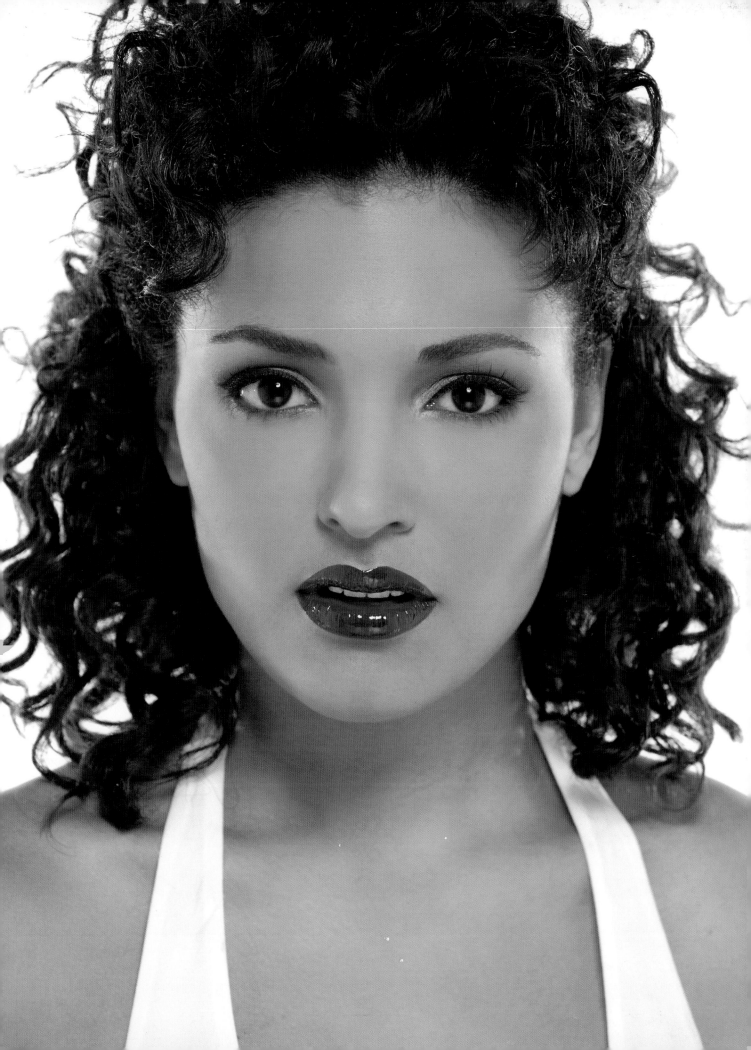

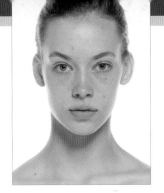

copper mist

There are so many ways to wear a smoky eye. I love this version because it is a nice twist. The copper shade really brings out those blue eyes! Because it's so subtle, it's easy to wear, even when you want to be a drama queen for daytime. Play with this application and feel free to try this technique with other fun shades.

Here's how to get this look:

eyes

1. Using your #22 highlighting brush, apply a shimmer champagne eye shadow powder to your lid and brow bone. (Remember, when I say brow bone, I mean the area just under the arch of your brow.) Start with champagne because even though you're doing a smoky eye, you want it to be a bit softer.

2. It's time to curl your eyelashes and apply the first layer of mascara to your top lashes. (See page 42 to review how to curl properly.)

3. Using your #11 midtone brush and a matte midtone eye shadow and starting from the outside corner of your crease, glide your brush across to the inside corner. Use a matte taupe shadow (a shade just a bit darker than your skin tone) so that you get soft definition.

4. Use your #28 blending brush (the one that is always clean and ready to blend with) and blend your midtone so that there are no hard edges.

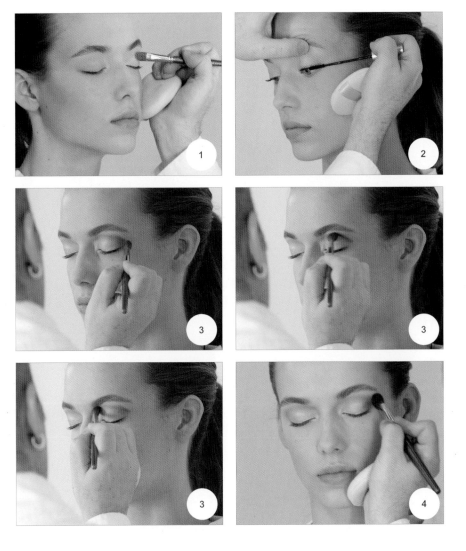

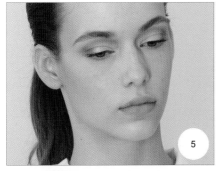

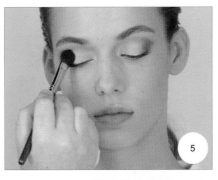

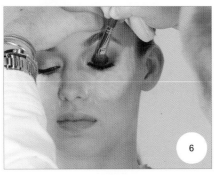

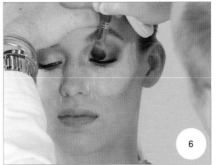

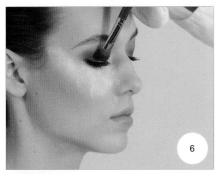

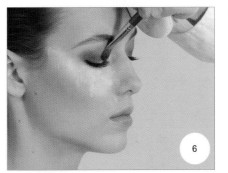

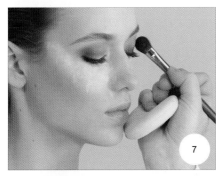

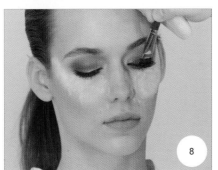

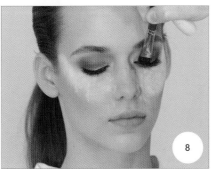

5. Grab your #30 contour brush and some midtone eye shadow and define the outer third of your eyelid. Follow with your #28 brush to blend.

6. With your #27 shadow brush, apply a shimmery copper eye shadow starting at the base of your lash line and bring your color across and up to your crease. You are getting a higher concentration of color at the lash line, fading away as you work to the crease.

7. Use your #28 brush to blend your midtone so that there are no hard edges.

8. With your #18 eyeliner brush, grab some black eye shadow and lay it all along your top lash line for definition. As you apply, be sure to pull up with your brush to blend the color.

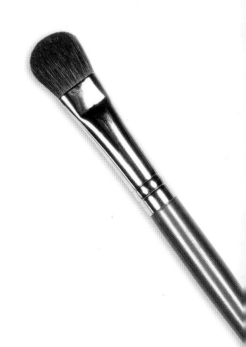

9. Now, grab your #30 contour brush and apply a shimmery burgundy eye shadow right along the lash line.

10. Follow all the shadows with your #28 blending brush to blend and create the perfect fade. Remember, your goal is to make the color darkest at the lash line, then slowly fading as you go up toward the brow.

11. Next, grab your #13 detail eye shadow brush and apply your midtone eye shadow all along your lower lash line. Once again, start your application from the outside corner, sweeping it across to the inside corner.

12. With your #18 brush, lay black eye shadow right into the base of your lower lashes.

13. Follow with your #13 brush and retrace all along your lower lash line, again from the outside corner toward the inside corner, with a touch of the shimmery burgundy to blend it all together and create more smoke.

14. Now, with a black eyeliner, line the waterline of your lower lid. (Remember, the waterline is the inner rim above the lower lash line.) This will add just a little bit more drama to your smoky eye.

15. Now it's time for another layer of mascara on your top lashes and a layer on your lower lashes. After you finish the rest of your makeup, add yet another layer to the top lashes. Remember, with this look lush lashes are very important, so you want to really layer your mascara on your top lashes. (See page 44 to review how to layer your mascara properly.)

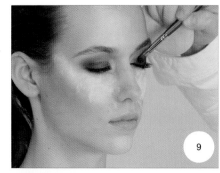

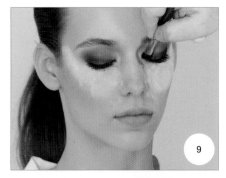

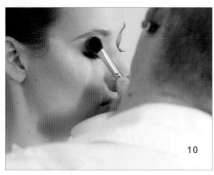

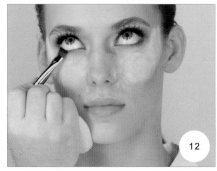

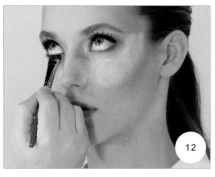

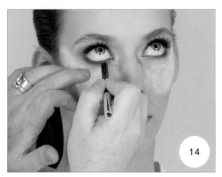

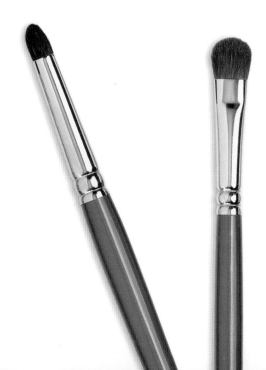

cheeks

1. Because the eyes are so dramatic in this look, your cheeks need to be soft. You only need a bit of bronzer for definition. Using your #73 bronzer/blush brush, apply your matte bronzer, beginning at the back of your cheekbone and sweeping it forward toward the apple of your cheek. Then take the brush back toward your ear. This lays your color in place.

2. Now take your brush and use it in the opposite direction (up and down) to blend. Be sure to blend well, or it won't look natural.

3. Don't forget to add a little at the temples to help shape your face. Sweep the bronzing powder up around the temples and eye sockets. This always gives the face more color and gives you a glow.

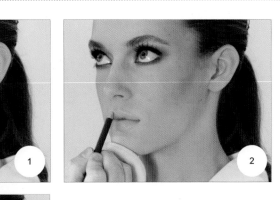

lips

1. Here, you want your lips to be soft, but well defined. Start by concealing your lip and lip line. This gives you the perfect pale canvas for your subtle lip look.

2. Using a pale pink lip pencil, line your lips. Begin with a V in the "cupid's bow," or center curve, of the lips. Bring the liner up and around the curves of your cupid's bow.

3. Next, starting at the outer corners, move toward the center with your pencil.

4. On the lower lip, first accentuate the lower curve of the lip. Then begin from the outer corners, moving toward the center. Remember to use your entire lip: Take the color to the almost invisible line just at the edge of the colored part of your lips.

5. Make sure you fill in your entire lip with your lip pencil. This will help your lip liner look more natural and your lip color last longer.

"it's so subtle, it's easy to wear, even when you want to be a drama queen for daytime."

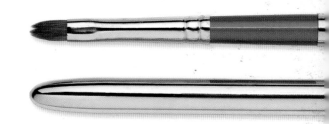

6. Using a #80 lip brush, blend your liner before you apply your lip gloss. This will also make it look more natural.

7. End with a sweep of the perfect pale pink lip gloss to make your lips shiny, fuller looking, and sexy. Make sure you apply your gloss with your #80 lip brush because if you apply gloss with a brush, it will look shinier.

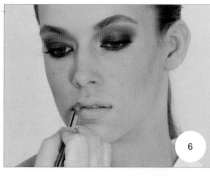 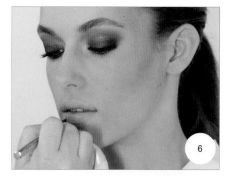

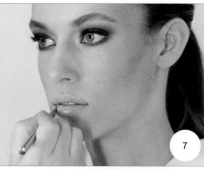 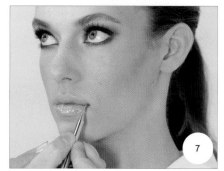

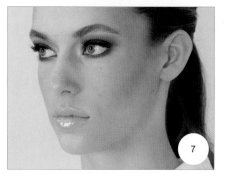

"try this technique with other fun shades."

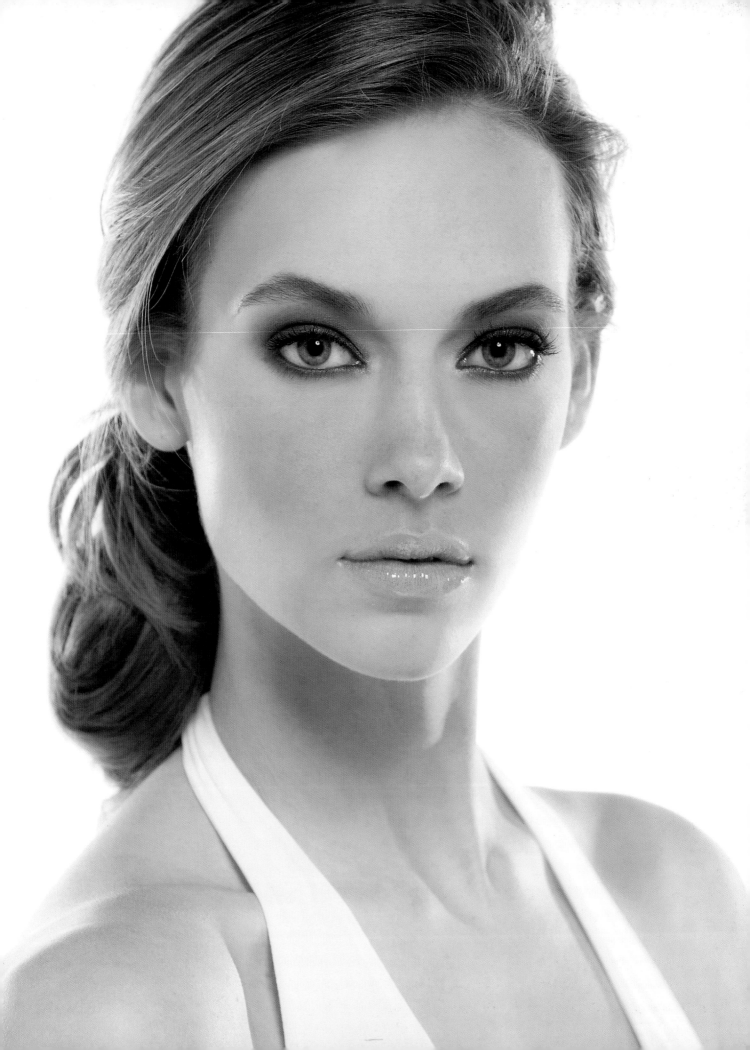

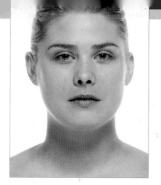

stand out in the crowd

The eyes are the windows to the soul, so why not draw attention to your soul? This look is definitely the way to get everyone's attention. Defined eyes, subtle cheeks, and shiny lips—talk about perfection! This is smoky without going too dark. Pay attention to the play of textures, which is part of what makes this look work. Go ahead and enjoy a night out where everyone in the room wants to meet you!

Here's how to get this look:

eyes

1. Using your #22 highlighting brush, apply a matte beige eye shadow just to your brow bone. (Remember, when I say brow bone, I mean the area just under the arch of your brow.)

2. With a #27 eye shadow brush (because you will be applying your color to a large area), apply a dark matte taupe midtone eye shadow. Start at the base of your upper lash line and bring the color up and over your entire lid, all the way up to just under your brow bone. By starting along your lash line and working your way upward, you will get the highest concentration of color where you laid your brush first, making your color deeper at the lash line.

3. Again using your #27 brush, apply more midtone eye shadow in a half-moon shape all along the crease to create more definition.

4. Use your #28 blending brush (the one that is always clean and ready to blend with) and blend your midtone so that there are no hard edges.

5. It's time to curl your eyelashes and apply the first layer of mascara to your top lashes. (See page 42 to review how to curl properly.)

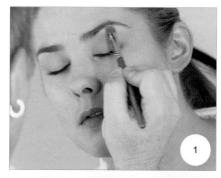

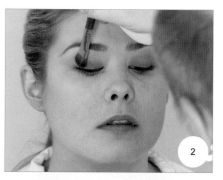

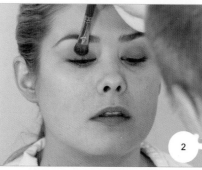

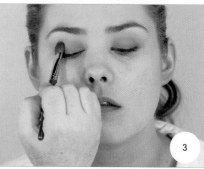

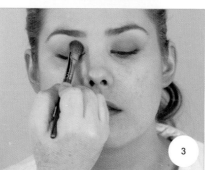

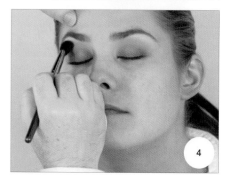

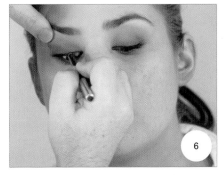

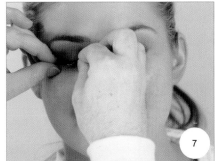

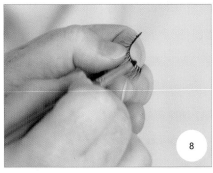

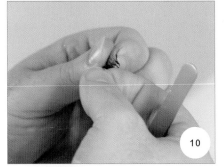

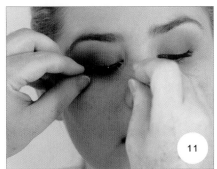

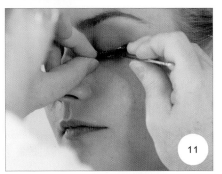

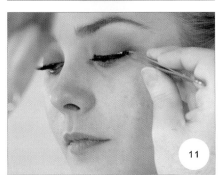

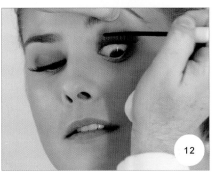

6. Now it's time to get ready to apply false eyelashes! First, with your black eyeliner, draw a thin line across your upper eyelid right along your lash line. This helps you know where to place your false eyelashes and helps conceal the lash band. This way, even if you don't get the false lash in place directly against your natural lashes, no one will know because the liner will ensure that no skin shows between your natural lashes and the false ones.

7. Measure and trim the outside end of your false eyelashes to fit the width of your eyelid. Usually strip lashes, when used straight from their container, are too wide for most eyes. Trimming them will help them fit better and feel much more comfortable.

8. Paint the lash band with black gel or liquid liner to also help in hiding it once it's on.

9. Apply eyelash glue to the false eyelashes all along the band.

10. Allow the glue to dry for a minute so that it will get tacky (slightly sticky). As you allow it to dry a bit, roll the lash to help shape it to fit your lid better.

11. Now place the lash right on top of your eyeliner. Using the handle end of a pair of tweezers, push the lash right up against your natural lash line.

12. Once the glue has dried, apply a coat of mascara to blend your natural lashes with the false ones.

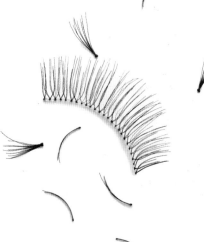

"talk about perfection!"

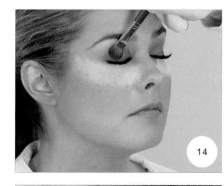 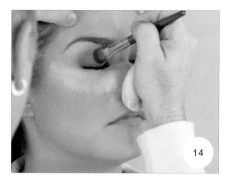

13. Because you are about to use a very dark color, using your #76 powder brush, apply a bit of powder under the eye to catch any spills. That way, when you are finished, you can just brush the powder and the shadow drippings away and still have flawless skin.

14. Now with your #27 shadow brush and using a dark shimmery gray eye shadow, start at the base of your lash line and bring your color up and over your entire lid to your crease. This gives you the most intense color right at your lash line.

15. Again, use your #27 brush to apply more of the dark shimmery gray eye shadow in a half-moon shape all along your crease and on your lid. Pat it on to give you more intense color application.

16. Use your #28 blending brush (the one that is always clean and ready to blend with) and blend your contour so that there are no hard edges.

17. With your #30 contour brush, apply another layer of gray eye shadow right along your lash line.

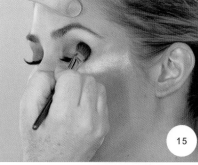 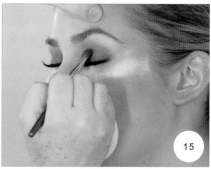

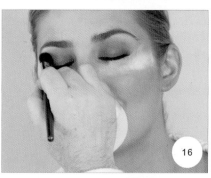 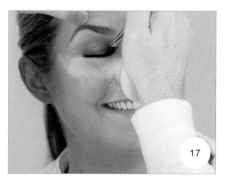

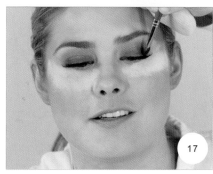 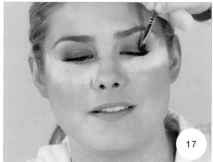

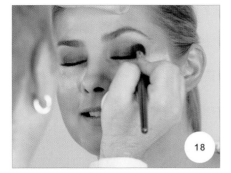

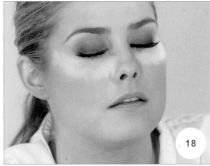

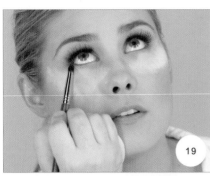

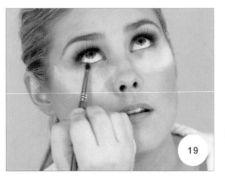

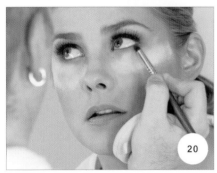

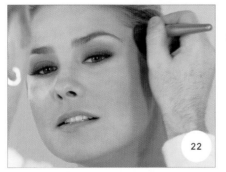

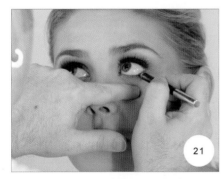

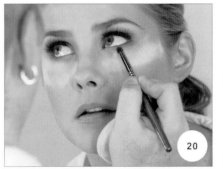

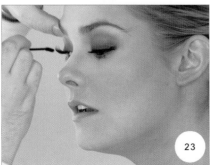

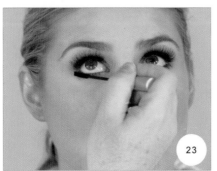

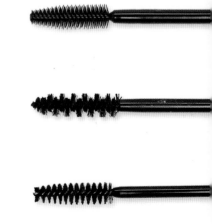

18. Follow with your #28 brush to blend.

19. Now, grab your #13 detail eye shadow brush and apply your midtone eye shadow all along your lower lash line. Once again, start your application from the outside corner, sweeping it across to the inside corner.

20. With that same detail eye shadow brush, apply a layer of your contour color right over your midtone all along your bottom lash line. By layering on your midtone, then your contour on top of it, you are creating a gradation of color, making your lower lash line definition look more natural and blended.

21. Now with a black eyeliner, line the water- line of your lower lid. (Remember, the waterline is the inner rim above the lower lash line.) This will add just a little bit more drama to your smoky eye.

22. With your #76 brush, remove all the pow- der under your eyes, and with the pow- der will go all the shadow fallout.

23. Finally, apply a layer of mascara to your bottom lashes.

cheeks

1. Using your #73 bronzer/blush brush, apply your matte bronzer. Begin at the back of your cheekbone and sweep it forward toward the apple of your cheek. Then take the brush back toward your ear. This lays your color in place.

2. Now take your brush and use it in the opposite direction (up and down) to blend. Be sure to blend well, or it won't look natural.

3. Don't forget to add a little at the temples to help shape your face. Sweep the bronzing powder up around the temples and eye sockets. This always gives the face more color and gives you a glow.

4. Also, feel free to blend some bronzer along your jawbone. This also helps create that glow and defines your face.

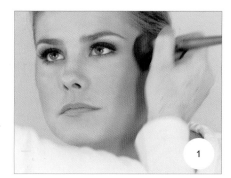

lips

1. End with a quick sweep of the perfect sheer peach lip gloss to make your lips shiny, fuller looking, and sexy. Make sure you apply your gloss with your #80 lip brush because if you apply gloss with a brush, it will look shinier.

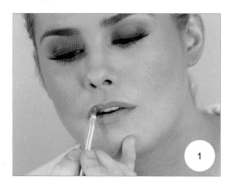

"go ahead and enjoy a night out where everyone in the room wants to meet you!"

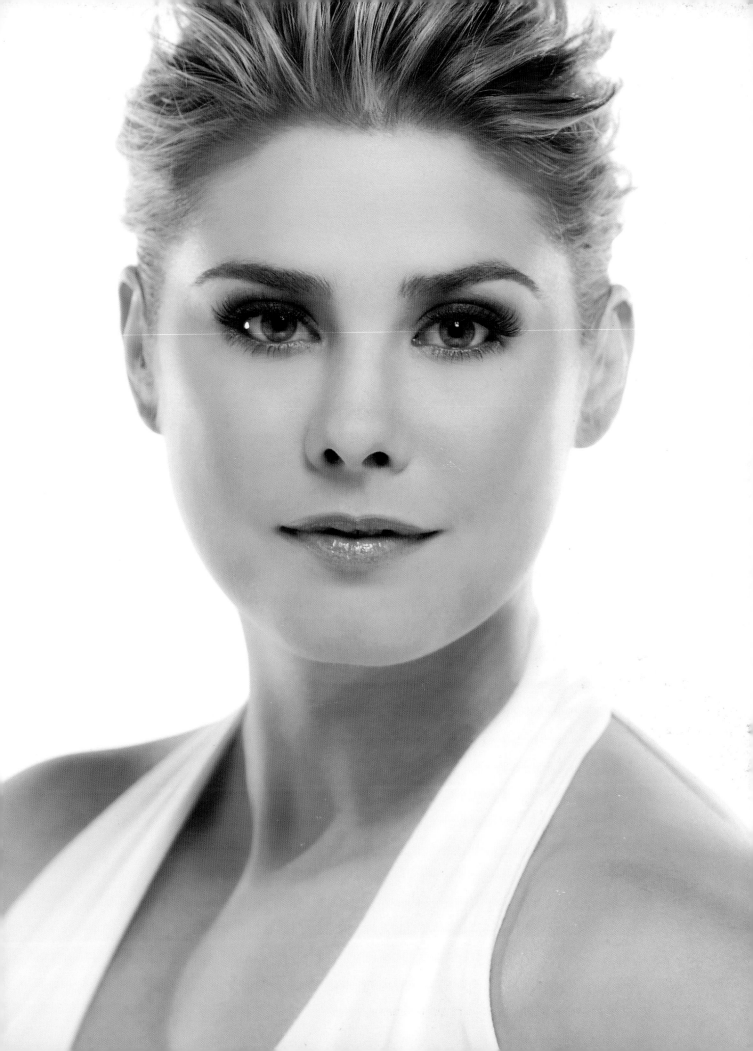

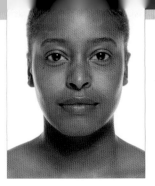

alter ego

There are so many times when you want to try something totally out of your comfort zone but are too afraid. That's when it's time to call on your alter ego. You know, the one that is scared of nothing. Give her a name and paint her up and take her out! She is not afraid of color, especially when it is applied in a way that is foolproof and attention-grabbing. You know what you want, so go for it!

Here's how to get this look:

eyes

1. With your #22 highlighting brush, apply a matte flesh eye shadow to your brow bone. (Remember, when I say brow bone, I mean the area just under the arch of your brow.)

2. Now grab your #14 detail highlighting brush and apply a shimmery acid-green crème-to-powder shadow to the inner third of your lid. With this look, you are going to do a lot of layering of crème and powder to make the color pop.

3. Next, with your #22 brush, apply a light shimmery blue crème-to-powder eye shadow to the outer two-thirds of your eyelid.

4. With the same brush, apply a shimmery acid-green eye shadow powder directly on top of the crème you applied earlier.

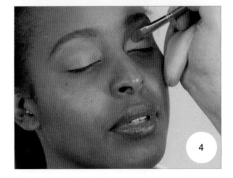

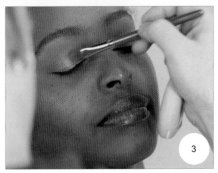

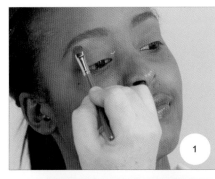

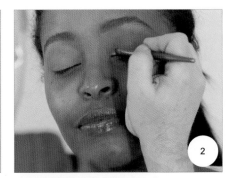

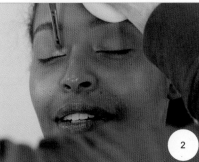

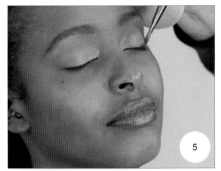

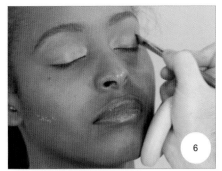

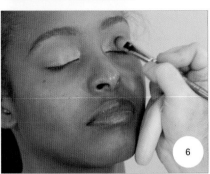

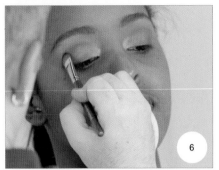

5. Again with your #22 brush, apply a matte dark blue crème-to-powder eye shadow, starting at the outer lash line and blending upward.

6. Now create a half-moon shape all along the crease to get a defined crease.

7. Next, grab your #27 shadow brush and layer a dark shimmery blue eye shadow powder over your crème. Start at the lash line and blend it up toward the crease and across the outer two-thirds of your lid.

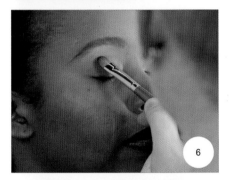

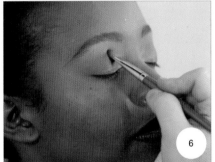

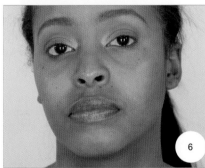

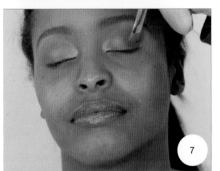

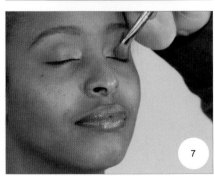

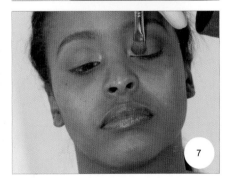

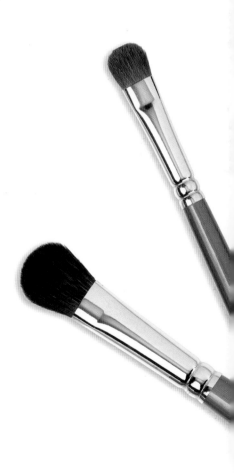

8. Now pat on more in a half-moon shape all along your crease.

9. Using your #28 eye shadow blending brush, blend everything together to get that perfect fade.

10. With your #28 brush, grab a little midtone eye shadow, a matte ginger, and blend it onto the inner third of your crease. This helps ground all your bright color.

11. To give your lash line a little more punch, start by lining your upper lash line with a black eyeliner. Begin at the inside corner, taking it all the way to the outside corner. Keep it really close to your lash line. You want it to be thinnest on the inside, then to slowly get just the slightest bit thicker as you get to the outside corner.

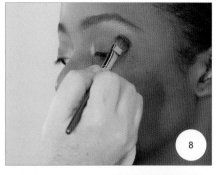

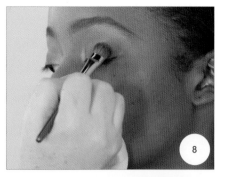

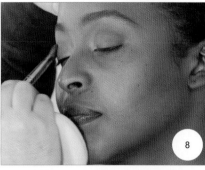

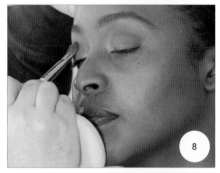

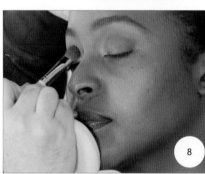

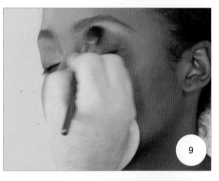

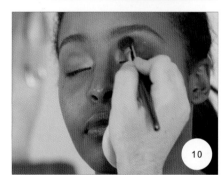

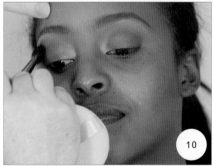

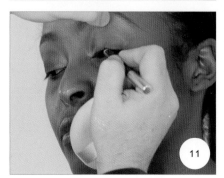

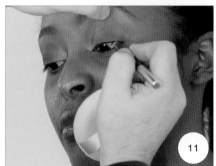

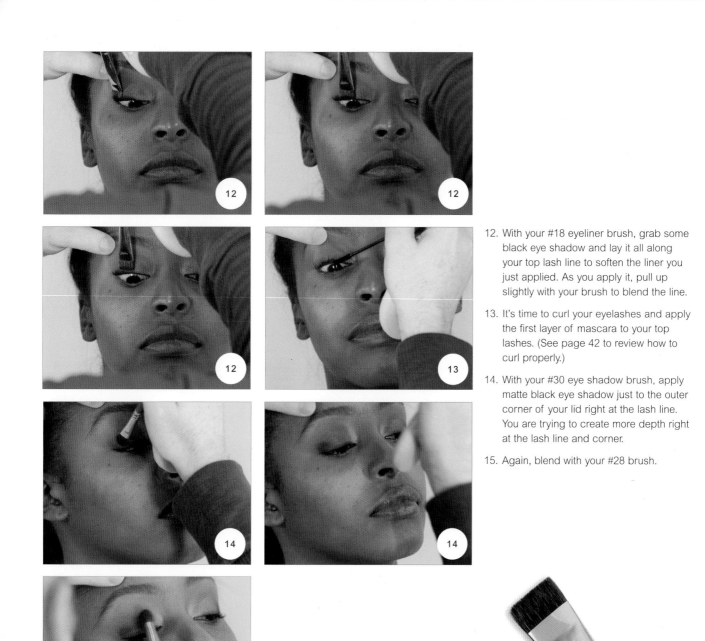

12. With your #18 eyeliner brush, grab some black eye shadow and lay it all along your top lash line to soften the liner you just applied. As you apply it, pull up slightly with your brush to blend the line.

13. It's time to curl your eyelashes and apply the first layer of mascara to your top lashes. (See page 42 to review how to curl properly.)

14. With your #30 eye shadow brush, apply matte black eye shadow just to the outer corner of your lid right at the lash line. You are trying to create more depth right at the lash line and corner.

15. Again, blend with your #28 brush.

"you know what you want, so go for it!"

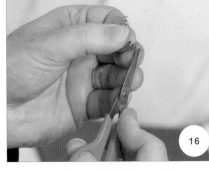

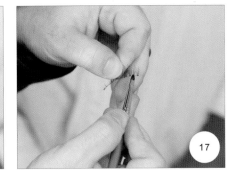

16. It's time for some false eyelashes. Measure and trim the outside end of your false eyelashes to fit the width of your eyelid. Strip lashes, when used straight from their container, are too wide for most eyes. Trimming them will help them fit better and feel more comfortable.

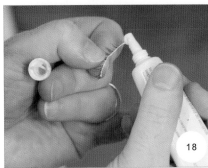

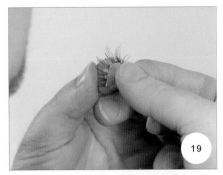

17. Paint the lash band with black gel or liquid liner to also help in hiding it once it's on.

18. Apply eyelash glue to the false eyelashes all along the band.

19. Allow the glue to dry for a minute so that it will get tacky (slightly sticky). As you allow it to dry a bit, roll the lash to help shape it to fit your lid better.

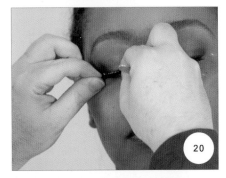

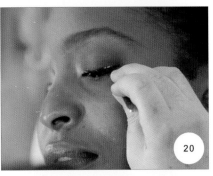

20. Now place the lash right on top of your eyeliner. Using the handle end of a pair of tweezers, push the lash right up against your natural lash line.

21. Using your #14 detail highlighting brush, highlight the inside corner of the lower lash line with your shimmery acid-green eye shadow.

22. Now grab your #13 detail eye shadow brush and apply a matte ginger midtone all along your lower lash line. Once again, start your application from the outside corner, sweeping it across to the inside corner.

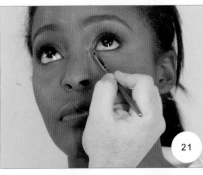

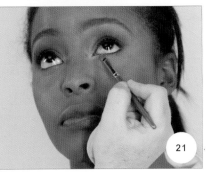

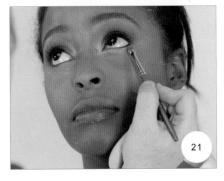

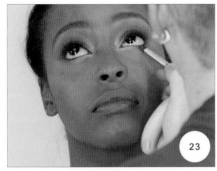

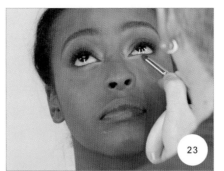

23. With that same detail eye shadow brush, apply a layer of your dark shimmery blue contour color right over your midtone all along your bottom lash line. By layering on your midtone, then your contour on top of it, you are creating a gradation of color, making your lower lash line definition look more natural and blended.

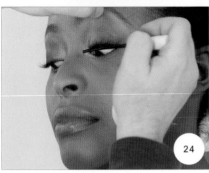

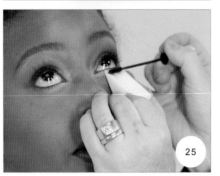

24. Once the glue has dried, apply a coat of mascara to blend your natural lashes with the false ones.

25. Finish your eyes with a layer of mascara on your bottom lashes.

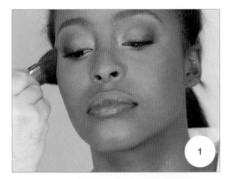

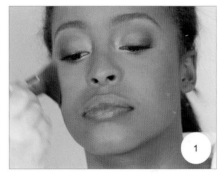

cheeks

1. Using your #73 bronzer/blush brush, apply your matte bronzer. Begin at the back of your cheekbone and sweep it forward toward the apple of your cheek. Then take the brush back towards your ear. This lays your color in place.

2. Now take your brush and use it in the opposite direction (up and down) to blend. Be sure to blend well, or it won't look natural.

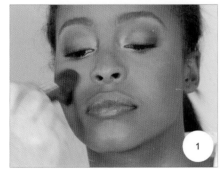

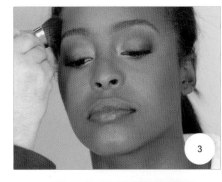

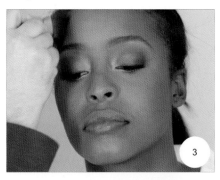

3. Don't forget to add a little at the temples to help shape your face. Sweep the bronzing powder up around the temples and eye sockets. This always gives the face more color and gives you a glow.

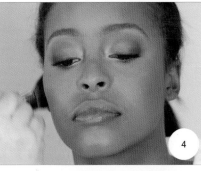

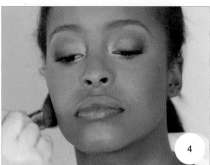

4. Also, feel free to blend some bronzer along your jawbone. This also helps create that glow and defines your face.

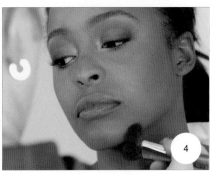

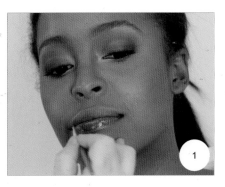

lips

1. End with a quick sweep of the perfect sheer raisin lip gloss to make your lips shiny, fuller looking, and sexy. Make sure you apply your gloss with your #80 lip brush because if you apply gloss with a brush, it will look shinier.

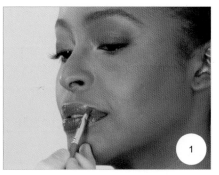

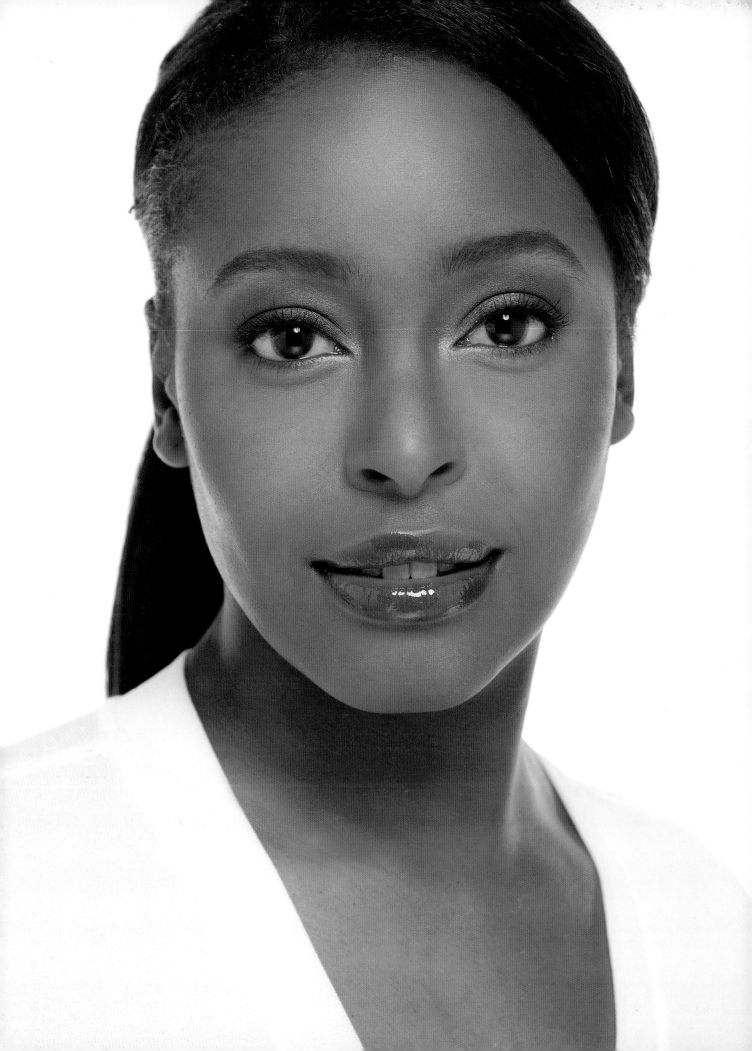

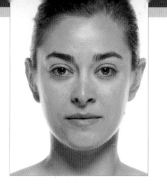

spiced beauty

Talk about spicing up your look! Using warm russet colors will really bring out your eye color. Surrounding your eyes with warmth will just make them glow. After all, girls, everyone could use a little spice in her life! Experiment with colors you may have never considered before. You can see what it did for our model; now see what it can do for you.

Here's how to get this look:

eyes

1. With a #27 eye shadow brush (because you will be applying your color to a large area), apply a dark matte taupe midtone eye shadow. Start at the base of your upper lash line and bring the color up and over your entire lid, all the way up to just under your brow bone. (Remember, when I say brow bone, I mean the area just under the arch of your brow.) By starting along your lash line and working your way upward, you will get the highest concentration of color where you laid your brush first, making your color deeper at the lash line.

2. Use your #28 blending brush (the one that is always clean and ready to blend with) and blend your midtone so that there are no hard edges.

3. It's time to curl your eyelashes and apply the first layer of mascara to your top lashes. (See page 42 to review how to curl properly.)

4. Because you are about to use a very dark color, using your #76 powder brush, apply a bit of powder under the eye to catch any spills. Then, when you are finished, you can just brush the powder and the shadow drippings away and still have flawless skin.

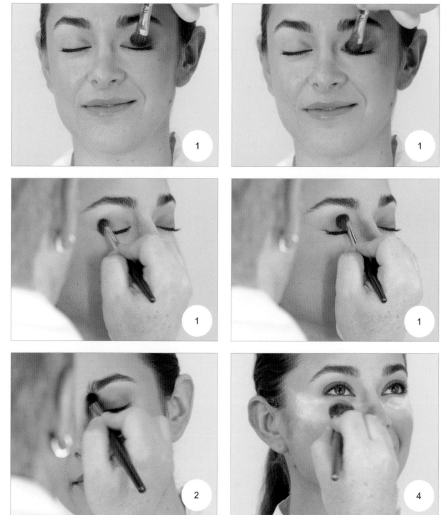

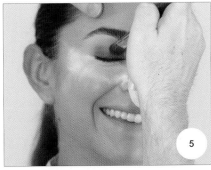

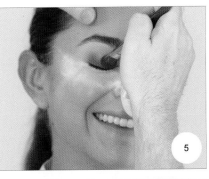

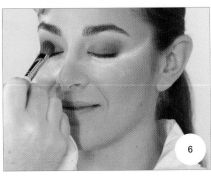

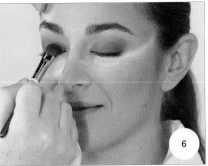

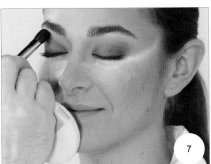

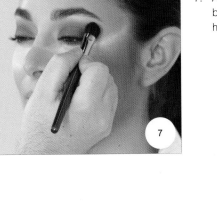

5. With your #27 brush, using a shimmery terra-cotta eye shadow, start at the base of your lash line and bring your color up and over your entire lid up to your crease. Again, this is giving you the most intense color right at your lash line.

6. Use your #27 brush to apply more shimmery terra-cotta eye shadow in a half-moon shape all along your crease and on your lid. Pat it on to give you more intense color application.

7. Again, use your #28 blending brush to blend your contour so that there are no hard edges.

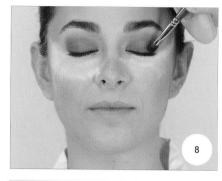
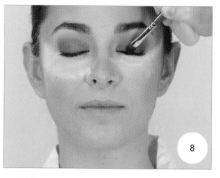

8. With your #30 contour brush, apply shimmery burgundy eye shadow right along your lash line.

9. Follow with your #28 brush to blend.

10. Now it's time to get ready to apply false eyelashes! First, using your #18 eyeliner brush and black eye shadow, draw a line across your upper eyelid right along your lash line. This helps you know where to place the false eyelashes and helps conceal the lash band. This way, even if you don't get the false lashes in place directly against your natural lashes, no one will know because the liner will ensure that no skin shows between your natural lashes and the false ones.

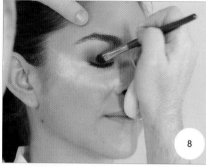
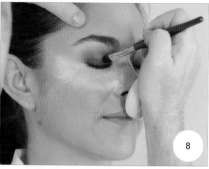

11. Measure and trim the outside end of your false eyelashes to fit the width of your eyelid. Usually strip lashes, when used straight from their container, are too wide for most eyes. Trimming them will help them fit better and feel more comfortable.

12. Paint the lash band with black gel or liquid liner to also help hide it once it's on.

13. Apply eyelash glue to the false eyelashes all along the band.

14. Allow the glue to dry for a minute so that it will get tacky (slightly sticky). As you allow it to dry a bit, roll the lash to help shape it to fit your lid better.

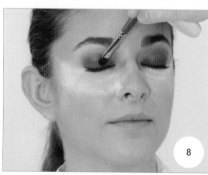
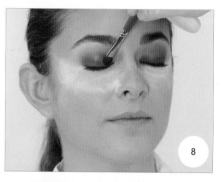

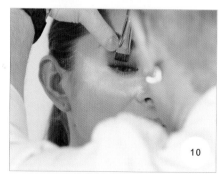
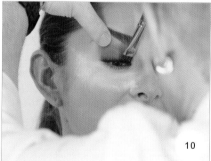

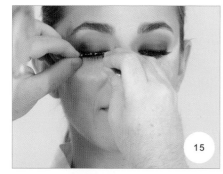

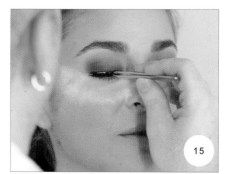

15. Now place the false lash right on top of your eyeliner. Using the handle end of a pair of tweezers, push the lash right up against your natural lash line.

16. Once the glue has dried, apply a coat of mascara to blend your natural lashes with the false ones.

17. With your #76 brush, remove all the powder under your eyes, and with the powder will go all the shadow fallout.

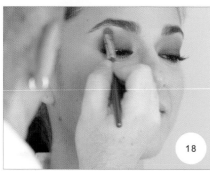

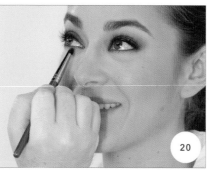

18. Using your #22 highlighting brush, apply a matte beige eye shadow just to your brow bone. You do this last to create a more defined edge to the smoky lid.

19. Now grab your #13 detail eye shadow brush and apply your midtone eye shadow all along your lower lash line. Once again, start your application from the outside corner, sweeping it across to the inside corner.

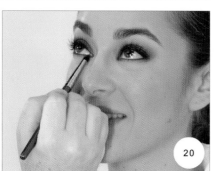

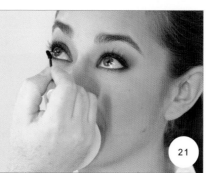

20. With that same detail eye shadow brush, apply a layer of your contour color right over your midtone all along your bottom lash line. By layering on your midtone, then your contour on top of it, you are creating a gradation of color, making your lower lash line definition look more natural and blended.

21. Finally, apply a layer of mascara to your bottom lashes.

"warm russet colors will really bring out your eye color."

cheeks

1. Using your #73 bronzer/blush brush, apply your matte bronzer. Begin at the back of your cheekbone and sweep it forward toward the apple of your cheek. Then take the brush back toward your ear. This lays your color in place.

2. Now take your brush and use it in the opposite direction (up and down) to blend. Be sure to blend well, or it won't look natural.

3. Don't forget to add a little at the temples to help shape your face. Sweep the bronzing powder up around the temples and eye sockets. This always gives the face more color and gives you a glow.

4. Also, feel free to blend some bronzer along your jawbone. This also helps create that glow and defines your face.

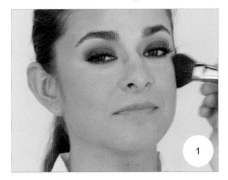
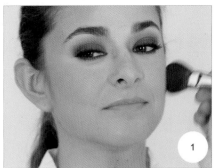

lips

1. You want your lips to be soft, but still well defined. Start by concealing your lip and lip line. This gives you the perfect pale canvas for your subtle lip look.

2. End with a quick sweep of the perfect sheer raisin lip gloss to make your lips shiny, fuller looking, and sexy. Make sure you apply your gloss with your #80 lip brush because if you apply gloss with a brush, it will look shinier.

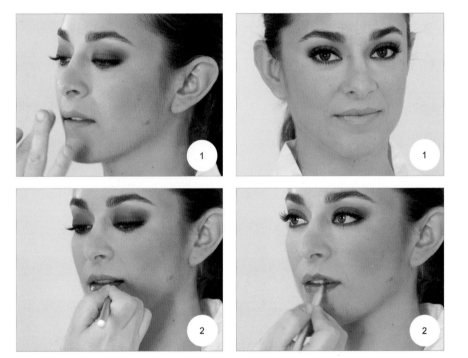

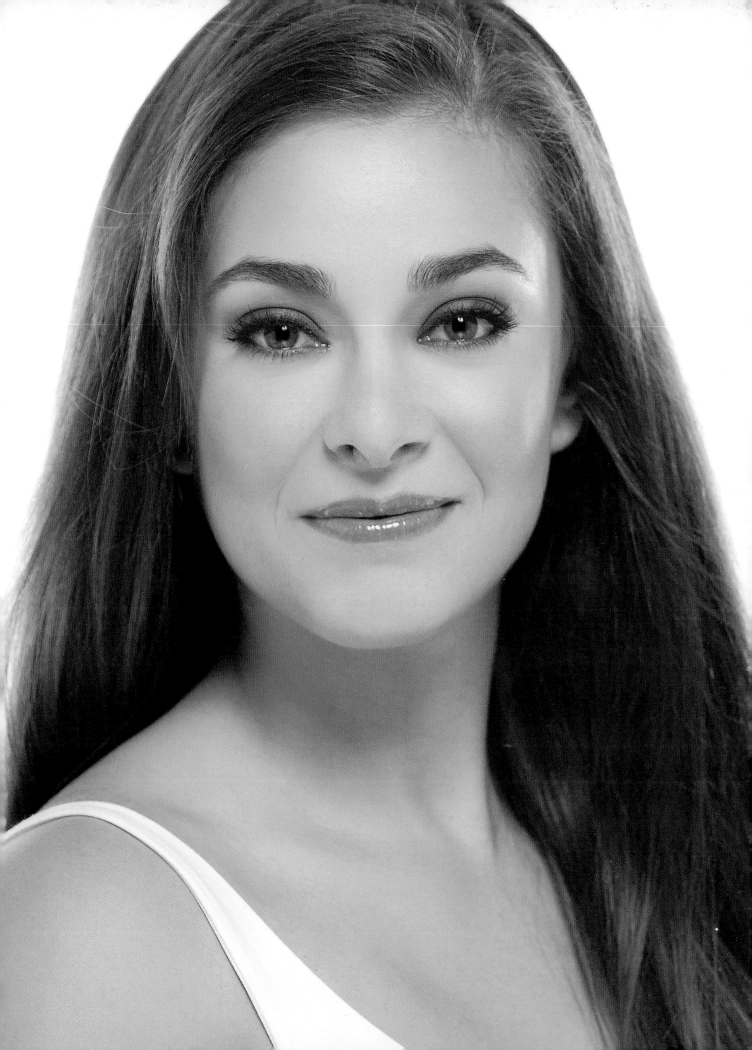

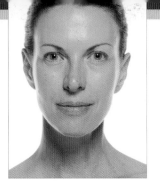

goodnight kiss

Talk about luscious lips—these lips are just crying to be kissed. But of course you won't want anyone to mess them up! This is a perfect look for when you want your lips to be the star of the evening. It's a great way to pair a dramatic eye and a dramatic lip, while still allowing your lips to stand out. Don't be afraid to play with color on your lips. Beauty is ageless.

Here's how to get this look:

eyes

1. Using your #22 highlight brush, apply a shimmery champagne eye shadow powder to your lid and brow bone. (Remember, when I say brow bone, I mean the area just under the arch of your brow.) You'll use the champagne first because even though you're doing a smoky eye, you want it to be soft.

2. Using your #11 midtone brush and a matte midtone eye shadow and starting from the outside corner of your crease, glide your brush across to the inside corner. Use a matte taupe shadow (a shade just a bit darker than your skin tone) so that you get soft definition.

3. Next, use your #28 blending brush (the one that is always clean and ready to blend with) and blend your midtone so that there are no hard edges.

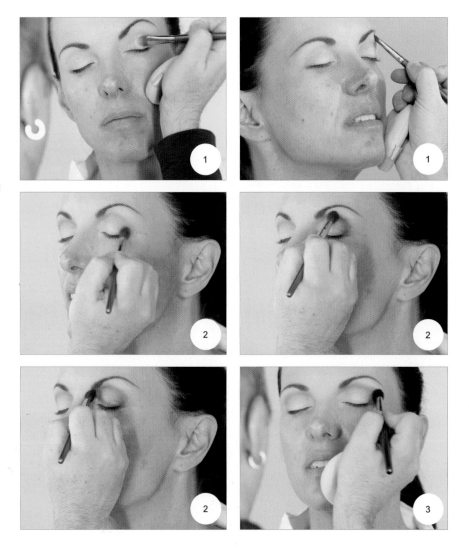

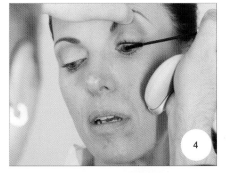

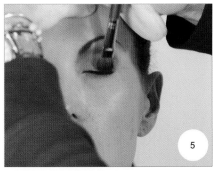

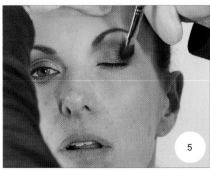

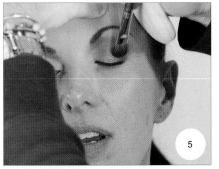

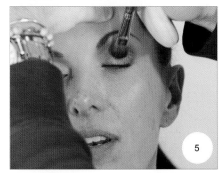

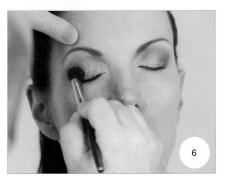

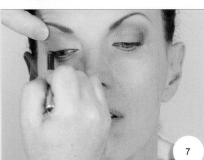

4. It's time to curl your eyelashes and apply the first layer of mascara to your top lashes. (See page 42 to review how to curl properly.)

5. Now, with your #27 shadow brush, apply a shimmery dark gray eye shadow; starting at the base of your lash line, bring your color up and over your entire lid up to your crease. This gives you the most intense color right at your lash line.

6. Use your #28 brush to blend your contour so that there are no hard edges.

7. Now it's time to put on your false eyelashes. First, with your black eyeliner, draw a thin line across your upper eyelid right along your lash line. This helps you know where to place the false lashes and helps conceal the lash band. This way, even if you don't get the false lash in place directly against your natural lashes, no one will know because the liner will ensure that no skin shows between your natural lashes and the false ones.

8. Next, using your #18 brush, set your liner with a matte black shadow.

9. Measure and trim the outside end of your false eyelashes to fit the width of your eyelid. Usually, strip lashes, when used straight from their container, are too wide for most eyes. Trimming them will help them fit better and feel more comfortable.

10. Paint the lash band with black gel or liquid liner to help disguise it once it's on.

11. Apply eyelash glue to the false eyelashes all along the band.

12. Allow the glue to dry for a minute so that it will get tacky (slightly sticky). As you allow it to dry a bit, roll the lash to help shape it to fit your lid better.

13. Now, place the lash right on top of your eyeliner. Using the handle end of a pair of tweezers, push the lash right up against your natural lash line.

We'll return to your eyes after the glue has dried.

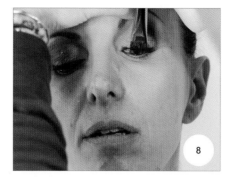

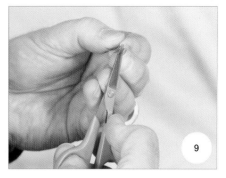

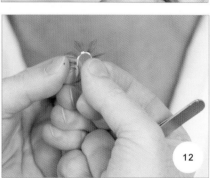

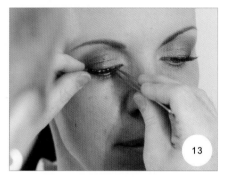

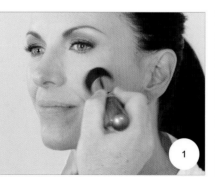

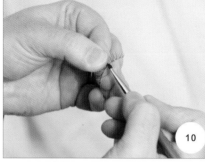

cheeks

1. Now it's time for a gorgeous glow! You are going to achieve this by layering your blush and using the perfect amount of bronzer. Start with a great crème-to-powder blush. Using your #64 crème blush brush, apply a bright apricot blush to the apple of the cheek, starting at the front of your apple and working toward the back.

2. Follow with a light dusting of loose or pressed powder.

We'll add bronzer in a moment.

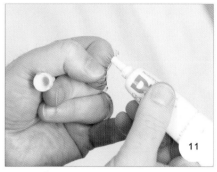

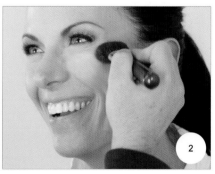

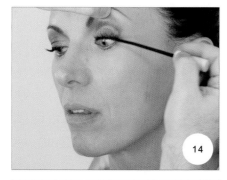

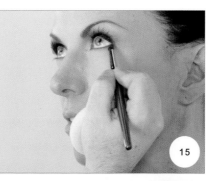

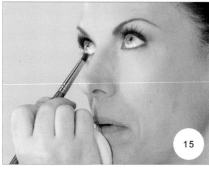

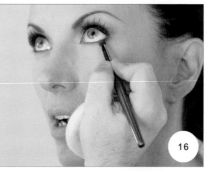

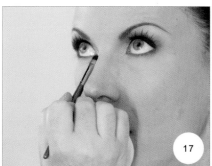

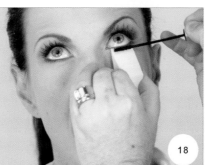

eyes

Here are the final touches for your eyes.

14. Now that the glue has dried, apply a coat of mascara to blend your natural lashes with the false ones.

15. Now grab your #13 detail eye shadow brush and apply your midtone eye shadow all along your lower lash line. Once again, start your application from the outside corner, sweeping it across to the inside corner.

16. With that same detail eye shadow brush, apply a layer of your contour color right over your midtone all along your bottom lash line. By layering on your midtone, then your contour on top of it, you are creating a gradation of color, making your lower lash line definition look more natural and blended.

17. Using your #14 detail highlighting brush, highlight the inside corner of the lower lash line. Because there is so little color to this look, this brightens the eye and opens it up to give you a wide-eyed effect.

18. Finish your eyes with a layer of mascara on your bottom lashes.

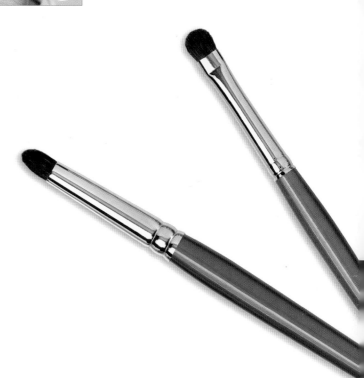

cheeks

Here are the final steps for your cheeks.

3. Using your #73 bronzer/blush brush, apply your matte bronzer. Begin at the back of your cheekbone and sweep it forward toward the apple of your cheek. Then take the brush back toward your ear. This lays your color in place.

4. Now take your brush and use it in the opposite direction (up and down) to blend. Be sure to blend well, or it won't look natural.

5. Don't forget to add a little at the temples to help shape your face. Sweep the bronzing powder up around the temples and eye sockets. This always gives the face more color and gives you a glow, and that is what this look is all about.

6. Also, feel free to blend some bronzer along your jawbone. This also helps create that glow and defines your face.

7. Now to reinforce that flush, smile and apply your powder blush (the perfect bright sheer apricot color) with your #73 brush on the apple of your cheek, starting at the front of your apple and working toward the back.

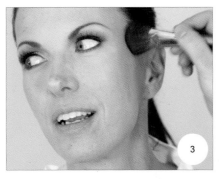

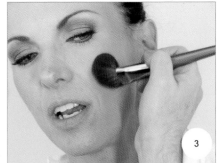

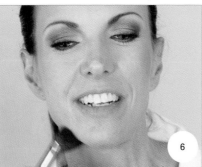

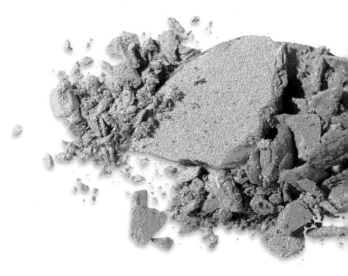

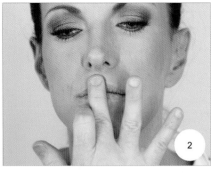

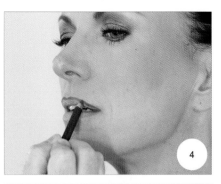

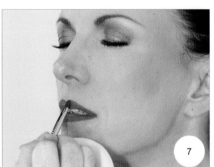

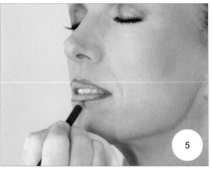

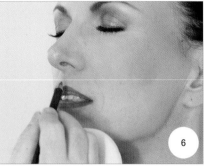

lips

1. This lip is bright and sophisticated. To help it look its most perfect, you need to prep your lips first. Because your lips will be a focus, you really want them to appear sumptuous and smooth, so before you start your color application, moisturize them with lip balm. This will help the color go on smoothly and evenly. After the balm has had a bit of time to soak in, blot off the excess with a tissue so that it won't shorten the staying power of your lipstick.

2. Now, using concealer, conceal your lip and along your lip line.

3. Grab your bright pink lip pencil and begin with a V in the "cupid's bow," or center curve, of the lips. Bring the liner up and around the curves of your bow.

4. Next, starting at the outer corners, move toward the center with your pencil.

5. On the lower lip, first accentuate the lower curve of the lip. Then begin from the outer corners, moving toward the center. Remember to use your entire lip: Take the color to the almost invisible line just at the edge of the colored part of your lips.

6. Now fill in your entire lip with your lip pencil, except just the very center. This will help your lip color last and stay in place because lip liner has a drier texture than lipstick.

7. With your #80 lip brush, blend your lip liner so that it is even and smooth.

"don't be afraid to play with color on your lips."

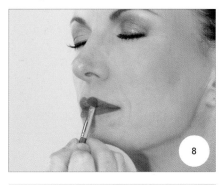
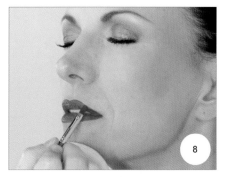

8. Using your lip brush, apply your fuchsia lipstick to your entire lip, making sure you blend well over your lip liner.

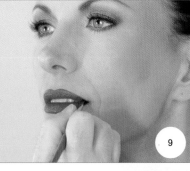
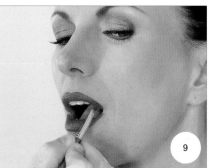

9. Now take a tissue and blot your lips. This will remove the moisture from the lipstick, but leave a layer of pigment. Then apply another layer of lipstick. Adding these three layers (one of liner and two of lipstick) will help your color be true and intense, as well as last longer.

10. End with a quick sweep of the perfect pink lip gloss to make your lips shiny, fuller looking, and sexy. Make sure you apply your gloss with your #80 lip brush because if you apply gloss with a brush, it will look shinier.

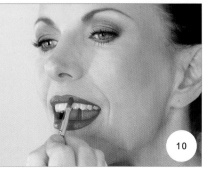

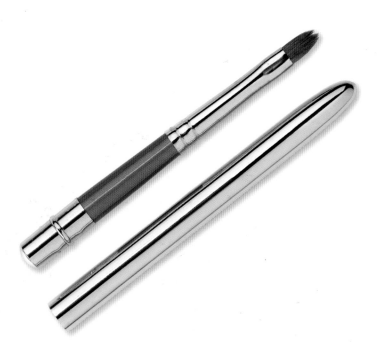

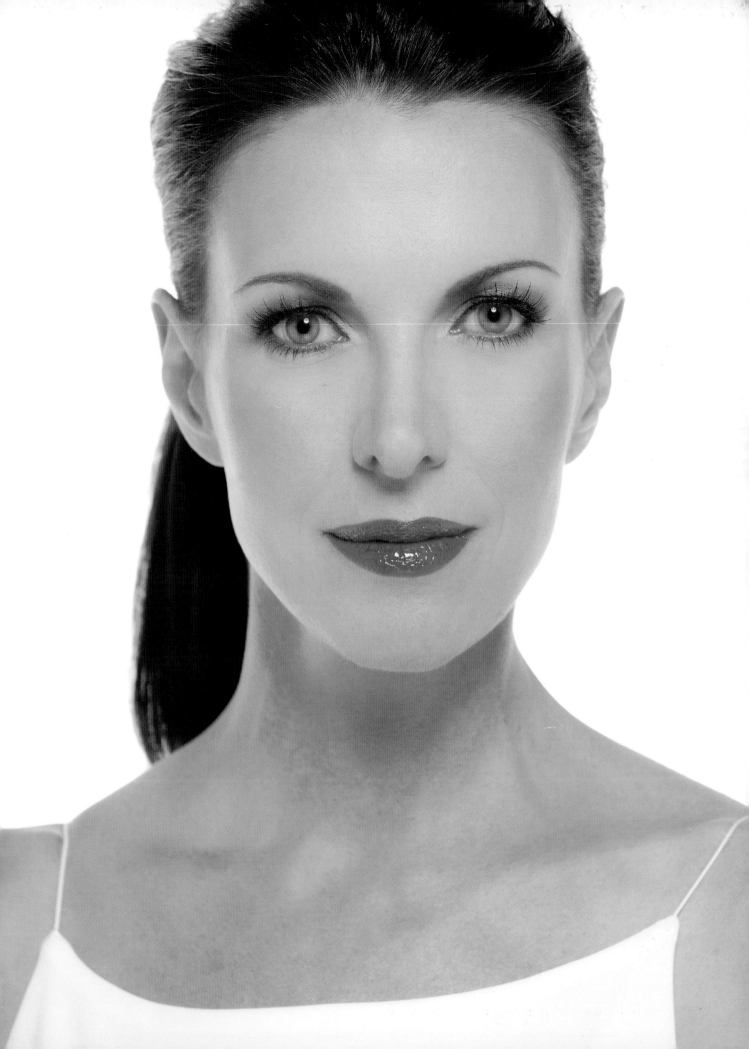

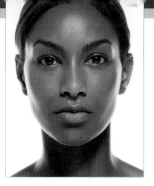

sultry splash

Here's a look that proves that sometimes even grays can bring out the amber in your eyes. I paired my smoky gray shadows with ginger shades so that the warmth of the ginger shadow brings out all the warmth in the iris of your eyes. Sultry is not only about a look but also about a state of mind. So get your face and mind in a sultry state and make it *your* night.

Here's how to get this look:

eyes

1. Using your #22 highlighting brush, apply a shimmery gold eye shadow just to your brow bone. (Remember, when I say brow bone, I mean the area just under the arch of your brow.)

2. It's time to curl your eyelashes and apply the first layer of mascara to your top lashes. (See page 42 to review how to curl properly.)

3. Using your #11 midtone brush and a matte midtone eye shadow and starting from the outside corner of your crease, glide your brush across to the inside corner. Use a matte ginger shadow (a shade just a bit darker than your skin tone) so that you get soft definition.

4. Use your #28 blending brush (the one that is always clean and ready to blend with) and blend your midtone so that there are no hard edges.

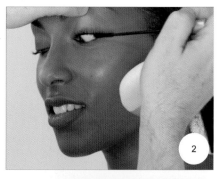

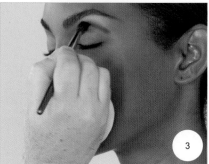

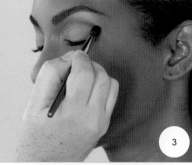

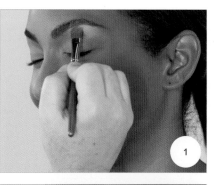

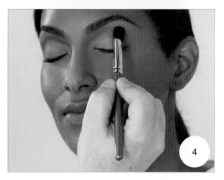

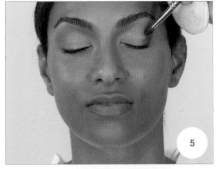

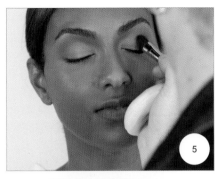

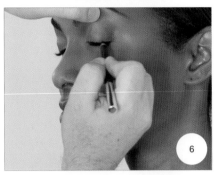

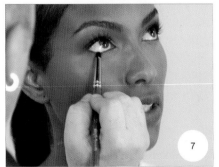

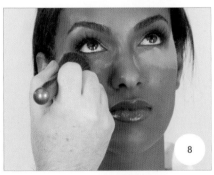

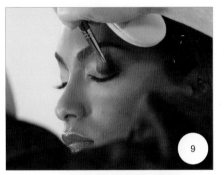

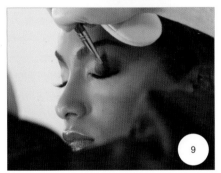

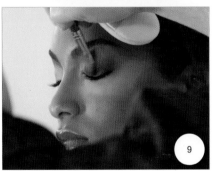

5. Grab your #30 contour brush and some midtone eye shadow and define the outer third of your eyelid. Follow with your #28 brush to blend.

6. With your black eyeliner pencil, line all across your top lash line. This will help create more depth of color at your lash line, which is very important for this look.

7. Now grab your #13 detail eye shadow brush and apply your midtone all along your lower lash line. Once again, start your application from the outside corner, sweeping it across to the inside corner.

8. Because you are about to use very dark colors, using your #76 powder brush, apply a bit of powder under the eye to catch any spilled shadow. This way, when you are finished, you can just brush the powder and any shadow drips away and still have flawless skin.

9. With your #27 shadow brush, apply your shimmery dark gray eye shadow. Start at the base of your lash line and bring your color across and up to your crease. You are getting a higher concentration of color at the lash line, fading away as you work toward the crease.

10. Follow again with your #28 brush to blend your contour color.

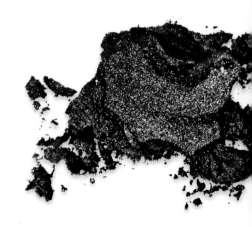

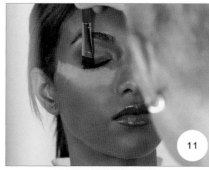

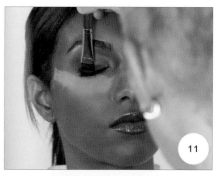

11. Now to create true intensity at your lash line, using your #18 brush, grab some matte black eye shadow and lay your brush at your lash line. Then pull upward to blend. Do this all the way across your upper lash line.

12. With your #27 brush, apply more shimmery gray eye shadow in a half-moon shape all along your crease.

13. Finish by blending everything with your #28 blending brush.

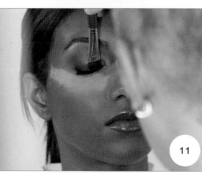

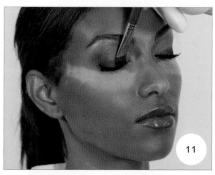

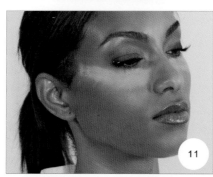

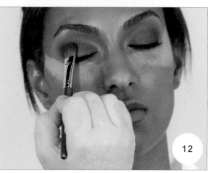

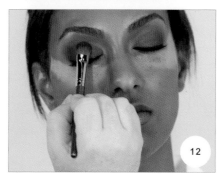

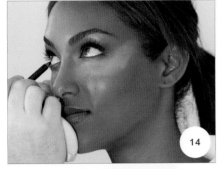

14

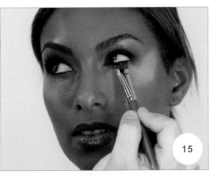

15

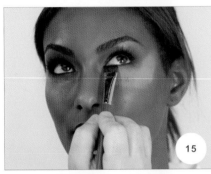

15

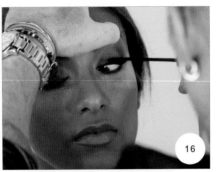

16

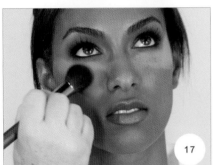

17

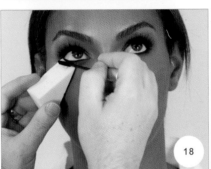

18

14. Now with a black eyeliner pencil, line the waterline of your upper and lower lid. (Remember, the waterline is the inner rim above the lower lash line and underneath the upper lash line.) This will add a little bit more drama to your smoky eye.

15. With your #18 brush, lay black eye shadow right into the base of your lower lashes, from corner to corner.

16. Apply another layer of mascara to your top lashes. (See page 44 to review how to layer your mascara properly.) You want to apply it before you remove the powder below your eye, so that if there is any dark powder on your lashes from applying your shadow, the powder can catch it.

17. Now, with your #76 brush, remove the powder from under your eye, and with it will go any the shadow fallout.

18. Apply mascara to your bottom lashes.

cheeks

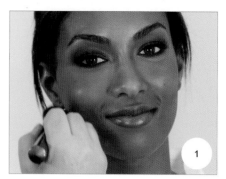

1. With this look you want a flushed cheek. You are going to achieve this by layering your blush. Start with a great crème-to-powder blush. Using your #64 crème blush brush, apply a bright apricot blush to the apple of the cheek, starting at the front of your apple and working toward the back.

2. Follow with a light dusting of loose or pressed powder.

3. Now to reinforce that flush, smile and apply your powder blush (the perfect bright sheer apricot color) with your #74 bronzer/blush brush on the apple of your cheek, starting at the front of your apple and working toward the back.

lips

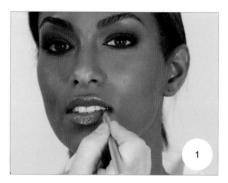

1. End with a quick sweep of the perfect sandy beige lip gloss to make your lips shiny, fuller looking, and sexy. Make sure you apply your gloss with your #80 lip brush because if you apply gloss with a brush, it will look shinier.

"sultry is not only about a look but also about a state of mind."

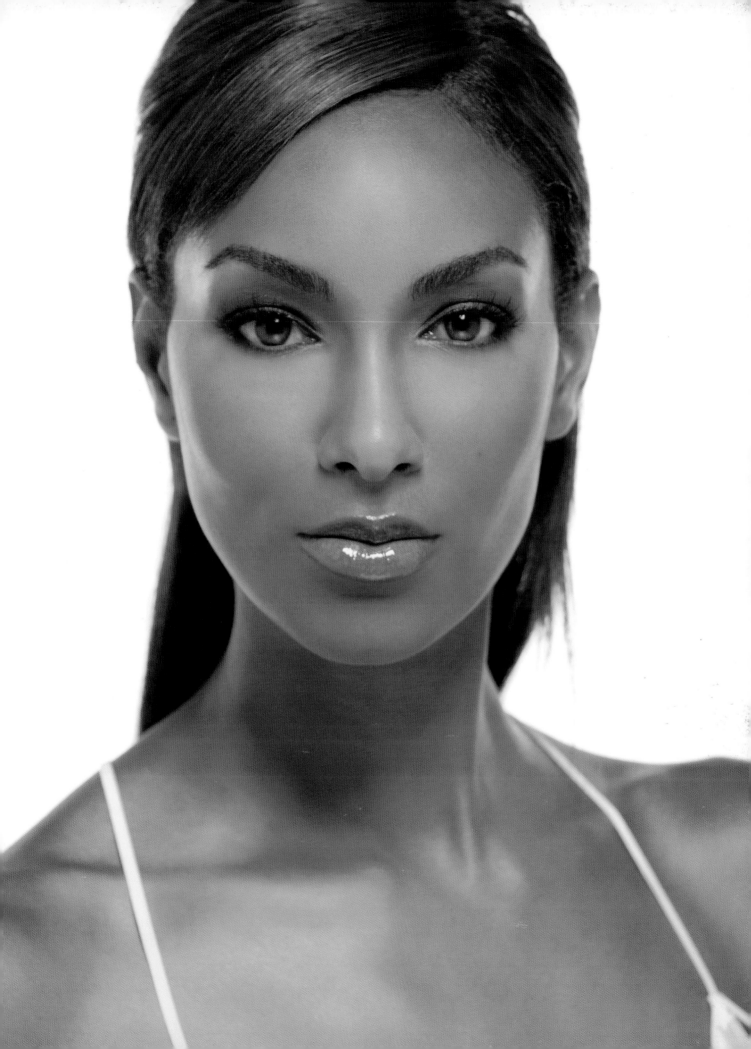

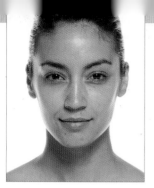

urban nights

When you want drama to be the theme of your evening, only this look will do. When someone says smoke, this look says fire! These defined, sultry eyes will be all the drama you need for your night out. Absolutely deep and dark at the base of the lashes and fading out from there, with bronzed cheeks and a nude mouth, this look says you are ready to go. Tonight is the perfect night for you to go for it, girl!

Here's how to get this look:

eyes

1. With your #22 highlighting brush, apply a matte beige eye shadow to your brow bone. (Remember, when I say brow bone, I mean the area just under the arch of your brow.)

2. Using your #11 brush and a matte mid-tone eye shadow and starting from the outside corner of your crease, glide your brush across to the inside corner. Use a matte caramel shadow (a shade just a bit darker than your skin tone) to get soft definition. Even though you are about to do a smoky eye, you want to start by creating crease definition.

3. Use your #28 blending brush (the one that is always clean and ready to blend with) and blend your midtone so that there are no hard edges.

4. Now grab your #13 detail eye shadow brush and apply your midtone all along your lower lash line. Start your application from the outside corner, sweeping it across to the inside corner.

5. It's time to curl your eyelashes and apply the first layer of mascara to your top lashes. (See page 42 to review how to curl properly.)

6. For this look, you really want the most intense color to be right at your lash line, but you still want it to blend outward. So with your black eyeliner, line all along your top lash line from corner to corner.

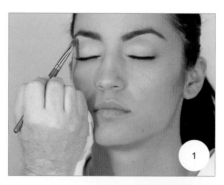

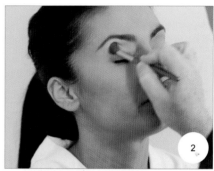

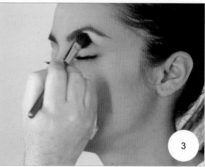

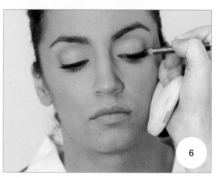

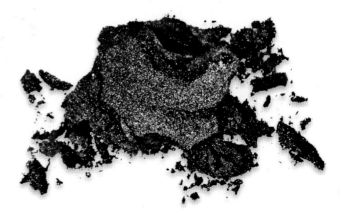

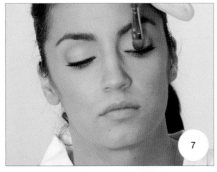

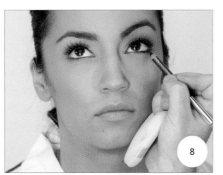

7. Now grab another #22 brush and smudge your liner. By lining and smudging first, you'll create a really intense lash line that still looks blended.

8. Again, with your pencil, line all along your lower lash line and follow with your brush to blend.

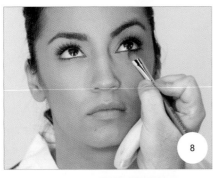

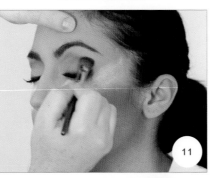

9. Because you are about to use very dark colors, using your #76 powder brush, apply a bit of powder under the eye to catch any spills. Then, when you are finished, you can just brush the powder and the shadow drippings away and still have flawless skin.

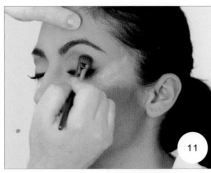

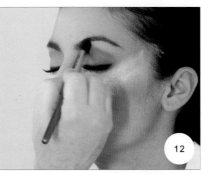

10. With your #27 eye shadow brush (because you will be applying your color to a large area), apply your matte caramel midtone eye shadow. Start at the base of your upper lash line and bring the color up and over your entire lid, all the way up to just under your brow bone. By starting along your lash line and working your way upward, you will get the highest concentration of color where you laid your brush first, making your color deepest at the lash line.

11. Using the same brush, apply your midtone color in a half-moon shape all along your crease, patting the color on for more color concentration.

12. Again use your #28 blending brush to blend your midtone so that there are no hard edges.

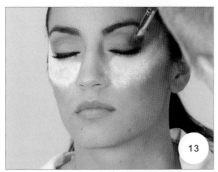

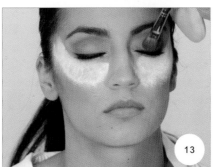

13. With your #27 shadow brush, apply your shimmery dark gray eye shadow, starting at the base of your lash line and bringing your color across and up to your crease. Once again, you are getting a higher concentration of color at the lash line, fading away as you work to the crease.

14. Follow again with your #28 brush to blend your contour color.

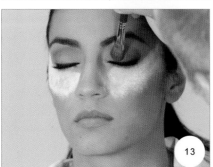

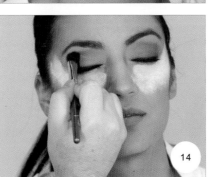

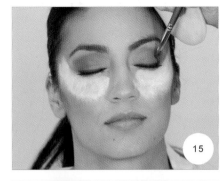 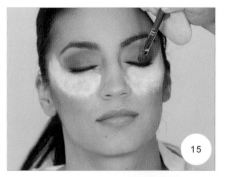

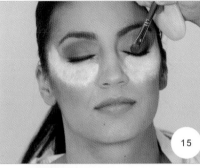 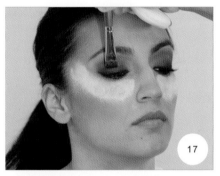

15. Grab your #30 brush and apply more shimmery dark gray eye shadow all along the lower half of your eyelid to create more depth.

16. Of course, follow with your #28 brush to blend.

17. Now to create true intensity at your lash line, using your #18 brush, grab some matte black eye shadow and lay your brush at your lash line. Then pull upward to blend. Do this all the way across your upper lash line.

18. Finish by blending everything with your #28 blending brush.

19. Now, with a black eyeliner pencil, line the waterline of your upper and lower lid. (Remember, the waterline is the inner rim above the lower lash line and underneath the upper lash line.) This will add just a little bit more drama to your smoky eye.

20. For a little more definition, reinforce the highlight on your brow bone with your #22 brush and a matte beige shadow. (Remember that for this look, you used *two* #22 brushes one to apply your highlight and one to smudge your eyeliner.)

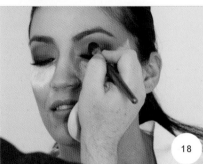 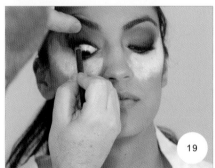

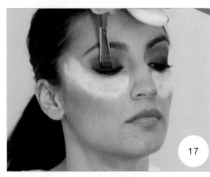 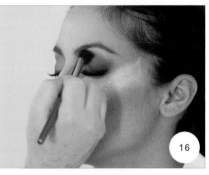

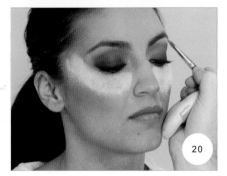

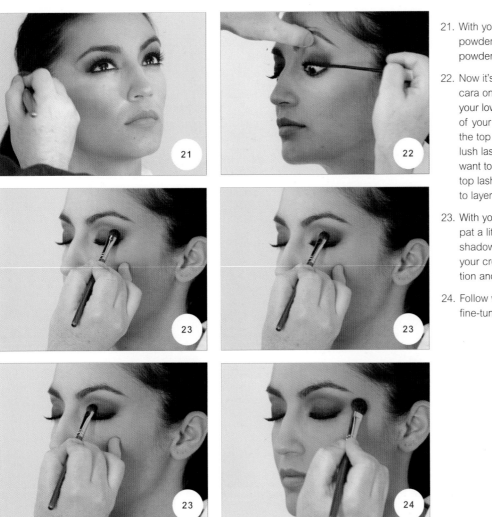

21. With your #76 brush, remove all the powder under your eyes, and with the powder will go any eye shadow fallout.

22. Now it's time for another layer of mascara on your top lashes and a layer on your lower lashes. After you finish the rest of your makeup, add yet another layer to the top lashes. Remember, with this look lush lashes are very important, so you want to really layer your mascara on your top lashes. (See page 44 to review how to layer your mascara properly.)

23. With your #30 brush for more control, pat a little more shimmery dark gray eye shadow in a half-moon shape right along your crease. You want a bit more definition and blending.

24. Follow with your #28 blending brush to fine-tune your blend.

cheeks

1. Using your #73 bronzer/blush brush, apply your matte bronzer. Begin at the back of your cheekbone and sweep it forward toward the apple of your cheek. Then take the brush back toward your ear. This lays your color in place.

2. Now take your brush and use it in the opposite direction (up and down) to blend. Be sure to blend well, or it won't look natural.

3. Don't forget to add a little at the temples to help shape your face. Sweep the bronzing powder up around the temples and eye sockets. This always gives the face more color and gives you a glow.

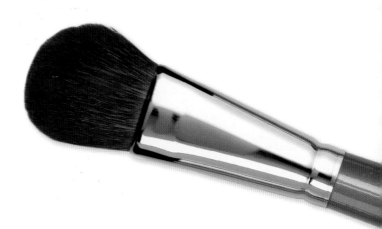

lips

1. You want your lips to be soft, but still well defined. Start by concealing your lip and lip line. This gives you the perfect pale canvas for your subtle lip look.

2. Now, using a barely there nude lip pencil, line your lips. Begin with a V in the "cupid's bow," or center curve, of the lips. Bring the liner up and around the curves of your bow.

3. Next, starting at the outer corners, move toward the center with your pencil.

4. On the lower lip, first accentuate the lower curve of the lip. Then begin from the outer corners and move toward the center. Remember to use your entire lip: Take the color to the almost invisible line just at the edge of the colored part of your lips.

5. Make sure you fill in at least halfway toward the center of your lip. This will help your lip liner look more natural and your lip color last longer.

6. Using a #80 lip brush, blend your liner before you apply your lipstick. This will make it look more natural.

7. Using your lip brush because it gives you better application and helps color last longer, fill in your entire lip with the perfect nude lipstick. Make sure you blend really well over your lip liner.

8. End with a quick sweep of the perfect sheer peach lip gloss to make your lips shiny, fuller looking, and sexy. Make sure you apply your gloss with your #80 lip brush because if you apply gloss with a brush, it will look shinier.

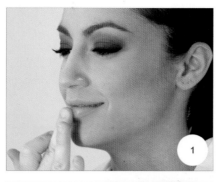

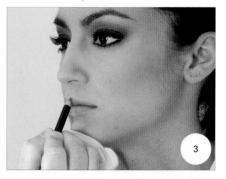

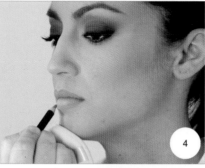

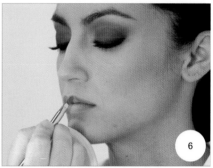

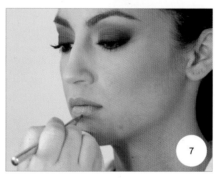

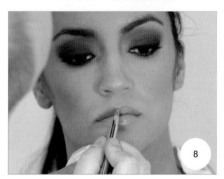

"when someone says 'smoke,' this look says 'fire!'"

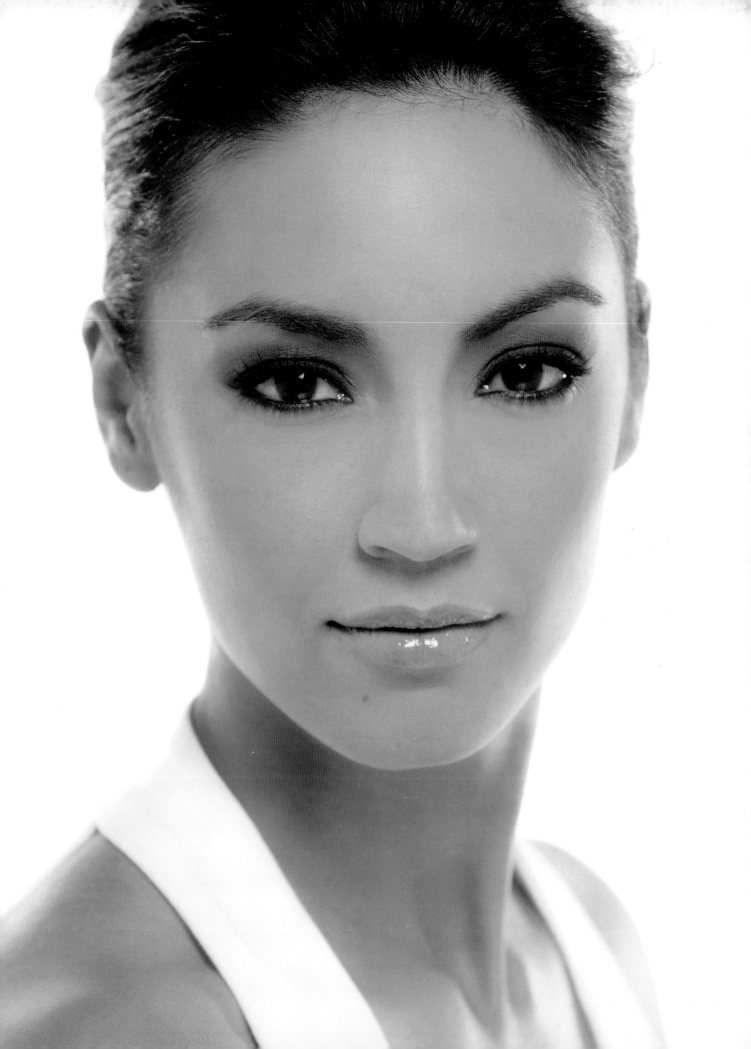

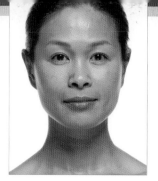

unforgettable nights

Sometimes you just need to take a classic and give it a complete twist. Here is a twist to a smoky eye that I think will be a blast for your next night out. I love mixing colors and using a different color on the top of your lid with another color at your lower lash line. But make sure that the darker of the two shades is *always* on your top lid. I know you will love the effect of mixing colors and playing with this application. Now go have an unforgettable night, but don't forget who showed you how to make it unforgettable!

Here's how to get this look:

eyes

1. Using your #14 detail highlighting brush, apply a crème-to-powder shimmery beige eye shadow to your lid, but only right along your lash line. You are going to layer crème and powder to make your lid more dramatic.

2. With the same brush, apply a shimmery champagne eye shadow powder directly on top on the crème you applied to your lid.

3. For this look, you want the highlight on your lid to be more dramatic than your brow bone. To achieve this, use your #22 brush and apply a matte beige eye shadow on your brow bone. The fact that it is matte and a bit darker will make it look more subtle.

4. Using your #11 midtone brush and a matte midtone eye shadow and starting from the outside corner of your crease, glide your brush across to the inside corner. Use a dark matte taupe shadow (a shade just a bit darker than your skin tone) so that you get soft definition.

5. Use your #28 blending brush to blend your midtone so that there are no hard edges.

6. Grab your #30 contour brush and some midtone eye shadow and define the outer third of your eyelid. Follow with your #28 brush to blend.

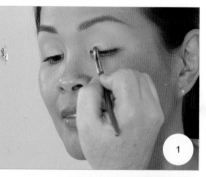

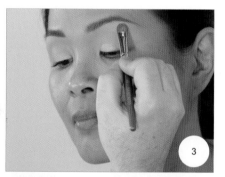

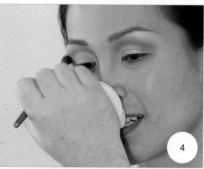

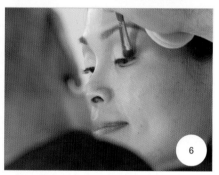

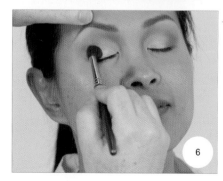

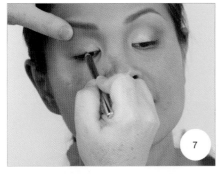 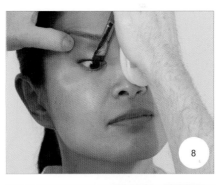

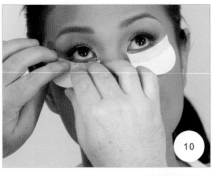 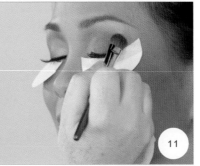

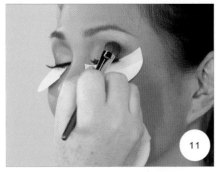 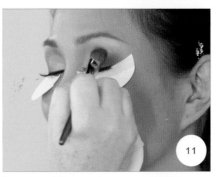

7. To give your lash line a little more punch, start by lining your upper lash line with a black eyeliner. Begin at the inside corner, taking it all the way to the outside corner. Keep it really close to your lash line. You want it thinnest on the inside. Slowly get just the slightest bit thicker as you get to the outside corner.

8. With your #18 eyeliner brush, grab some black eye shadow and lay it all along your top lash line to soften the liner you just applied. As you apply it, pull up slightly with your brush to blend the line.

9. It's time to curl your eyelashes and apply the first layer of mascara to your top lashes. (See page 42 to review how to curl properly.)

10. To help prevent color from falling under your eye area and darkening what you want to make look flawless, you can use shadow shields to catch the powder.

11. With your #27 eye shadow brush, pat dark shimmery green eye shadow in a half-moon shape all along your crease and the outer half of your lid.

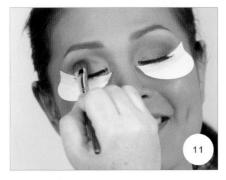 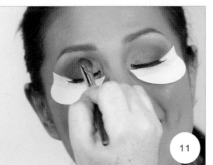

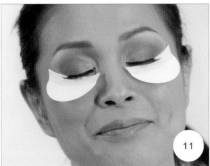

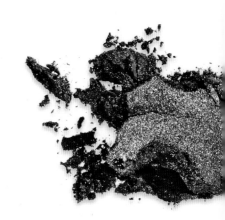

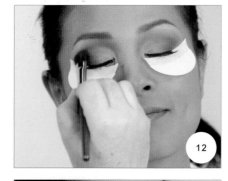

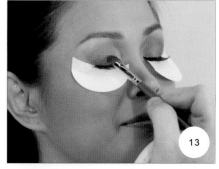

12. Now blend your shadow with your #28 blending brush.

13. Using your #30 eye shadow brush, pat more dark shimmery green shadow along your lash line. Remember when you pat shadow on instead of wiping it on, it lays more color down for more intensity.

14. Once again, use your #28 blending brush to blend.

15. Reinforce your brow highlight with your #22 brush and additional matte beige eye shadow.

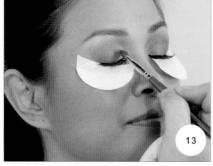

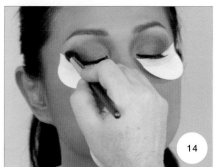

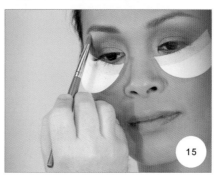

"now go and have an unforgettable night!"

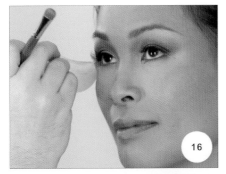

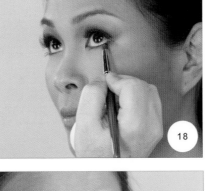

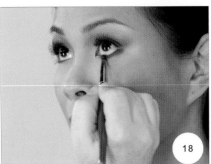

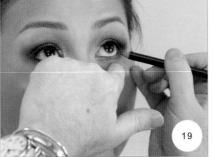

16. Now remove your shadow shields and all the powder they're holding.

17. Grab your #13 detail eye shadow brush and apply your midtone eye shadow all along your lower lash line. Again, start your application from the outside corner, sweeping it across to the inside corner.

18. With that same detail eye shadow brush, apply a dark shimmery burgundy shadow right over your midtone all along your bottom lash line from corner to corner. By layering on your midtone, then your contour on top of it, you are creating a gradation of color, making your lower lash line definition look more natural and blended.

19. Now with a dark burgundy eyeliner pencil, line the waterline of your lower lid. (Remember, the waterline is the inner rim above the lower lash line.) This will add just a bit more drama.

20. Now for another coat of mascara on your top lashes and a coat on your lower lashes. After you finish the rest of your makeup, add yet another coat to your top lashes. (See page 44 to review how to layer your mascara properly.)

cheeks

1. Now it's time for a gorgeous glow! You are going to achieve this by layering your blush and using the perfect amount of bronzer. Start with a great crème-to-powder blush. Using your #64 crème blush brush, apply a bright apricot blush to the apple of the cheek, starting at the front of your apple and working toward the back.

2. Follow with a light dusting of loose or pressed powder.

3. Using your #73 bronzer/blush brush, apply your matte bronzer. Begin at the back of your cheekbone and sweep it forward toward the apple of your cheek. Then take the brush back toward your ear. This lays your color in place.

4. Now take your brush and use it in the opposite direction (up and down) to blend. Be sure to blend well, or it won't look natural.

5. Don't forget to add a little at the temples to help shape your face. Sweep the bronzing powder up around the temples and eye sockets. This always gives the face more color and gives you a glow, and that is what this look is all about.

6. Also, feel free to blend some bronzer along your jawbone. This also helps create that glow and defines your face.

7. Now to reinforce that flush, smile and apply your powder blush (the perfect bright sheer apricot color) with your #73 brush on the apple of your cheek, starting at the front of your apple and working toward the back.

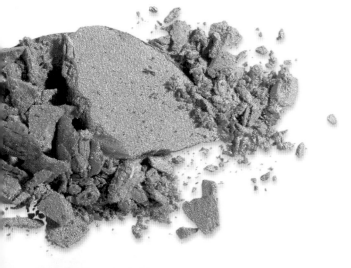

lips

1. You want your lips to be soft and natural. To help create this effect, start by concealing your lip and lip line. This gives you the perfect pale canvas for your subtle lip look.

2. Then, using a taupe nude lip liner, line your lips. Begin with a V in the "cupid's bow," or center curve, of the lips. Bring the liner up and around the curves of your bow.

3. Next, starting at the outer corners, move toward the center bow.

4. On the lower lip, first accentuate the lower curve of the lip. Then begin from the outer corners, moving toward the center. Remember to use your entire lip: Take the color to the almost invisible line just at the edge of the colored part of your lips.

5. Now, using the same pencil, fill in halfway toward the center of your lips. This will help your lip color last longer and make it easier to blend your liner.

6. Using a #80 lip brush, blend your liner before you apply your lip gloss.

7. End with a quick sweep of the perfect sandy beige lip gloss to make your lips shiny, fuller looking, and sexy. Make sure you apply your gloss with your #80 lip brush because if you apply gloss with a brush, it will look shinier.

Now you know how to apply makeup to take your look from calm and casual to smoldering. But what if you want to start light and build intensity as the day turns into night? Turn to chapter 8 and you'll see exactly how to build on your original look to turn up the heat!

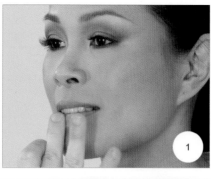
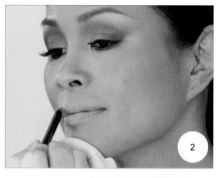
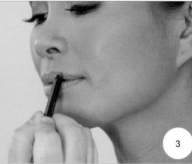
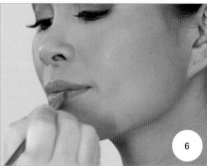
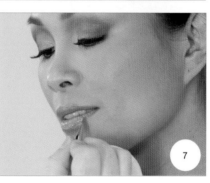
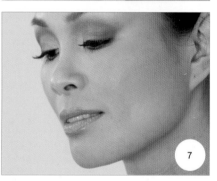
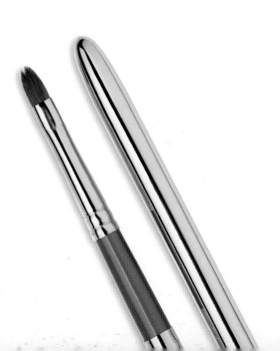

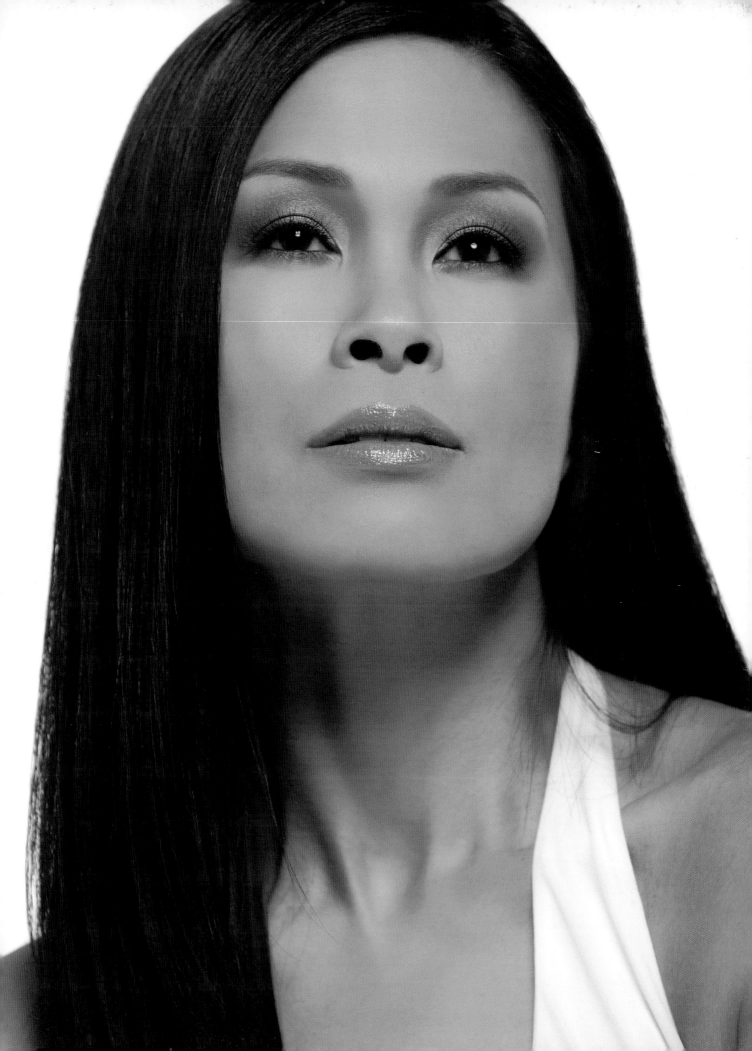

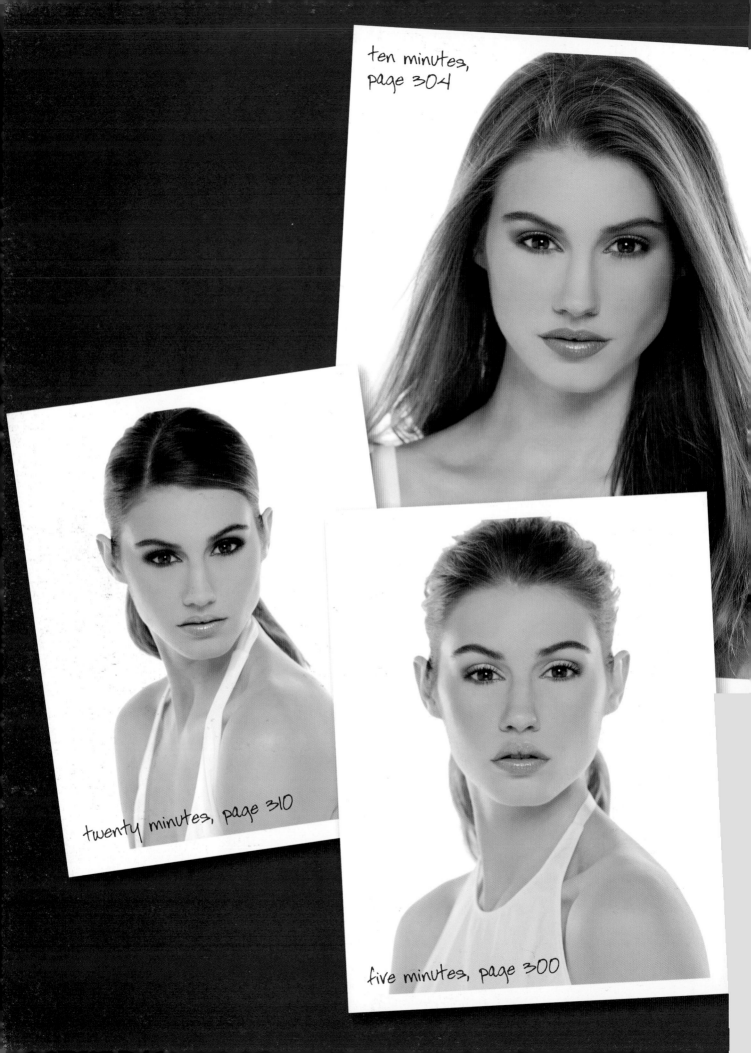

ten minutes,
page 304

twenty minutes, page 310

five minutes, page 300

8

everything adds up to fabulous

I believe most women think that changing their look, even if it's just for an evening, is all about reinventing the wheel. But in reality, it may just mean adding 5 more minutes to the amount of time you're already spending getting ready. You will be surprised what you can do with that extra 5 minutes!

This chapter illustrates just what I am talking about. I am building one look off of another. I am starting with a simple, beautiful, easy-to-achieve 5-minute look and then building it from there. Because I'm building the looks using the same model, this will show you very clearly what adding that extra 5, 10, or 15 minutes can do.

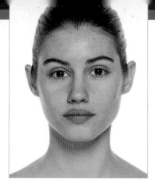

5 minutes to glamorous

Girls, I hope that by now I've convinced you that getting your glam on isn't about spending hours in front of your makeup mirror. It's about using the right tools, choosing the right types and shades of makeup, and applying them quickly, cleanly, and professionally, just the way I've shown you. It will take you just 5 minutes to create this look. And things will just get better from here!

eyes

1. Using your #22 highlighting brush, apply a crème-to-powder shimmery beige eye shadow to your lid (just from the lash line to your crease). You are going to layer crème and powder to make your lid more dramatic.

2. With the same brush, apply a shimmery champagne eye shadow powder directly on top of the crème you applied to your lid and to your brow bone. (Remember, when I say brow bone, I mean the area just under the arch of your brow.)

3. It's time to curl your eyelashes and apply the first layer of mascara to your top lashes. (See page 42 to review how to curl properly.)

4. Using your #11 midtone brush and a matte midtone eye shadow and starting from the outside corner of your crease, glide your brush across to the inside corner. Use a matte taupe shadow (a shade just a bit darker than your skin tone) so that you get soft definition.

5. Use your #28 blending brush (the one that is always clean and ready to blend with) and blend your midtone so that there are no hard edges.

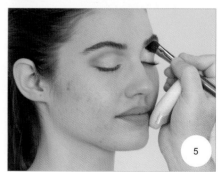
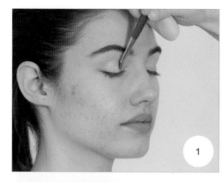
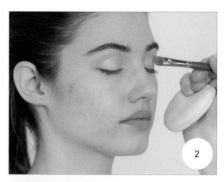
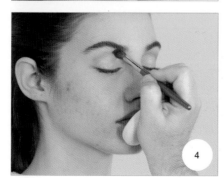
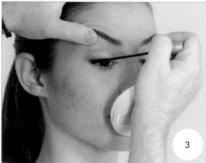
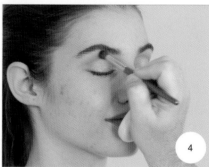

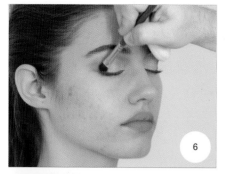

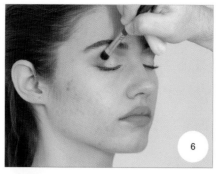

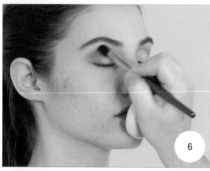

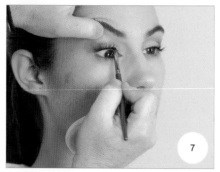

6. Grab your #30 contour brush and some of your midtone eye shadow and define the outer third of your eyelid. Follow with your #28 brush to blend. This just starts your lid definition.

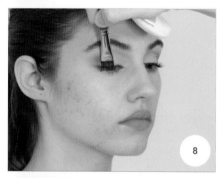

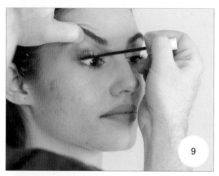

7. For lash line definition, use your #41 detail eyeliner brush and push black eye shadow into the base of your lash line.

8. With your #18 eyeliner brush, grab some black eye shadow and lay it all along your top lash line for definition. As you apply it, pull up slightly with your brush to blend the line.

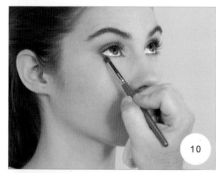

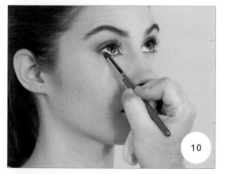

9. Apply another layer of mascara to your top lashes. (See page 44 to review how to layer your mascara properly.)

10. Now grab your #13 detail eye shadow brush and apply your midtone eye shadow all along your lower lash line. Once again, start your application from the outside corner, sweeping it across to the inside corner.

11. Using your #14 detail highlighting brush, highlight the inside corner of the lower lash line. Because there is so little color to this look, this step really brightens the eye and opens it up to give you a wide-eyed effect.

12. Finish with a layer of mascara on your bottom lashes.

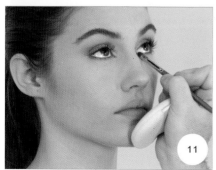

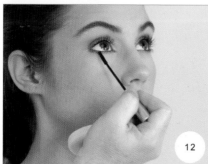

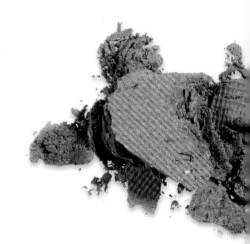

cheeks

1. Using your #73 bronzer/blush brush, apply your matte bronzer. Begin at the back of your cheekbone and sweep it forward toward the apple of your cheek. Then take the brush back toward your ear. This lays your color in place.

2. Now take your brush and use it in the opposite direction (up and down) to blend. Be sure to blend well, or it won't look natural.

3. Don't forget to add a little at the temples to help shape your face. Sweep the bronzing powder up around the temples and eye sockets. This always gives the face more color and gives you a glow.

4. Also, feel free to blend some bronzer along your jawbone. This also helps create that glow and defines your face.

5. Now to create a beautiful flush, smile and apply your powder blush (the perfect bright sheer peach color) with your #73 brush on the apple of your cheek, starting at the front of your apple and working towards the back.

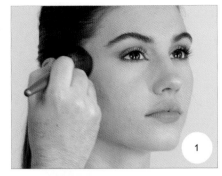
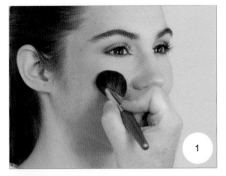
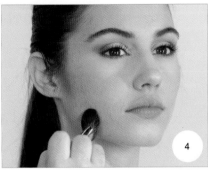
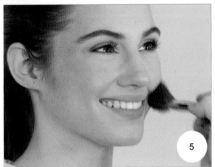

lips

1. Prep your lips for the lip color; apply a generous amount of lip balm. Press and rub your lips together to evenly distribute the balm. Lastly, grab a tissue and blot off excess balm.

2. End with a quick sweep of the perfect sheer peach lip gloss to make your lips shiny, fuller looking, and sexy. Make sure you apply your gloss with your #80 lip brush because if you apply gloss with a brush, it will look shinier.

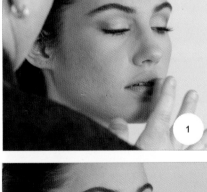
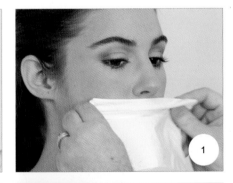
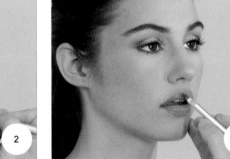

"it takes just 5 minutes to get your glam on."

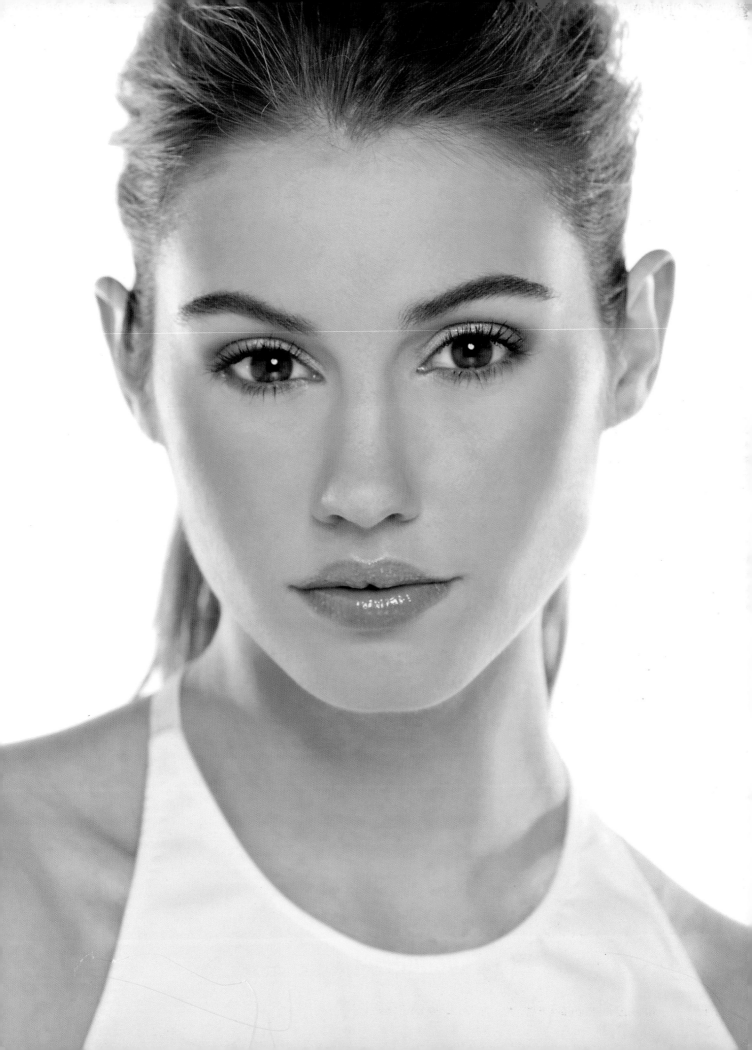

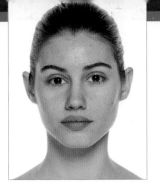

add 5 more minutes and you'll get noticed

Time to up the ante with a more dramatic eye, a bit more color on your cheeks, and a sexy lip. Believe it or not, you only need 5 more minutes to get this luscious look! Can you say hot?!

eyes

1. To give your lash line a little more punch, start by lining your upper lash line with a black eyeliner. Begin at the inside corner, taking it all the way to the outside corner. Keep it really close to your lash line. You want it thinnest on the inside, slowly getting just the slightest bit thicker as you get to the outside corner.

2. With your #18 eyeliner brush, grab some black eye shadow and lay it all along your top lash line to soften the liner you just applied. As you apply it, pull up slightly with your brush to blend the line.

3. Because you are about to use a very dark color, using your #76 powder brush, apply a bit of powder under the eye to catch any spills. Then, when you are finished, you can just brush the powder and any shadow drips away and still have flawless skin.

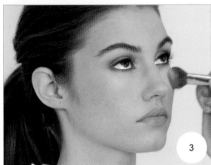

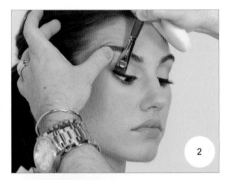

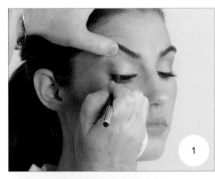

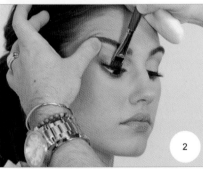

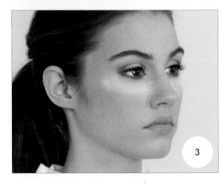

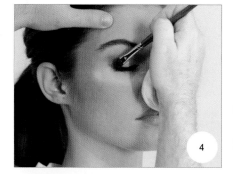

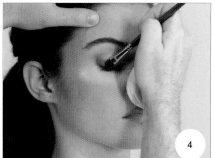

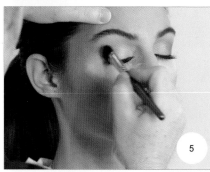

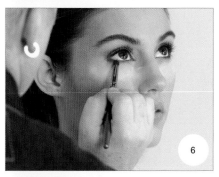

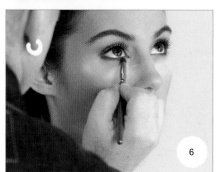

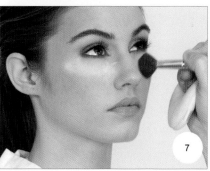

4. With your #30 contour brush, apply a matte dark brown eye shadow on the outer third of your eyelid and up into the crease. You are layering it over the midtone that you applied earlier so it starts to create a blend.

5. Follow again with your #28 brush to blend your contour color.

6. Now with your #13 detail eye shadow brush, apply a layer of your contour color right over the midtone that you applied earlier all along your bottom lash line. By layering on your midtone, then your contour on top of it, you are creating a gradation of color, making your lower lash line definition look more natural and blended.

7. With your #76 brush, remove the powder from under your eye, and with it will go any shadow fallout.

8. Now it's time for another layer of mascara on your top lashes and a layer on your lower lashes. After you finish the rest of your makeup, add yet another layer to your top lashes. Remember, with this look, lush lashes are very important, so you want to really layer your mascara on your top lashes. (See page 44 to review how to layer your mascara properly.)

We'll add more drama to your eyes later in the look.

"can you say hot?!"

lips

1. Using a barely-there nude lip pencil, line your lips. Begin with a V in the "cupid's bow," or center curve, of the lips. Bring the liner up and around the curves of your bow.

2. Next, starting at the outer corners, move toward the center with your pencil.

3. On the lower lip, first accentuate the lower curve of the lip. Then begin from the outer corners, moving toward the center. Remember to use your entire lip: Take the color to the almost invisible line just at the edge of the colored part of your lips.

4. Make sure you fill in at least halfway toward the center of your lip. This will help your lip liner look more natural and your lip color last longer.

5. Using a #80 lip brush, blend your liner before you apply your lipstick. This will make it look more natural.

6. Again, using your lip brush (because it gives you better application and helps color last longer), fill in your entire lip with the perfect peachy nude lipstick. Make sure you blend really well over your lip liner.

We'll end with a layer of lip gloss at the end of this look.

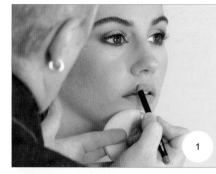
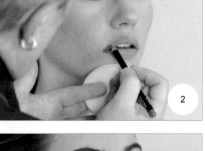
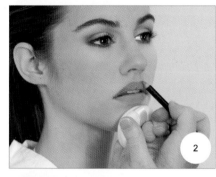
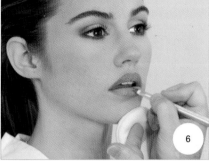
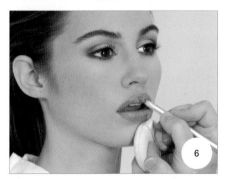

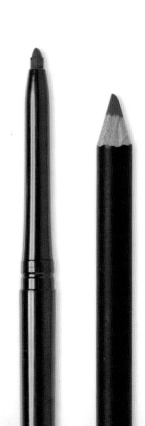

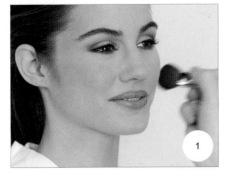

cheeks

1. It's time for a little extra color! Grab your #73 bronzer/blush brush and smile. Apply your powder blush (the perfect bright sheer peach color) on the apple of your cheek, blending back toward the area that you bronzed. This technique gives your face that fresh flush that is so perfect.

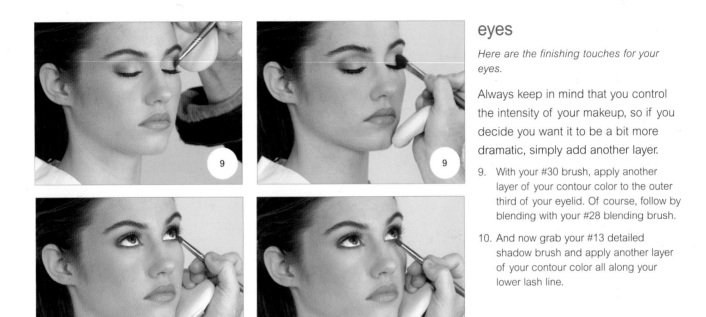

eyes

Here are the finishing touches for your eyes.

Always keep in mind that you control the intensity of your makeup, so if you decide you want it to be a bit more dramatic, simply add another layer.

9. With your #30 brush, apply another layer of your contour color to the outer third of your eyelid. Of course, follow by blending with your #28 blending brush.

10. And now grab your #13 detailed shadow brush and apply another layer of your contour color all along your lower lash line.

lips

Here is the final step for your lips.

7. End with a quick sweep of the perfect sheer peach lip gloss to make your lips shiny, fuller looking, and sexy. Make sure you apply your gloss with your #80 lip brush because if you apply gloss with a brush, it will look shinier.

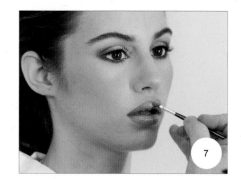

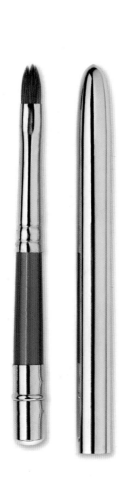

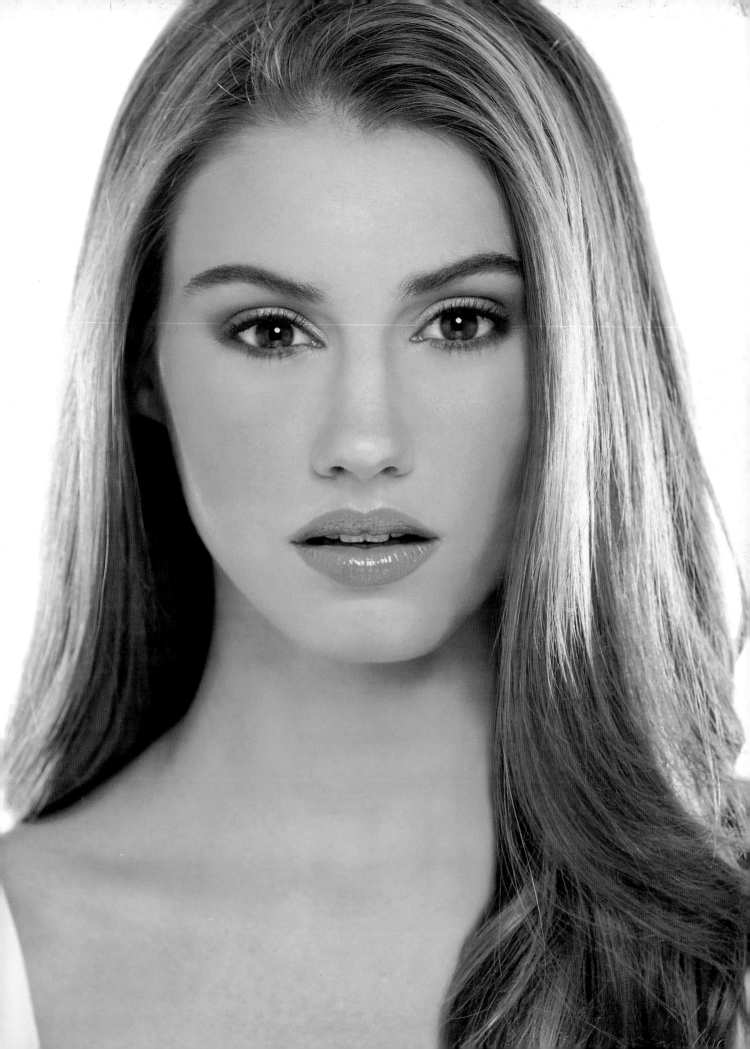

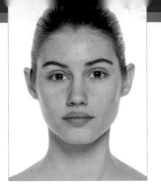

day into night

Wait, you only need 10 more minutes and you're ready for your night out! You won't believe how easy it is to take your look from fabulous to "Don't I know you?" You're already prepped, so just try it!

eyes

1. Because you are about to use a very dark color, using your #76 powder brush, apply a bit of powder under the eye to catch any spills. Then, when you are finished, you can just brush the powder and any spilled shadow away and still have flawless skin.

2. With your #27 eye shadow brush (because you will be applying your color to a large area), apply your matte taupe midtone eye shadow; start at the base of your upper lash line and bring the color up and over your entire lid, all the way up to just under your brow bone. By starting along your lash line and working your way upward, you will get the highest concentration of color where you laid your brush first, making your color deepest at the lash line.

3. Use your #28 blending brush (the one that is always clean and ready to blend with) and blend your midtone so that there are no hard edges.

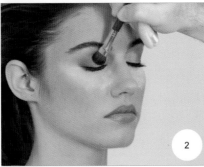

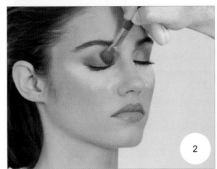

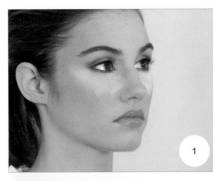

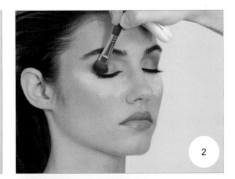

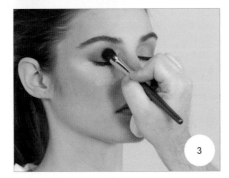

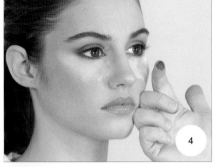

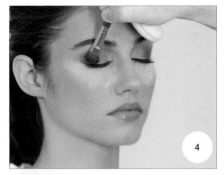

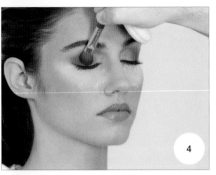

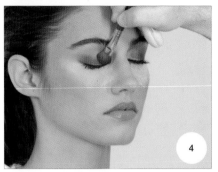

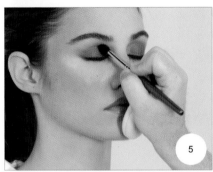

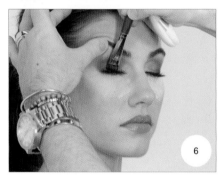

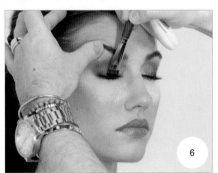

4. With your #27 eye shadow brush, apply your shimmery dark burgundy eye shadow. Start at the base of your lash line and bring your color across and up to your crease. Once again, you are getting a higher concentration of color at the lash line, then fading away as you work toward the crease.

5. Follow again with your #28 brush to blend your contour color.

6. Now to create true intensity at your lash line, using your #18 brush, grab some matte black eye shadow and lay your brush at your lash line. Then pull upward to blend. Do this all the way across your upper lash line.

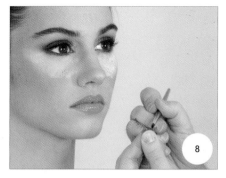

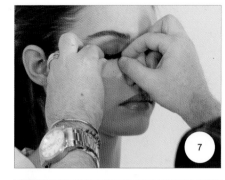

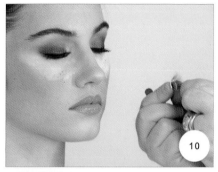

7. It's time to add the ultimate drama: false eyelashes! Measure and trim the outside end of your false eyelashes to fit the width of your eyelid. Strip lashes, when used straight from their container, are usually too wide for most eyes. Trimming them will help them fit better and feel more comfortable.

8. Paint the lash band with black gel or liquid liner to help hide it once it's on.

9. Apply eyelash glue to the false eyelashes all along the band.

10. Allow the glue to dry for a minute so that it will get tacky (slightly sticky). As you allow it to dry a bit, roll the lash to help shape it to fit your lid better.

11. Now place the lash right on top of your eyeliner. Using the handle end of a pair of tweezers, push the lash right up against your natural lash line.

12. With your #76 brush, remove all the powder under your eyes. With the powder will go any shadow fallout.

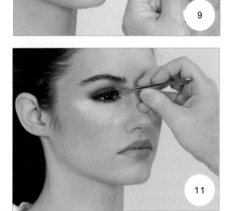

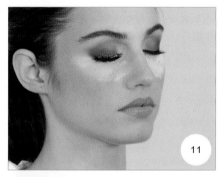

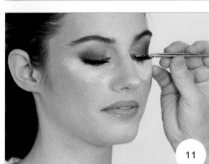

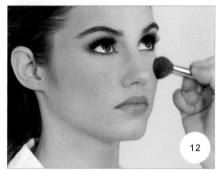

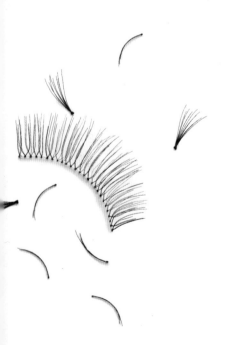

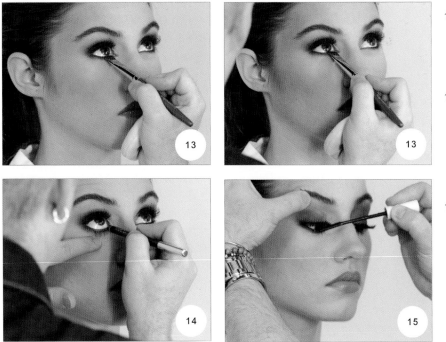

13. With your #18 brush, lay black eye shadow right into the base of your lower lashes, from corner to corner. This creates lots of drama without making a really thick smudged line.

14. With a black eyeliner pencil, line the waterline of your upper and lower lid. (Remember, the waterline is the inner rim above the lower lash line and underneath the upper lash line.) This will add a little bit more drama to your smoky eye.

15. Since the glue has now dried, apply a layer of mascara to your top lashes, blending them into the false ones and making it all look much more natural.

cheeks

1. With a powder brush, grab some loose powder and buff or blend your cheek color to make it look more subtle. With this look, you're actually downplaying the color you added earlier. This eye needs less cheek color, not more.

lips

1. You want your lips to be soft and natural. To help create this effect, start by concealing your lip and lip line. This gives you the perfect pale canvas for your subtle lip look.

2. End with a quick sweep of the perfect sandy beige lip gloss to make your lips shiny, fuller looking, and sexy. Make sure you apply your gloss with your #80 lip brush because if you apply gloss with a brush, it will look shinier.

See how easy it is to build from one look to the next? You can change your look from day to night or casual to smoldering simply by adding to the baseline you've already created. It's all about feeling gorgeous in your own skin, and sweetheart, I can tell you, you *are!* Bringing out your own true beauty is what this book is all about.

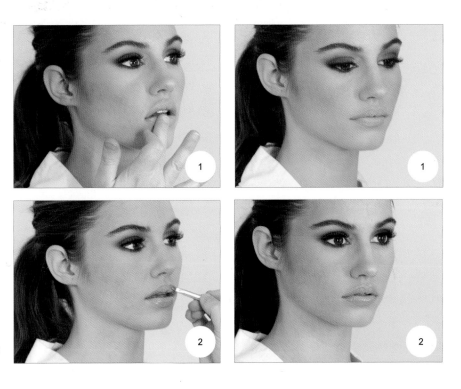

"just 10 more minutes and you're ready for your night out!"

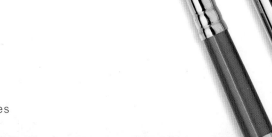

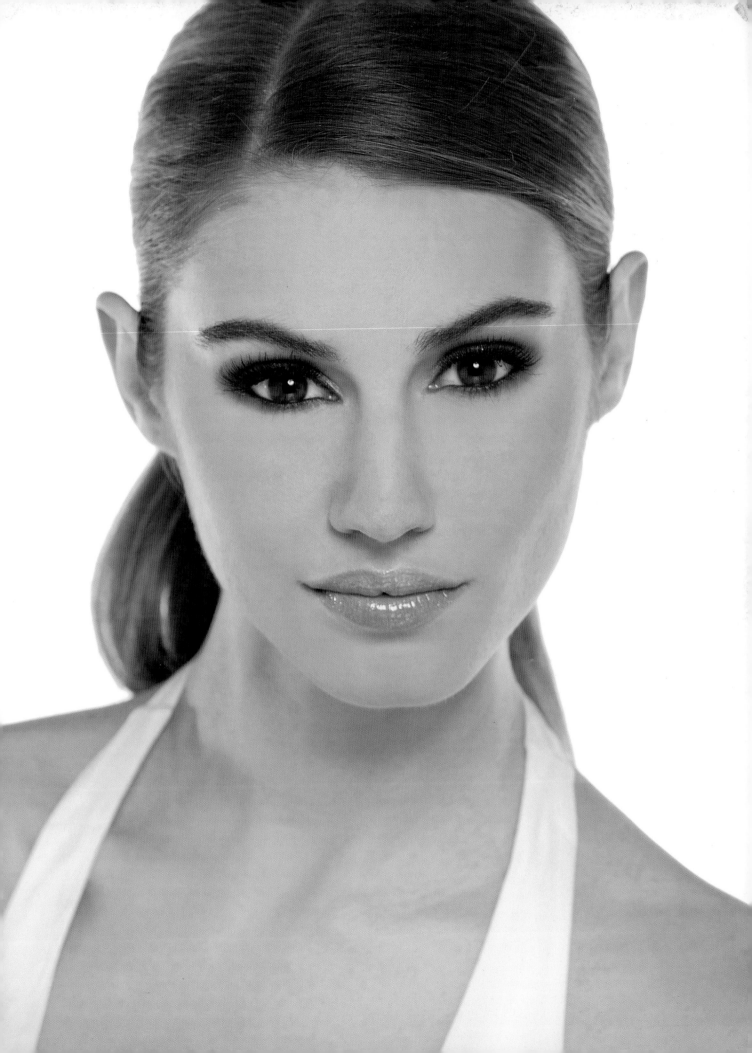

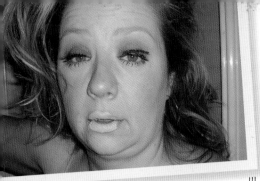

talk about inspiration!!! my favorite picture ever!!! it makes me smile!!! missy!!!

afterword: who me? no, you!

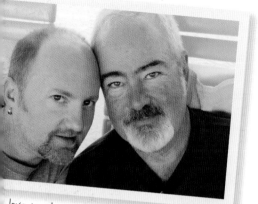

love is always inspiring!!! chip!!!

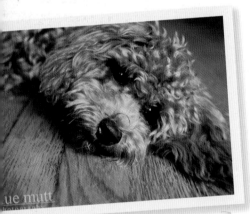

ue mutt

and they call it puppy love!!! gigi!!!

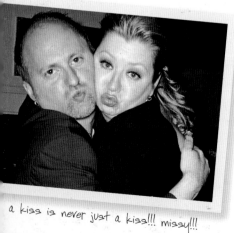

a kiss is never just a kiss!!! missy!!!

We all get inspiration from different places. For me, it comes from people, places, and movies. My first beauty inspiration was my grandmother. She didn't exactly apply her makeup perfectly, but you could see the way it physically transformed her, inside and out. She never went anywhere without putting her prettiest face forward. Friends whom I've had fun giving many different looks to—some serious and some not—all inspired me. So do people walking down the street prancing around in looks that make them feel confident. And, as you know, confidence is the most important aspect of true beauty.

Growing up, many movies set the standard for my vision of the ideal beauty. Many of the actresses in the movies were far from perfect beauties by society's standards yet all were gorgeous to me. I have discovered over the years I always find that "flaws" add to someone's beauty, not detract from it. They make a woman striking and her own version of beautiful. In looking at my work, you can see, for me, it's all about pretty. My favorite look from my favorite movies, of course, is a dramatic eye and a nude lip, mixed with glowing skin, which has become my signature.

Places inspire me with their beauty, the color in the surroundings, the culture, and the buildings. I love when you arrive in another country or city and are bombarded with amazing visuals, the things that make that particular place special—very much like the features that make you special. With that said I guess you could actually say what I love most about places is the people who make them place special.

I would love for you to find what inspires you. What excites you. What makes you smile. This book is not about me telling you what is pretty. I do not care who you are, where you live, or what your life entails. I want you to understand that everyone is pretty. It is just a matter of you discovering what makes you different and special and embracing your pretty.

my gang!!! pam, mayolo, missy, david, and susie!!!

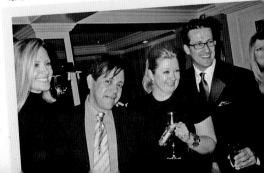

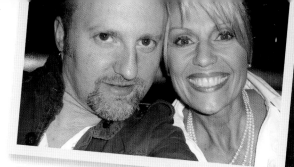

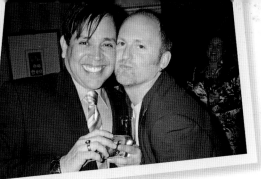

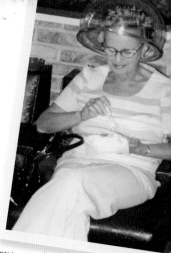

Pretty is as pretty does. We have all heard it our entire lives. My hope is that this book helps you play and discover your very own pretty, that it helps you discover a new look for your fun night out, or a new technique to draw attention to your favorite feature. More importantly, that it helps you discover the inner you.

With each and every book that I have written the most important point that I have always tried to get across is "love who you are today and every-day." Don't worry about who you think you should be or who society says you should be. "Love you." Trust me, I know it is easier said than done, especially because we are constantly bombarded with images of what society thinks is beautiful. I promise you, when you love you, everyone else will follow suit. Remember, everyday is just another opportunity for you to be the most beauti-ful you that you can be.

with tons of love—

Robert Jones

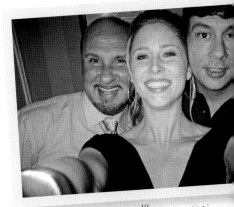

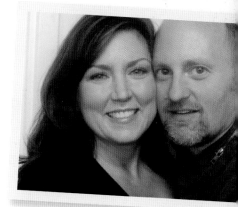

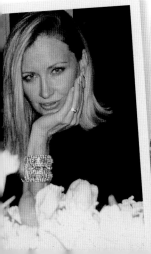

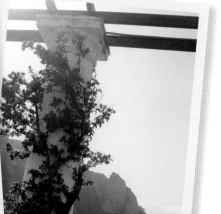

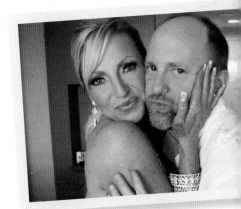

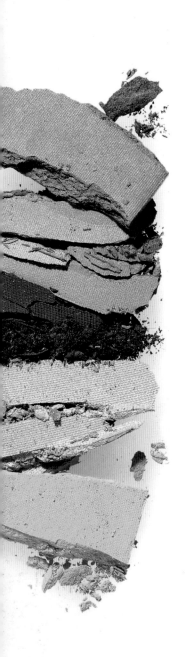

acknowledgments

So many people to thank, so little time!!!!

I need to thank my family, chosen and blood, that have always been there for me (Missy, Mayolo, Debbie, Donna, Roger, Randy, Julianne, Pam, David, Tracey, Poppi, Michael, Christopher). Most of all, Chip McFadin, my love and my rock.

The entire Fair Winds Press family. Especially Will Kiester, my hero, for always being in my corner and rescuing me. Cara Connors, Meg Sniegoski, and Daria Perreault for putting up with my kind of crazy.

Jennifer Grady, Megan Lakanen, and John Gettings for taking care of all the details. And everyone there who has touched any of my projects.

Ellen Phillips, what can really be said BUT thank you for getting me even when I don't get myself, and can you believe this is our fifth book together.

Al Zuckerman, what an incredible man and friend, the best agent in the business.

Larry Travis for giving it his all.

Elaine Moock and Sunni Smyth, for being the keepers and cheerleaders of my crazy.

Maryanne and John McCormack, two very special people who touched my life very early on and showed me that with hard work and talent any dream can come true.

Thank you to all you girls out there who have supported me in my mission to help you be the most beautiful you that you can be.

And thank God for giving me the strength and the ability to trust in the universe's grand plan for me.

about the author

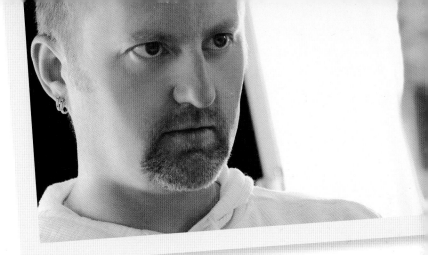

Robert Jones did not necessarily start out on this career path. Robert showed promise as an artist as early as age 6 and was pushed, or maybe we should say, encouraged to pursue painting and drawing. He competed and won a scholarship to study at a prestigious art school at age 11. After seven long years of intense art training he wanted more and decided to get more. From there he attended a performing arts high school where he majored in theater. It is there he first dabbled in makeup, applying painting principles to the face. Growing up with three sisters he always had the opportunity to prove he was naturally gifted at working with hair. He was also able to put that talent to use in school performances. Upon graduating, his advisors expressed their belief that he should pursue his natural gifts. From there he attended school and worked to get his license to do hair.

After a number of years in a salon, he once again wanted more. With his life motto "just jump and figure out how to make it work later," he got the opportunity to work with new models at an agency. From there one thing lead to another and the rest is history. During more than 20-something years in the beauty industry he has traveled the world working with so many amazing people.

His work has appeared in countless magazines such as *Allure, Vogue, Marie Claire, InStyle, Shape, Life and Style, Glamour, Brides,* and *Elle.* He has worked with celebrities such as Cindy Crawford, Claire Danes, Selena Gomez, Eve Best (his favorite, he loves her), Sheryl Crow, Laura Linney, Natascha McElhone, Delta Burke, Diahann Carroll, and many others. He has worked with beauty clients such as Mary Kay, Almay, Olay, Avon, Nexxus, Clinique, Chanel, Prescriptives, and Christian Dior; fashion clients such as Neiman Marcus, Bergdorf Goodman, Saks Fifth Avenue, and Bloomingdales, just to name a few.

He has a signature line of brushes and beauty tools available online at robertjonesbeauty.com that will be in stores soon. Robert also has an online makeup academy that can help anyone become the makeup expert that he or she wishes to be at robertjonesbeautyacademy.com. This is his fifth book; he is also the author of the four best-selling books, *Makeup Makeovers, Makeup Makeovers: Weddings, Looking Younger,* and *Makeup Makeovers: Beauty Bible.*

He has lived in Europe and New York, but now has chosen to be back in Texas with his other half Chip and fur baby Gigi, as much as possible, especially because work keeps him in the travel mode constantly.